Fungi Pathogenic for Humans and Animals

MYCOLOGY SERIES

Edited by

Paul A. Lemke

Department of Botany,
Plant Pathology, and Microbiology
Auburn University
Auburn, Alabama

Other Volumes in Preparation

Fungi Pathogenic for Humans and Animals

(IN THREE PARTS)
PART B
Pathogenicity and Detection: II

EDITED BY
Dexter H. Howard
Department of Microbiology and Immunology
School of Medicine, University of California
Los Angeles, California

with the assistance of
Lois F. Howard
Department of Medicine
School of Medicine, University of California
Los Angeles, California

MARCEL DEKKER, INC.   New York and Basel

Library of Congress Cataloging in Publication Data
(Revised for volume 3 pt. B:II)
Main entry under title:

Fungi pathogenic for humans and animals.

(Mycology series ; v. 3)
Includes bibliographies and indexes.
Contents: pt. A. Biology – pt. B., I-II. Pathogenicity
and detection.
1. Fungi, Pathogenic--Collected works. I. Howard,
Dexter H., [date].   II. Howard, Lois F.
III. Series.
QR245.F86   616.9'69   82-18240
ISBN 0-8247-1875-5 (pt. A)
    0-8247-1144-0 (pt. B:I)
    0-8247-7081-1 (pt. B:II)

MARCEL DEKKER, INC.
270 Madison Avenue, New York, New York 10016

Current printing (last digit):
10 9 8 7 6 5 4 3 2 1

PRINTED IN THE UNITED STATES OF AMERICA

Introduction to the Series

Mycology is the study of fungi, that vast assemblage of microorganisms which includes such things as molds, yeasts, and mushrooms. All of us in one way or another are influenced by fungi. Think of it for a moment—the good life without penicillin or a fine wine. Consider further the importance of fungi in the decomposition of wastes and the potential hazards of fungi as pathogens to plants and to humans. Yes, fungi are ubiquitous and important.

Mycologists study fungi either in nature or in the laboratory and at different experimental levels ranging from descriptive to molecular and from basic to applied. Since there are so many fungi and so many ways to study them, mycologists often find it difficult to communicate their results even to other mycologists, much less to other scientists or to society in general.

This Series establishes a niche for publication of works dealing with all aspects of mycology. It is not intended to set the fungi apart, but rather to emphasize the study of fungi and of fungal processes as they relate to mankind and to science in general. Such a series of books is long overdue. It is broadly conceived as to scope, and should include textbooks and manuals as well as original and scholarly research works and monographs.

The scope of the Series will be defined by, and hopefully will help define, progress in mycology.

Paul A. Lemke

Foreword

Reports of mycosis as a primary or secondary disease are rising rapidly. This increase is due to greater clinical awareness and improved diagnostic skills and to increased use of immunosuppressive drugs. Knowledge of their nutrition, physiology, and geographic distribution is essential for the understanding of fungal pathogens. Also, the understanding of phagocytic mechanisms in host response and the efficacy of vaccines plays an important role in the better management of mycosis. In addition to increased understanding of the pathogens, improved techniques for in vitro and in vivo detection and routine clinical laboratory procedures for the isolation and conservation of the pathogens are urgently needed to combat diagnostic and therapeutic difficulties. This book, the last of three parts in a series, clearly meets that need.

The authors are prominent figures in their field, with long records of research achievement. Professor Howard, an internationally renowned mycologist, has made a major contribution to our knowledge of host-parasite interactions and the physiology of fungal pathogens. He is also a noted teacher who has trained many young scientists in the field. Both microbiologists and clinicians will find this book most useful and will appreciate its thorough coverage of basic and practical problems relating to mycoses.

K. J. Kwon-Chung
Clinical Mycology Section
Laboratory of Clinical Investigation
National Institute of Allergy and Infectious Diseases
National Institutes of Health
Bethesda, Maryland

Preface

The original plan for a comprehensive coverage of the zoopathogenic fungi called for a division of the work into three parts. The first part was to include chapters on the basic biology of the fungi with special consideration of classification, morphology, and physiology. The second part was to cover aspects of pathogenicity such as mechanisms of pathogenesis, host responses (cellular and humoral), toxins, and antigens. The last part was to have dealt with practical matters of detecting the fungi in nature and in clinical materials and with certain applications such as vaccines and antifungal drugs.

In gathering the material, it became clear that the topical divisions would have produced volumes of exaggerated disproportion. Far too much on the basic biology was at hand and some of the topics in pathogenicity required preparations that exceeded practical deadlines. Therefore, rearrangements were made. The third volume of the series, labeled Part B:II, now contains two sections and an Addendum. The first of these sections contains chapters on pathogenesis, including aspects of basic biology that have a direct relation to mechanisms of tissue invasion, namely, cell wall composition, subcellular particles, and enzymes involved in in vivo survival or tissue destruction. In addition, the rearrangement has allowed for an updated coverage of cellular defense mechanisms involving phagocytic cells and, in an Addendum, a reconsideration of the genus *Exophiala,* a particularly troublesome member of the dematiaceous group.

The second section of Part B:II is more or less as originally planned and covers such practical matters as epidemiology, detection of fungi in tissue, growth of fungi in culture, and the development of fungal vaccines.

And thus the work is completed. I gratefully acknowledge the indispensable assistance of Mrs. Lois F. Howard, who checked all bibliographical material, read all of the manuscripts, and tried to maintain consistency throughout the three parts of the work. I also thank Ms. Bette Y. Tang for the numerous typings and retypings of edited manuscripts. Some support for this venture has been supplied by research grant AI 16252 from the National Institute of Allergy and Infectious Diseases, National Institutes of Health, which is used to fund the Collaborative California Universities-Mycology Research Unit (CCU-MRU).

I am especially grateful to the group of splendid authors who collaborated with me to produce this volume.

Dexter H. Howard

Contents

ix

Contributors

Jill Adler-Moore, PhD, Department of Biological Sciences, California State Polytechnic University, Pomona, California

Winnifred B. Atkins, Mycology Department, American Type Culture Collection, Rockville, Maryland

G. S. de Hoog, PhD, Centraalbureau voor Schimmelcultures, Baarn, The Netherlands

Jacob Fleischmann, MD, Department of Medicine, UCLA School of Medicine, Los Angeles, California

John N. Galgiani, MD, Section of Infectious Diseases, Veterans Administration Medical Center, and Department of Internal Medicine, University of Arizona, College of Medicine, Tucson, Arizona

Nancy K. Hall, PhD, Department of Pathology, University of Oklahoma Health Sciences Center, Oklahoma City, Oklahoma

Dexter H. Howard, PhD, Department of Microbiology and Immunology, UCLA School of Medicine, Los Angeles, California

Shung C. Jong, PhD, Mycology Department, American Type Culture Collection, Rockville, Maryland

Howard W. Larsh, PhD, Department of Botany and Microbiology, University of Oklahoma, Norman, Oklahoma

Robert I. Lehrer, MD, Department of Medicine, UCLA School of Medicine, Los Angeles, and VA Medical Center, West Los Angeles, California

Masahiko Okudaira, MD, DMSc, Department of Pathology, School of Medicine, Kitasato University, Kanagawa, Japan

Errol Reiss, PhD, Division of Mycotic Diseases, Center for Infectious Diseases, Centers for Disease Control, Atlanta, Georgia

Glenn D. Roberts, PhD, Department of Laboratory Medicine, Mayo Medical School, Rochester, Minnesota

Contents of Part A

Contents of Part B: I

Fungi Pathogenic for Humans and Animals

Part One
PATHOGENESIS

1

Nutrition, Physiology, and Metabolism of Zoopathogenic Fungi

Dexter H. Howard / UCLA School of Medicine, Los Angeles, California

I. INTRODUCTION

A. History

1. Nutrition and Physiology

   a. The Concept of a Pure Culture: Exact knowledge about the nutrition and physiology of fungi developed from efforts to cultivate them artificially. Experiments on the
culture of various microfungi, e.g., *Mucor, Botrytis,* and *Aspergillus,* were conducted as
early as 1710 by Antonio Micheli [59], and the cultivation of larger fungi such as the
mushrooms was practiced long before that [3]. However, solid information on the
nutritional needs of microfungi came forth only after the concept of a pure culture
arose in the nineteenth century when such cultures became essential to establishment
of distinctive features that could be used as bases for nomenclature and classification
[232]. The requirements for a pure culture are a sterile nutrient medium which can be
inoculated with a single cell of the organism to be studied and kept from contamination with other microorganisms in the environment. Failure to provide these essentials
would, in the words of Oscar Brefeld, "lead only to nonsense and overgrowth by
Penicillium glaucum" ("da kommt nur Unsinn und *Penicillium glaucum* heraus") [60].

   b. Insights Gained from Experiments on Spontaneous Generation: No single subject so captivated the attention of experimentalists as did the controversy over the
spontaneous generation of microbes in putrid fluids [126]. The necessity of preparing
fluids devoid of living animalcules was mandatory to these studies, and the boiling of
liquids susceptible to putrefaction in order to rid them of life (to sterilize them) became
the common practice among investigators in the eighteenth century. This practice continued into the midnineteenth century and was augmented by plunging media-containing
vessels into boiling solutions of sodium chloride or calcium chloride to achieve even
higher temperatures for sterilization. The need for higher temperatures arose from the
occasional failure of plain boiling to sterilize. This failure was often the result of the
presence of spore-forming bacteria in some of the decoctions used to study spontaneous
generation [428]. John Tyndall and Ferdinand Cohn recognized the source of these
failures and independently devised "systems of discontinuous sterilization" which became
known as "tyndallization" [92]. The system employed a period of heating, which
destroyed all vegetative forms, followed by a period of storage at room temperature during which spores that were not destroyed by the heat germinated into vegetative cells.
A second heating then killed these freshly hatched germlings. The cycles of heating and
storage could be repeated many times, but usually three sufficed. The relative merits
of dry and moist heat in sterilization were determined by Koch and Wolffhügel [60]
and by Koch et al. [60]. Such studies led ultimately to replacement of boiling salt
solutions for sterilization which was a cumbersome procedure. The replacement method
was steam under pressure. This principle had been incorporated in Denys Papin's
"digester or engine for softening bones" which was modified in the late nineteenth
century into devices that became known as autoclaves [3,60,85].
   Early experiments on spontaneous generation also influenced the methods for stopper-
ing containers used in microbiological studies. In the nineteenth century, the controversy
over spontaneous generation focused on whether air was necessary to vivify or enliven a
properly sterilized organic infusion. In the very early experiments of F. Schulze [60],
air was made to pass through strong acid before it entered the flasks of heated infusions.
These experiments were hard for others to repeat unequivocally and they were followed

by those of Theodor Schwann in which air was allowed to enter flasks of sterilized infusions only after it had been heated [60]. Proponents of spontaneous generation objected to the experiments of Schulze and to those of Schwann on the basis that the vigorous chemical and physical means used to rid the air of potential germs could just as likely have destroyed its nonviable but vivifying ability. H. Schroeder and T. von Dusch countered this objection by filtering the air that entered experimental flasks through cotton wool [60]. It seems that William Roberts adopted this method in his studies on spontaneous generation by using plugs of cotton wool to stopper glass vessels containing sterilized infusions [92,107], and cotton-stoppered containers became universally employed for cultivation of microbes.

It was Pasteur who provided the simplest solution to the problem of allowing air into sterilized containers: He modified the necks of containers into S shapes whose convolution could not be ascended by those microbes contained in the air entering the flasks [60]. Such experimental containers provided the culmination of the arguments over the importance of air in activating sterilized infusions but were not practical for routine use in the culture of microorganisms.

c. Early Work on Fermentation: Early widespread efforts to cultivate microbes also grew from the desire to have a ready source of "infusorians" to study under the microscope [232]. The most common media were infusions of mixed microbial populations. Most studies of this sort dealt with putrescible or fermentable fluids sterilized by the various heating methods described in the preceding paragraph and then inoculated with a sample from an already fermented or putrefied material. The changes wrought in such fluids were considered by some to be due to the microbes that teemed in the fluids, but others were equally certain that microbes were the consequence, not the cause, of fermentation or putrefaction [232].

Pasteur's work on fermentation began with his conviction that alcoholic fermentation was caused by the round globular bodies found in a fermented brew, a fact asserted long before separately by Cagnard-Latour, by Kützing, and by Schwann [60]. From this conviction, Pasteur reasoned that one need only search the sediment of other sorts of fermentation to find therein the microbial form responsible for the change [108]. His assumption proved correct and a whole cascade of findings came from his successive search of fermented products for their germs. A part of the proof of his assumption was to passage some of the sediment to fresh, unfermented substrate, and by such successive passages, he undoubtedly achieved a profound enrichment of a particular kind of microbe. But no matter how often the passages were repeated, he clearly never had a pure culture in the acceptable sense. Pure cultures were actually obtained in fluid cultures by Joseph Lister, who employed a dilution method based on calculations made from estimates of the number of bacteria per microscopic field. The estimates came from experiments in which a specially constructed syringe equipped with a graduated screw device was employed [60]. But such methods were laborious, and pure cultures were only achieved efficiently with the development of solid substrates for cultivation.

d. The Development of Solidified Culture Media: The earliest efforts to use solid media involved natural products such as potato slices or carrot plugs, but such primitive methods would not allow exact studies on essential ingredients.

A series of observations that suggested how solidified substrates might be useful in efforts to derive clones of microbes was made by Salomonsen with clotted blood [353].

He noted that dark spots developed in glass cylinders containing blood undergoing putrefaction and that these spots contained nearly pure outgrowths of different kinds of bacteria. He used this observation as a basis for an extended series of experiments to achieve pure collection of putrefactive microbes by drawing blood into capillary tubes and breaking the tube where isolated spots occurred. He found that each spot contained only one sort of bacterium. While instructive in reference to blood, Salomonsen's method did not have other obvious applications; however, it was an ingenious forerunner of the use of solid media for achieving pure cultures.

It is generally acknowledged that Vittadini was the first (1852) to use gelatin as a solidifying agent of the liquid media with which he attempted to grow *Beauveria bassiana* [3,60]. This same solidifying agent was employed by Oscar Brefeld in his extensive studies on pure cultivation of fungi [60]. The method was adopted by Klebs in work with bacteria and used by Koch in his development of the poured-plate method for purification of bacteria. It was for such work in Koch's laboratory that Frau Hesse, the wife of one of his co-workers, suggested the use of agar-agar as a substitute for gelatin [3,60]. She obtained samples from friends in the Dutch East Indies, where agar is used in preparations of jams [60]. Agar is one of those marvelous innovations that was fundamental to rapid advances in knowledge about the microbial etiology of infectious diseases.

Two new devices were developed during the major methodological advances described in the preceding paragraphs. Each has added enormously to the ease of nutritional work. The first was the van Tieghem cell for microscopical observation of hanging-drop cultures [3]. This technique, which gradually developed into the slide cell chamber, of which there are several modern-day examples [e.g., 27], has facilitated observations of microscopic features of fungi. The second device was the "small modification" that Petri made in Koch's plate method of cultivation. No other culture chamber was so universally and immediately adopted as was Petri's marvelous dish [295].

e. Early Work on Nutrition: Among those working with fermentation, it was common practice to add albuminoid (proteins such as gelatin, casein, etc.) to the mixtures under study [108]. Justus von Liebig and others believed that these substances acted as the agency of fermentation. Pasteur, however, regarded them as merely food for the yeast of alcoholic fermentation or the bacterium of lactic acid fermentation. When, therefore, he replaced the albuminoid material with an inorganic source of nitrogen, such as ammonium tartrate, and observed fermentation to take place, he concluded that the chemical theory of Liebig and his school was wrong and that the biological theory developed independently by Cagnaird-Latour, by Kützing, and by Schwann must be correct. Actually Pasteur inadvertently avoided a contradiction of his assertion [3]. Liebig, who was a good experimentalist, could not grow yeasts in Pasteur's inorganic liquid medium. Pasteur and Liebig were to have resolved the argument by experiments performed before a commission chosen to judge the matter, but Liebig's death interrupted the intended resolution of the controversy. It is now well known that strains of *Saccharomyces cerevisiae* require growth factors, e.g., biotin, pantothenic acid, inositol, and nicotinic acid, for growth in synthetic media. This need was met by Pasteur's large starting inoculum but not by Liebig's smaller one. The true resolution of this aspect of the Pasteur-Liebig debate was not supplied until Wildier's work on inoculum size and initiation of growth by yeast cells in a sugar-containing synthetic medium [445]. He showed that the factor, which he called bios, necessary for initiation of growth from small inocula was present in meat extract, commercial peptones, and in boiled wort of germinated barley. Subsequent studies by others gradually established the nature of the many growth-promoting substances in bios [3].

As well as good fortune in using a large inoculum, Pasteur had included an additive to his fluid medium that was crucial. The ash that was an ingredient of the medium was the ashes of incinerated yeasts and supplied to the medium phosphates, potassium, magnesium, iron, and other essential inorganic ions. The addition was one of the critical innovations of the medium that accounted for its success and again reflects the genius of Pasteur's experimental approach to the fermentation problem [108].

One of Pasteur's first students was Jules Raulin who wrote his doctoral thesis on "Études chimiques sur la végétation" [315]. He continued to work on this project after leaving Pasteur's tutelage and eventually he published his results. Raulin began with an ammonium-sugar-salts (i.e., yeast ash) medium that Pasteur had designed for *Penicillium*. From this, Raulin devised a synthetic medium that was suited to the growth of *Aspergillus niger*. A long series of experiments ensued in which Raulin noted the effects of the addition of various substances. These studies established an excellent model for physiological investigations of fungi [3].

These, then, are the basic features of the history of artificial cultivation of microbes. Such antecedents form the basis for development of knowledge about the nutrition and physiology of fungi. Certain other historical events in reference to the pathogenic fungi will be noted by way of introduction to the selected topics covered in this chapter.

2. Metabolism

The metabolism of fungi is known in detail. Some of the interest in metabolic processes of fungi derives from the fact that they produce industrially useful metabolites, but to a considerable extent the wealth of current information is the result of the exquisite tools which fungi provide for dissecting the biochemical bases of life processes. The extraordinary plasticity of fungi has allowed the creation of mutants that are essential to understanding the details of metabolic pathways. The manipulation of fungi in pursuit of finite information on their metabolism has often revealed fascinating examples of adaptability. A recent example will serve to document this point. A physiological adaptation to the loss of amino acid transport ability has been described in *Neurospora crassa* [100]. In this study, data were presented that showed that a strain of *N. crassa* devoid of constitutive amino acid transport ability could nevertheless utilize arginine, which it could not transport, as a sole source of nitrogen. Under the proper condition of nitrogen starvation and the presence of arginine, the transport-deficient mutant produced an extracellular enzyme that removed the α-amino group from the amino acid. The α-amino group was released as ammonium ions, which then served as the nitrogen source. Thus, microbial model systems have been applied to areas of biology because of their advantage of genetic manipulation, and such applications have resulted in a vast store of information on microbial metabolism.

a. *Chemical Composition of Fungi:* The earliest investigations on fungal chemistry dealt with chemical composition. This sort of information accumulated over the years until by 1890 Zopf and, a few years later, Zellner presented compilations of the cumulative knowledge [452,453]. Interest in the chemical composition of zoopathogenic fungi centers in two areas: (1) changes in constituents that accompany dimorphism (see Chap. 10, Part A, of this series), and (2) components that may be the basis for pathogenetic mechanisms (see Chaps. 1 and 5, Part B:1 of this series, and Chap. 2 of this volume).

b. Secondary Metabolites: Interest in secondary metabolities of fungi, i.e., those synthetic by-products that have no obvious role in the primary needs of the organism, as have proteins and nucleic acids, was actively pursued by Raistrich and his colleagues for over 30 years [3]. One of the earliest textbooks of industrial mycology was that of one of Raistrich's colleagues, George Smith [386], a volume recently revised and re-issued [287]. A particular group of such metabolites, the mycotoxins, has been considered in Chap. 10, Part B:I, of this series.

c. Carbohydrate Utilization: The degradation of carbohydrate was among the earliest activities of fungi to be explored experimentally. A vast store of knowledge accumulated gradually, and it remained for Foster to survey the chemical activities of fungi and to place this knowledge in perspective [130,131,132]. It has been established for yeasts and for filamentous fungi that a carbohydrate source is first converted to glucose, which is metabolized to pyruvate by the Embden-Meyerhof-Parnas (EMP) or the hexose monophosphate (HMP) pathway, or more uncommonly by the Entner-Douderoff (ED) pathway. Pyruvate is next incorporated into the tricarboxylic acid (TCA) cycle. The final stages of utilization include coupling to the respiratory chain which involves the cytochromes and transfer of electrons to molecular oxygen. The major features of carbohydrate metabolism have been summarized recently [16].

B. General Aspects

1. Autotrophs and Heterotrophs

Historically, microorganisms were divided into two principal classes on the basis of nutrition: the autotrophs, which can use completely inorganic substances, and the heterotrophs, which require organic nutrients. The insufficiency of this simple division to encompass the varieties of nutritional patterns among microbes has long been recognized [399] and has been replaced by a more comprehensive classification which takes into account the nature of the energy source and the nature of the principal carbon source while disregarding requirements for growth factors. According to this scheme, organisms that use light as an energy source are called phototrophic, whereas those that use chemical energy sources are called chemotrophic. Those organisms that use carbon dioxide as a principal carbon source are referred to as autotrophic, and those that use organic compound for this purpose are heterotrophic. By appropriate combinations of these terms, one designates: photoautotrophs (plants, algae, and certain bacteria), photoheterotrophs (purple, nonsulfur-containing bacteria), chemoautotrophs (certain bacterial groups), and chemoheterotrophs (animals, protozoa, fungi, and most of the bacteria) [399].

2. The Chemoheterotrophy of Zoopathogens

All fungi, then, are chemoheterotrophic and accordingly must seek their carbon saprophytically from nonliving sources or in one or another type of symbiosis with other living things [229]. The form of symbiosis adopted by the zoopathogens is parasitism [399]. Apart from the principal carbon source, pathogenic fungi vary widely in their other nutritional requirements. Early studies revealed forms that needed only inorganic sources of nitrogen, such as nitrate or ammonium ions, others that had to be supplied with amino acids, and finally, some with requirements for organic nitrogen as well as a number of ancillary growth factors. Originally, it was thought that parasitism involved the loss of enzyme essential for the synthesis of microbial constituents, making it necessary to add complex ingredients to a culture medium [127,205]. Certainly some elegant examples of this sort of correlation can be found among the pathogenic bacteria and phytopathogenic fungi. But a moment's reflection quickly affirms that such a correlation is largely lacking among zoopathogenic fungi. Even parasites thought to be strictly anthropophilic and not to exist in any other location, e.g., *Malassezia furfur* or *Microsporum audouinii*, have requirements rather easily met in artificial culture media (Table 1). Admittedly, there are two pathogens that have so far defied efforts to cultivate them, viz., *Rhinosporidium seeberi* and *Loboa loboi*, and thus may presently be thought of as obligate parasites, but both seem to be acquired from exogenous sources [332] so that their in vitro cultivation may yet be achieved. In fact, as pointed out by Nickerson [269], almost a reverse correlation between pathogenicity and nutritional demands is observed in medical mycology, i.e., some of the most notable pathogens in vivo are the least demanding in vitro (Table 1). Therefore, the instructive lessons in this regard from bacteriology and phytopathology do not seem to obtain in medical mycology.

3. The Continued Interest in the Nutrition of Zoopathogens

Although clues as to the basis of pathogenicity were not immediately forthcoming from a study of the nutritional needs of pathogens, work on the subject is nevertheless of continuing interest. Such interest centers in three areas: (1) the practical demands for isolation and cultivation; (2) a sound basis for classification; and (3) the discovery of nutrient utilization which explains certain aspects of pathogenicity, e.g., dimorphism. These three areas will be considered in the ensuing portions of this chapter devoted to the nutrition of zoopathogens. In addition, selected topics from the area of physiology of the fungi pathogenic to humans and animals will be considered.

4. Antimetabolites as Therapeutics

The earliest efforts to develop drugs useful in the therapy of infectious diseases were directed toward selective toxicity, i.e., substances that would inhibit or kill microbes but leave the host unharmed. Initially, such efforts were largely empirical [85], but the discovery of sulfanilamide [374] and the eventual realization that its close structural relation to *p*-aminobenzoic acid was the basis of its mode of action as a metabolite antagonist led to many efforts to understand the metabolism of pathogens in order to discover key points of potential interruption. Unfortunately, this approach has yielded only small returns in the development of therapeutics [429] but has provided abundant information on the intermediary metabolism of microorganisms. It is clear from such studies [84,132,138,233,235,269,275,376,404] that the fundamental aspects of carbohydrate utilization and energy transfer are the same for pathogens as for saprophytes. Nevertheless, specific metabolic features of some parasites present features of compelling interest in that they hold promise of revealing features that may be related to pathogenicity. A few of these will be covered in succeeding portions of this chapter.

5. Summary

In summary, a comprehensive review of the nutrition and physiology of zoopathogenic fungi is not intended but rather the selective consideration of a few areas that have captured the interest of the author and appear to offer promise of providing exciting new information on the pathogenetic mechanisms employed by zoopathogenic fungi.

Table 1 The Nutritional Requirements of Selected Zoopathogens

Fungus	Disease	Pathogenicity	Nitrogen requirement	Growth factors	References
Blastomyces dermatitidis	Blastomycosis	Disseminated form highly fatal	Ammonium N	None	155,228,357
Coccidioides immitis	Coccidioidomycosis	Disseminated form highly fatal	Ammonium N	None	342,404
Paracoccidioides brasiliensis	Paracoccidioidomycosis	Disseminated form highly fatal	Ammonium N[a]	Thiamin[b]	15,155,314
Candida albicans	Candidiasis	Commensal to highly pathogenic	Ammonium N	Biotin	280
Cryptococcus neoformans	Cryptococcosis	Disseminated form may be fatal	Ammonium N	Thiamin	231
Microsporum audouinii	Ringworm	Moderately pathogenic but not fatal	Ammonium N (amino acids stimulate growth)	Thiamin Riboflavin Nicotinic acid	334
Malassezia furfur	Pityriasis versicolor	Very slight interaction with host	Amino acids	Thiamin Oleic acid	29,157,158 266,317

[a]There are some strains of Paracoccidioides brasiliensis (e.g., VIC Pb9) which are methionine auxotrophs [314,359].

[b]The thiamin requirement of Paracoccidioides brasiliensis [15] was not confirmed by Gilardi and Laffer [155], but I have found in keeping with the unpublished but mentioned results of San-Blas and Cova [359] that laboratory strains require it for yeast form growth at 37°C (D. H. Howard, unpublished observations).

Source: Adapted from Nickerson [269] and from Ainsworth [2].

II. NUTRITION

As was pointed out in the preceding section, the study of the nutritional needs of zoopathogens has served three fundamentally different purposes. The first was to design media that would be selectively useful in the cultivation of pathogens from the host and from natural sources. A second purpose arose from early studies on nutrition that showed the nutrient requirements for growth could be used as a means for classification of morphologically similar or identical forms. Finally, the search for explanations of particular traits such as dimorphism or tissue tropism was often centered at the outset in descriptions of nutritional control of those traits. Each of these purposes will be considered in the ensuing subdivisions of this section on Nutrition. The exact nutritional requirements of several of the fungi that cause systemic and inoculation mycoses have been compiled by Gilardi [154]. From an earlier study, Nickerson and Williams [273] report similar data for a number of dermatophytes and a few other pathogens. Tabular data of this sort offer interesting bases for comparative discussion (Table 1) but must be used cautiously. Quite apart from strain variation with respect to specific nutrients, e.g., the cysteine requirement of yeast cells of *Histoplasma capsulatum* (q.v.), there are unexplained instances of misinformation. An instructive example of this sort of thing was traced by Gilardi and Laffer [155]. As they record, Levine and Ordal reported that the mycelial phase of *Blastomyces dermatitidis* did not require any vitamins [228], while Holliday and McCoy [163A] detected a requirement for biotin. Levine and Ordal had used cotton-plugged agar slants in their work, which could have allowed contamination with biotin from the cotton or the agar. Agar contains 0.002 μg of biotin per gram, enough to satisfy the requirement of *B. dermatitidis* [155]. Subsequent work with washed agar by Salvin [357] and in liquid synthetic media [155] strengthens the assertion of Levine and Ordal that *B. dermatitidis* has no vitamin requirements (Table 1). There is no current explanation for the contradiction, and one must always be prepared to confirm nutritional data whenever the facts are or become a key issue.

A. Cultivation

1. Culture Media

Culture media used in the study of fungi are of four general sorts.

   a. Nonreproducible Media: Media such as hay infusions, carrot plugs, potato slices, or sterilized soil are valuable for certain purposes, but the substance of which they are composed varies and thus cannot be reproduced accurately. Culture media of this class are used in medical mycology for very specific purposes. A few examples include: the use of polished rice for distinguishing *Microsporum audouinii* and *M. canis* [86]; the use of soil and hair filaments to foster cleistothecial development by mating strains of dermatophytes [215]; the use of blood- or egg-containing media in culturing the parasitic phase of dimorphic pathogens, especially *Histoplasma capsulatum* [67,214,423]; the widespread use of corn meal agar or similar decoctions to foster chlamydospore (chlamydoconidia) development in *Candida albicans* [27]; the use of soil extract agar in studies on mating behavior of dermatophytes [215]; the use of sterilized soil for maintenance of stock cultures (see Chap. 4 of this volume); and the use of potato dextrose agar with some of the Mucorales (see Chap. 2, Part A, of this series) and as a medium for preservation of stock cultures by freezing [286].

b. Reproducible Media of Unknown Composition: The work of Oscar Brefeld alluded to in the Introduction provided the essential knowledge from which media designed to provide pure cultures could be concocted [3]. Preparations of this kind were elegantly employed in the definitive studies of Raimond Sabouraud on the dermatophytes. The medium that he devised consisted of 4% crude maltose (Brute de Chanut) or glucose (Massée de Chanut) and 1% granulated French peptone (Granulée de Chassaing) [2,382]. These ingredients were available from Maison Cogit, 36 Boulevard St. Michel, Paris [382], but the company went out of business during World War I [2,106]. Various substitutes were proposed [2,435,436,437] and the current product bears little resemblance to its progenitor yet continues to bear the name "Sabouraud's agar" or "Sabouraud's dextrose agar." Variations from Sabouraud's original recipe generally call for simple glucose-peptone combinations in agar [432] and frequently omit the adjustment of the pH to 5.6 [382] which Sabouraud incorporated as a selective device to discourage bacterial growth from skin samples. There are now a very large number of culture media prepared from more or less standardized commercial reagents such as glucose and peptone. The general assumption has been that use of such commonly available reagents for construction of culture media would result in greater standardization and more uniform experimental results, but there are anecdotal examples of variety in lots of a given peptone. More important, however, is the well-established fact that there are considerable differences among the "peptones" used to construct the various glucose-peptone agars that go under the name of Sabouraud's glucose medium [283]. Thus, reproducible media such as glucose-peptone may yet suffer from unsuspected variation among different laboratories because of the different commercial peptones employed.

c. Synthetic Media: These are media prepared from pure chemicals of known constitution that can be reproduced precisely regardless of the commercial source. It would of course be very desirable to have such a medium for all medically important fungi. Such a medium does not exist, but a number of examples of synthetic media with limited but important uses have been developed. A few examples will be given.

Historically, the earliest use of a medium that could be called synthetic was that used by Raulin whose work was alluded to in the Introduction to this chapter [315]. He developed a recipe for a medium comprised of 11 constituents, all of known chemical composition. Another early example of a synthetic medium still widely employed is that of Czapek's as modified initially by Dox and subsequently by Thom [382].

Coccidioides immitis has been grown on chemically defined media. There have been quite a few recipes and modifications for this purpose [e.g., 88,339,342], but the one used most extensively is Smith's asparagine liquid medium [385]. This medium has been widely adopted for work on antigens of both *C. immitis* and *Histoplasma capsulatum* [199]. Several defined media have been suggested for special studies with *H. capsulatum* [206,252,303].

d. Selective Media: Certain nutritional and metabolic attributes of zoopathogens have allowed for the design of both selective and differential media that help in cultivation and identification. With one exception, these are not specific for a given species but rather only select for fungi from among other microbial types or zoopathogens of a certain kind.

From the outset, advantage has been taken of the fact that fungi are rather more resistant to acid pH than are bacteria. Sabouraud adjusted the pH of his maltose-peptone medium to 5.6 to discourage the overgrowth of cultures from skin, hair, and nails by bacteria [350]. This goal was also achieved in the same way by Waksman in his glucose-peptone medium used for counting fungi in the soil [432]. The same purpose is now

Table 2 Assimilations, Hydrolytic Activity, and Physiological Attributes Used as a Basis of Classification of Human and Animal Pathogenic Fungi

Activity	Fungi	Reference
Aminopeptidases	*Blastomyces dermatitidis*	226
	Candida albicans	200,226,260
	Cryptococcus neoformans	226
	Dermatophytes	74
	Histoplasma capsulatum	226
	Histoplasma duboisii	226
	Histoplasma farciminosum	226
	Paracoccidioides brasilensis	226
	Sporothrix schenckii	226
Canavinine resistance	*Cryptococcus neoformans* (serotypes)	219
Carbohydrate assimilation	Yeasts	46,47,57,91,188, 221,223,231,338, 371,454
Carotenoid pigment	*Rhodotorula*	296
Citrate utilization	*Candida* spp.	281
Creatinine assimilation	*Cryptococcus neoformans*	30
	Sporothrix schenckii	395,397
Cycloheximide resistance	*Cryptococcus neoformans* (serotypes)	352
	Zoopathogens (general)	151,210,249,250, 351
Esterase	Dermatophytes	372
5-FC resistance	*Candida* spp.	281
Gelatin hydrolysis	*Candida* spp.	244
	Cladosporium spp.	135
	Cryptococcus neoformans	344
	Dematiaceous fungi	344
	Dermatophytes	344
	Histoplasma capsulatum	36
	Histoplasma spp.	41,344
	Paracoccidioides brasiliensis	344
	Sporothrix schenckii	344
Glycine utilization	*Candida* spp.	281
	Cryptococcus neoformans	219,352
Lactate dehydrogenase	*Candida* spp.	31,32,33
Lipid hydrolysis	Dermatophytes	255
	Malassezia (Pityrosporum)	157,158
L-malic acid dehydrogenase	*Blastomyces dermatitidis*	348
	Candida spp.	31,32,33
	Cryptococcus neoformans	30
Nitrate reduction	*Cryptococcus* spp.	325
Peroxidase	Dermatophytes	372
Phosphatases	*Candida* spp.	282,361,388
	Paracoccidioides brasiliensis	449

Table 2 (continued)

Activity	Fungi	Reference
pH tolerance	*Candida* spp.	281
Proteolysis[a]	*Candida* spp.	56,153,238, 349,392
	Cladosporium spp.	135
	Dermatophytes	254,258
Safrinine resistance	*Candida* spp.	281
Salt tolerance	*Candida* spp.	281
Selenite reduction	*Candida* spp.	125
Sorbose assimilation	*Candida* spp.	281
Sulfite reduction	*Candida* spp.	270
Telurite reduction	*Candida* spp.	125
Tetrazolium reduction	*Candida* spp.	175,293
Tyrosine utilization	*Candida* spp.	344
	Cryptococcus neoformans	344
	Dematiaceous fungi	344
	Dermatophytes	344
	Histoplasma spp.	41,344
	Paracoccidioides brasiliensis	344
	Sporothrix schenckii	344
Urea hydrolysis	*Candida* spp.	281,344
	Cryptococcus neoformans	344
	Cryptococcus spp.	370
	Dematiaceous fungi	344
	Dermatophytes	255,297,344
	Histoplasma spp.	41
	Paracoccidioides brasiliensis	344
	Sporothrix schenckii	344

[a]For a general review of proteinases of eucaryotic microorganisms, see Ref. 276. Additional citations will be found in Table 4.

most commonly fulfilled by incorporation of an antibacterial antibiotic, usually chloramphenicol [249]. Moreover, the resistance of many zoopathogens to cycloheximide allows an even more selective medium to be designed by its incorporation (Table 2).

Guzotia Seed Agar [390] used in conjunction with an incubation temperature of 37°C is both selective and differential. One very useful recipe for this medium [377] employs an inhibitor (diphenyl), which together with a stringent nitrogen source (creatinine) limits the number of fungi capable of growing on it, and these limitations, together with the fact that *Cryptococcus neoformans* is one of a very few commonly encountered yeasts that possesses a phenoloxidase which converts di- or polyphenolic compounds to melanin, makes the Seed Agar highly differential as well as selective. Advantage of these facts has been taken in several epidemiological surveys [178,203, 367] and in rapid yeast identification in heavily contaminated specimens [171,265].

2. Isolations from the Host

The realization that fungi could cause infectious diseases of animals dates from just under 150 years ago. In 1835, Agostino Bassi [3,60] provided experimental evidence that the muscardine disease of silkworm was caused by *Beauveria bassiana*. A few years later in 1841, David Gruby isolated the fungus of favus *Trichophyton schoenlienii* on potato slices [332]. Although the mold had been observed in materials from patients by Remak in 1837, Gruby's work was the first example of the actual cultivation of a zoopathogen from the tissues of a host. The history of early work on the dermatophytes was presented in Chap. 6, Part A, of this series and has been briefly considered by Bulloch [60] and by Ainsworth [3]. The popularity of Sabouraud's medium was almost immediate [106] and a modified Sabouraud's agar has become the basic medium used in the recovery of most fungi from clinical materials [163,250]. The details of current approaches to cultivation of fungi in the clinical laboratory is a subject treated comprehensively by Glenn Roberts in Chap. 8 of this volume and will not be considered here.

3. Isolations from Nature

The ability to grow a particular microbe from a mixture of microorganisms was fundamental to progress in microbiology in the nineteenth century [232]. Pasteur's success in relating certain microbes to particular sorts of fermentation rested on the principle of enrichment or "Darwinization," as it was sometimes referred to in the very early literature. This principle was rather simply put by Beijerinck when he wrote, "Everything is everywhere, the environment only selects" [26]. Thus, Pasteur simply designed conditions such that microbes capable of utilizing a particular substrate outgrew other members of a mixed population. Enrichment culture techniques were used by both Beijerinck and Winogradsky to isolate species capable of carrying out particular physiological functions [e.g., 26,51,446]. The implication of the techniques was immediately obvious, and they have been widely adopted in microbiological research.

a. Selection by Baiting: The restriction of dermatophytes to the hair, skin, and nails generated interest in the ability of these fungi to grow on such products in vitro [122,240,273,421]. The keratinophilic nature of dermatophytes was thereby readily established, and the use of sterilized hair as a bait for isolating dermatophytes and other keratinophilic fungi from soil was a logical extension of these early observations [425, 426]. Precedence for baiting techniques is found in the work of Gordon and Hagen [159] who coated glass rods with paraffin, buried them in the soil, and dug them up at intervals and isolated from them pathogenic strains of *Nocardia asteroides*. The word "baiting" derives from Karling who in 1946 isolated Chytrids by placing various types of chitin and keratin on soil or in water [197]. Other sorts of baiting techniques have not been widely applied to zoopathogens [288].

b. Selection on Basis of Pathogenicity: One obvious feature of pathogens, i.e., their ability to cause disease, was adopted and expanded by Emmons to isolate systemic pathogens from exogenous sources [117,118,119,120,403]. The procedure has taken two forms. In the first form, rodents and other animals from endemic areas are trapped and their lungs cultivated on nutrient media. By this means, pathogens as well as interesting saprophytes inhaled by animals grow out and thereby help to delineate the geographic distribution of the fungi [117,119]. The second form of the procedure is to inject appropriately treated soil suspensions into mice and then to culture pieces of liver and spleen after a suitable incubation period [103, 117]. This method was used initially by Stewart and Meyer to isolate *Coccidioides immitis* from soil [403] and has been fundamental to gathering vast amounts of information on the natural sources of infection by systemic pathogens [5, 7, 8, 120].

c. *Growth from Single Cells: Cloning*: The realization that pure cultures were essential for solid advances in microbiology led to systematic efforts to grow cultures from single-cell inocula. As was indicated earlier, Oscar Brefeld provided methods for initiating cultures from single spores of *Aspergillus* and Lister achieved the same result with individual bacterial cells of *Streptococcus lactis*. Each used the principle of progressive dilution: Brefeld looked to see that the final drop in a dilution sequence contained a single spore [3], whereas Lister devised a mathematical probability approach to realize the end point of his dilutions [60]. The need to clone from a single representative before working with an isolate is fundamental to all nutritional and physiological work.

The fact that a single cell gives rise to a single clone of individuals is a basic attribute that allows the quantitative approach of assessing the numbers of individuals in a suspension of cells by determining the colony-forming units in that suspension. *Histoplasma capsulatum* in its yeast form has always presented a frustrating, but at the same time, fascinating problem to those who wished to make a quantitative plate count on the number of individuals in a suspension. The problem is that *H. capsulatum* in the yeast form does not clone on agar media. One may, of course, use the obvious alternative of incubating plates containing the dilution sequence at room temperature and then counting the mycelial colonies which arise. Although this option provides acceptable data, one must wait 10-14 days to be sure all of the colonies are visible. The fascinating question of why individual yeast cells of *H. capsulatum* cannot initiate yeast-form colonies on agar media is unanswered. This inability is noted in liquid cultures as well. Thus, Pine [299] reported no growth in liquid shake cultures inoculated with fewer than 5×10^4 cells. Addition of albumin to the medium allowed about 50-fold fewer cells to initiate growth. Salvin reported the same restriction on inoculum size (8×10^3) in stagnant liquid cultures under carbon dioxide [354, 356], and Scherr recorded a similar result in his work [366]. By redesigning the medium, Pine was able to obtain growth in stagnant liquid cultures with approximately 100 cells, but the success was negated by addition of agar [300] and results with solid media have always been very unsatisfactory.

The problem appears to be related to the nature of the medium. Toxicity of the peptones used was strongly indicated by McVickar's observations on exhaustive adsorption of peptone media [253]. However, some sort of growth factor availability must also be a consideration, since McVeigh and Morton had to use inocula of greater than 10^4 cells to get growth in a synthetic medium devoid of peptones [252]. Clearly, a single yeast cell of *H. capsulatum* can initiate continued growth because it does so in the cytoplasm of mouse macrophages in cell culture [177]. Moreover, a single viable aggregate is able to initiate an infection in a mouse [347].

A series of observations recently published by Burt and his colleagues has established that a siderophore of the hydroxamic acid type functions as a growth factor for *H. capsulatum* and that supplementation of media with hydroxamic acids allows for outgrowth of small inocula at 37°C [62, 63]. The data in the published reports from Burt's laboratory show that colony counts very close to theoretical expectations are achieved from inocula incubated at 37°C on siderophore-enriched agar plates. Thus, trapping and transport of iron by the siderophore may be the factor that, together with peptone toxicity, controls the ability of *H. capsulatum* to initiate growth from a single cell placed on an agar medium. If these observations are confirmed and combined with the peptone-toxicity results of others, it might be possible to design solid media that could be used for replica plating and other methods essential to an approach to the basic biology of *H. capsulatum*.

B. Classification

1. Yeasts

Pasteur's finding that fermentations were uniquely caused by distinctive microbes led eventually to the realization that utilization of a given set of carbohydrates could be used as a basis for taxonomic decisions. This realization found its most elegant early expression in the procedure devised by Beijerinck [25] for determining the assimilation of various substrates. He called the procedure an auxanographic method. Others soon adopted similar schemes of relating fermentative or assimilative abilities to species identification [71], but its modern form is best exemplified in the original work by Lodder on the classifications of yeasts [231]. The essence of the auxanogram was incorporated into the test as developed by Wickerham [443] and is the basis of all the new systems for rapid identification of clinically important yeasts [46,47,57,91,188, 221,223,338,371,454]. The logical extension of such rapid methods into automated systems has been made [168,278].

2. Dermatophytes

Pasteur's first three students were Jules Raulin, Phillippe van Tieghem, and Émile Duclaux. Each produced a doctoral thesis on a topic related to Pasteur's work on fermentation. Van Tieghem's thesis was entitled "Sur la fermentation de l'urée et d'acide hippurique" and was completed in 1864. That of Duclaux was titled "Sur l'absorption de l'ammoniaque et la production des acides volatile pendant la fermentation alcoolique" and appeared in 1865. I have already mentioned that Raulin continued to work on his thesis "Études chimiques sur la végétation," which he ultimately published in 1870 [315].

Duclaux set up his own laboratory, which became justly famous, and he ultimately became the successor to Pasteur as the Director of the Pasteur Institute in Paris. One of Duclaux's first students, Verujsky, studied the utilization of carbon compounds by dermatophytes [431]; this work has been judged to be one of the earliest studies on the metabolism of zoopathogens [273]. Subsequent work established the utilization of various carbohydrates and lipids as sole carbon sources by a variety of dermatophytes [Ref. 273 and literature cited therein]. Efforts have been made to take advantage of the selective ability of dermatophytes to utilize carbon sources as a basis for distinguishing among them [e.g., 298,373], but none of these efforts has matched the usefulness of such tests for yeasts.

Robbins et al. [337] and Burkholder and Moyer [61] were among the first to describe growth factor needs of the dermatophytes [273]. Building on their observations, Lucille Georg comprehensively examined the vitamin requirements of a number of species in the genus *Trichophyton* [144]. This work augmented by her observation of the histidine requirement of *T. megninii* [146] became the basis for a method for the classification of some dermatophytes in the genus *Trichophyton* [144,145,146, 147,148,149,150,151,152,413].

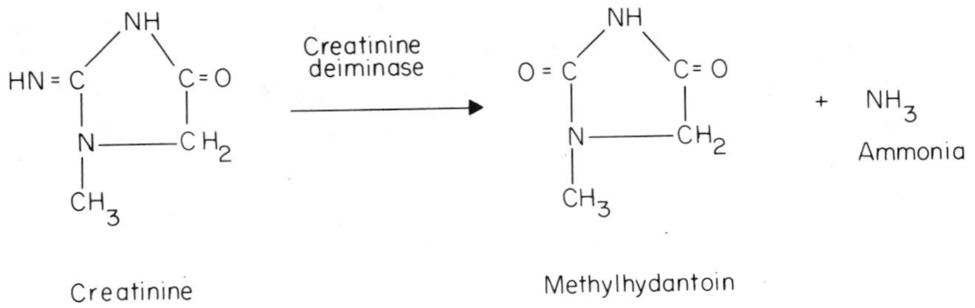

Figure 1 Conversion of creatinine to methylhydantoin and ammonia. (From Ref. 305.)

The investigations of Mosher et al. [262] on the nitrogen requirements of *Trichophyton mentagrophytes* was one of the earliest attempts to study nitrogen needs in a pathogenic fungus. This same subject was approached by Robbins and Ma in 1945 [336], and the utilization of single amino acids by dermatophytes has been examined from time to time [334,381]. More recently Hilger et al. [174] have examined the ability of *T. mentagrophytes* to utilize single amino acids as sole carbon and nitrogen sources. Observations of this sort have been reported with other pathogens, e.g., *Histoplasma* spp. [302]. However, even though these observations collectively are of intrinsic interest and in one or two instances have supplied a basis for morphogenetic studies [e.g., 18,167], on balance, the nitrogen utilization pattern of dermatophytes has not supplied a firm basis for differentiation among species with the single exception of the histidine requirement of *T. megninii* [146].

3. Specific Situations

a. Cryptococcus: In 1962, Staib showed that creatinine was assimilated by *Cryptococcus neoformans* [390,391]. The pathogenic species of *Cryptococcus*, *C. neoformans* var. *neoformans* (serotypes A and D) and *C. neoformans* var. *gattii* (serotypes B and C), use creatinine as a source of nitrogen but not of carbon [30,219,305]. Both varieties degrade creatinine in a single step which involves production of methylhydantoin and ammonia, a reaction catalyzed by creatinine deiminase (Fig. 1). Synthesis of the enzyme is repressed by ammonia in *C. neoformans* var. *neoformans* but not in *C. neoformans* var. *gattii*. Advantage of this difference was taken to devise a medium for separating the two varieties [219,305]. The medium contains creatinine and glucose with bromothymol blue as an indicator (CDB medium). Since the creatinine deiminase of *C. neoformans* var. *gattii* is not repressed by ammonia, the indicator registers an alkaline reaction due to ammonia which accumulates from creatinine degradation by this variety.

A modification of CDB medium has recently been published and, although the principle of its construction is quite different (in fact, has nothing to do with creatinine utilization), it will be explained here for the sake of continuity [219]. The modification involves the use of glycine as the sole carbon and nitrogen source in the medium and incorporates canavanine, an arginine analog. The indicator bromothymol blue is also incorporated into the medium (CGB medium). Strains of *C. neoformans* var. *gattii* (B and C serotypes) are not inhibited by the arginine analog, whereas all strains of serotype D and nearly 30% of serotype A *C. neoformans* var. *neoformans* are. The former variety can utilize glycine for both carbon and nitrogen needs, and since more carbon is required than nitrogen, the excess nitrogen accumulates as ammonia which alkalinizes the medium and changes the color of the indicator. With *C. neoformans* var. *neoformans,* the situation is different [257a]. Only 19% of serotype A isolates and 11% of serotype D isolates use glycine as a source of nitrogen and use it only poorly as a carbon source. All of the glycine-utilizing serotype D strains are sensitive to canavanine and as a result, they do not grow on CGB medium. The glycine-utilizing strains of the A serotype are either sensitive or resistant to canavanine. Only 19% of the glycine-utilizing A strains are sensitive to the analog whereas the other 81% are resistant. However, even these latter isolates fail to grow when the medium contains both glycine and canavanine. Thus, the CGB medium can be used to distinguish *C. neoformans* var. *neoformans* (no change in color of CGB medium) from *C. neoformans* var. *gattii* (CGB medium turns blue).

Another medium designed for the same purpose has been designed by Salkin and Hurd [352]. This medium (GCP) relies on exactly the same principles, i.e., a variable ability to utilize glycine and a selective inhibition of *C. neoformans* var. *neoformans* strains over *C. neoformans* var. *gattii* strains. However, the key differences in GCP medium are that a differential cycloheximide-resistance instead of canavanine-resistance is used as a selective device and the indicator is phenol red. A comparison of the relative merits of the CGB and the GCP media has been published recently [219].

b. Hair Penetration: It was pointed out in a preceding paragraph that early efforts to discover the nutritional predilection of ringworm fungi for keratin led to several studies on the utilization of keratinized substances in vitro by the dermatophytes [Ref. 273 and literature cited therein]. The pattern of erosion of hair filaments by keratinophilic fungi varies [122]. On the basis of such variation, Vanbreuseghem [425] suggested that the ability to utilize keratinized substrates could be used as a diagnostic method. Ajello and Georg recommended a hair perforation method for distinguishing atypical isolates of *Trichophyton mentagrophytes* and *T. rubrum; T. mentagrophytes* perforated hair whereas *T. rubrum* did not under the controlled conditions described by the authors [6,9]. More recently Padhye et al. [292] suggested that this hair perforation test could be usefully extended to distinguishing among various species of *Epidermophyton, Microsporum,* and *Trichophyton.*

c. Malassezia ovalis (Pityrosporum ovale): This yeast was the first fungus shown to require a fatty acid, oleic acid, for growth [29]. The relationship of this organism to *M. furfur* (syn., *Pityrosporum obiculare, P. furfur*) is not settled at present [332], but early efforts to cultivate it from the scales of pityriasis versicolor (tinea versicolor) were unavailing until fatty acids, in crude form, were added to the media [see Ref. 29 for a review of the literature]. Species of the genus *Malassezia* are the only yeasts requiring fatty acids found in common association with humans and animals [2,332].

C. Morphogenesis

Nutritional factors that influence the dimorphism of pathogens have been exhaustively studied and the results of such observations summarized on a number of occasions [e.g., 19,162,271,301,304,331,343,402]. In several instances, synthetic media have been devised to accommodate these needs. More recently, attention has been directed toward a study of metabolic control mechanism (see Chap. 9, Part A, of this series). A few examples of this sort of work will be described in subsequent sections of this chapter.

III. PHYSIOLOGY

A. Aeration

Fungi are aerobic. There are no reported examples of obligate anaerobes and the degree to which fungi may grow as facultative anaerobes varies widely. At one time it was considered that fungi could not survive without some oxygen [84]. However, a number of examples are now known where optimal growth takes place in environments of very low oxygen tension [115,116,173], and *Saccharomyces cerevisiae, S. steineri, Candida albicans, C. (Torulopsis) glabrata, Malassezia (Pityrosporum)* spp., and *Mucor rouxii* have been grown in rigidly controlled, oxygen-free atmospheres [124,162,405, 414,416]. It thus seems clear that oxygen-indifferent, facultatively anaerobic fungi resembling the lactic acid bacteria occur in nature [115,116,173].

It has been noted that high carbon dioxide levels generally inhibit the growth of fungi [84], but a number of examples are known of fungi that not only grow well but may even thrive under atmospheres high in carbon dioxide [115,116,408]. In research with zoopathogens, carbon dioxide is recognized as a factor that markedly affects morphogenesis, especially dimorphism. A few examples will suffice to document this well-reviewed topic [19,162,301,304,331,343,402]. The formation of macroconidia by *Trichophyton mentagrophytes* and *T. rubrum* is stimulated by growing cultures in an atmosphere of air with 12-24% (v/v) carbon dioxide [80], and this fact can be used in preparing properly sporulating examples for classroom use (D. H. Howard, unpublished observation), though admittedly the macroscopic features of such cultures is far from those typical of a fresh isolate. Carbon dioxide has long been recognized to sponsor the spherule form of growth of *Coccidioides immitis* in vitro [50,234,236] and cultures of *Sporothrix schenckii* more readily form blastoconidia when cultured under increased carbon dioxide tension [246,247,312,355]. A similar favorable effect on the conversion of *Histoplasma capsulatum* has been observed [22,58]. In fact, the yeast cell form of *H. capsulatum* was at one time thought to be a facultative anaerobe [354] in spite of De Monbreun's original statement to the contrary [102]. However, Pine's rigorously controlled experiments established that yeast cells of *H. capsulatum* would not grow under completely anaerobic conditions [299,300]. This also is true for *Blastomyces dermatitidis* and *Paracoccidioides brasiliensis* [155,323]. Nevertheless, the in vivo environment must be of reasonably low oxygen tension, and lowered oxidation-reduction potentials clearly foster yeast-like growth by a great variety of fungi [330,333]. Systemic pathogens subsist in environments of very low oxygen tension and such environments repress oxygen-induced enzymes, such as catalase, which might otherwise antagonize oxidative antimicrobial systems [179,180,181].

B. Growth

The rate of growth of the pathogenic fungi that customarily reproduce as yeasts (*Candida* and *Cryptococcus*) or those that have a yeast form in vivo and under special circumstances in vitro (*Histoplasma capsulatum, Blastomyces dermatitidis, Paracoccidioides brasiliensis,* and *Wangiella (Exophiala) dermatitidis*), has been examined on a number of occasions (Table 3). There is little doubt about the artificiality of the growth curves generated from such studies [242], but it is difficult to overcome the desire for precision in this regard, even though the in vivo growth rates must be much slower than those obtained under the optimum in vitro conditions. The study of certain biological features, e.g., cell wall structure, antigen production, or growth repression by immunological means,

Table 3   Generation Times of Some Zoopathogens or Related Forms

Fungus	T (°C)	Generation time (h)[a]	Reference
Blastomyces dermatitidis	37	10-14	375
		12-14[b]	
Candida albicans	24	1.7-3.6	94
Coccidioides immitis	37	48-96[c]	410
Cryptococcus albidus	23	2	419
Cryptococcus neoformans	37	3.8-4.0[d]	264
(A/D serotypes)[e]		2.4-3.0	326
Histoplasma capsulatum	37	10-12	316
		8-10	137
		12-13	375
Paracoccidioides brasiliensis	37	13-21	359
Sporothrix schenckii	35-37	1.2-4.8	72
Torulopsis glabrata	37	0.75	184,289
Wangiella (Exophiala) dermatitidis	25	4.5	341

[a]In dimorphic forms, the yeast T form is meant, except for Coccidioides immitis, in which the time from endospore to mature spherule is given.

[b]R. Cox (personal communication). Somewhat shorter generations times have been noted in tissue culture media [54], but the studies were not designed specifically as growth studies nor generation times recorded per se.

[c]Range seen among strains (M. Huppert, personal communication).

[d]Tissue culture media. There may be strain variation (J. Murphy, personal communication).

[e]The data given are for the A/D serotype. The B/C serotypes grow more slowly (K. J. Kwon-Chung, personal communication).

are influenced by in vitro culture conditions, and generally those optimum for growth should be chosen.

Certain aspects of the filamentous growth of pathogens have been implicit in the discussions of nutrition and physiology throughout this chapter [242]. Sporulation is an important aspect of filamentous growth. Generally, sporulation is sponsored by conditions that restrict growth [97]. A very large number of recipes for media have been suggested on the basis of such a generalization [45,250]. A medium that fosters sporulation of Histoplasma capsulatum is that of Coy Smith's [179,383]; simple water agar is useful in inducing sporulation of a number of the pathogens [250]. The needs for primary isolation from a host often involves selection of media that sponsor growth while the needs of identification, involving as they so often do spore morphology and ontogeny, may require transfer to specialized media designed to foster sporulation.

C. Hormones

Syngamy is regulated in a number of fungi by soluble substances that are mating-type specific. These substances are called hormones if they act on the same individual and pheromones if they work on different individuals. However, these distinctions are not always easily applied to fungi, and different authors have not consistently used the same designation for the same substance. Griffin [161] has presented a discussion of this matter and an overview of the various hormones that have been described. In keeping with his usage, I have adopted the term hormone in this brief consideration of the topic.

Hormones have been described in *Allomyces* (Chytridiomycetes), *Achlya* (Oomycetes), *Mucor, Blakeslea,* and *Phycomyces* (Zygomycetes), *Saccharomyces, Neurospora, Ascobolus,* and *Bombardia* (Ascomycetes), and in *Rhodosporidium* and *Tremella* (Basidiomycetes) [161]. In addition, soluble substances that are not mating-type specific but induce fruiting structures have been recognized [161]. Literature citations included in Griffin's overview of the subject provide additional sources of information [161].

Kwon-Chung presented evidence for a mating hormone in *Nannizzia incurvata* [215], but no further work on its characteristics has been published. The sexual stimulation of certain dermatophytes by mating types of *Arthroderma simii* [406,407] suggests the action of a hormone, but extended efforts to reveal such a substance have so far been unavailing as have those to find a hormone active between mating types of *A. benhamiae* (D. H. Howard, unpublished observations).

D. Light and UV-Irradiation

Many studies of the physiological effects of visible light on plant pathogenic fungi and on saprophytes have been published [69,225,418], but similar studies on fungi pathogenic for humans and animals are few [37,55]. Since a majority of the zoopathogens exist in nature, it would seem that important information might be gained by studying the effects of visible light on them.

The effects of UV-irradiation on zoopathogens have been studied more extensively than have those of visible light. The earliest example of this type of study is that of Emmons and Hollaender [121] who showed that when the spores of *Trichophyton mentagrophytes* are exposed to UV-radiation, besides the lethal effects, there were a strikingly large number of mutants among the survivors. The authors point out that the mutations were most numerous at wave lengths of 2537-2650 Å, and note that this range is the one at which nucleic acids have their most intense absorption band. They go on to state, "The greater efficiency in the 2,600 (Å) region, both in lethal and sublethal action, may indicate that the nucleic acid-containing components of the chromosomes are most susceptible to changes and that these changes in them may affect the inherited characters of the cell" [121]. This suggestion received direct confirmation a few years later when Avery, MacLeod, and McCarty [399] established that the transforming principle of the pneumococcus was a nucleic acid.

These early studies by Emmons and Hollaender were not immediately followed by similar work with other zoopathogenic fungi. The lethality of UV-irradiation for *Candida albicans* was recorded early on [237,420] and the mutagenicity for *C. tropicalis* was reported [415], but it was not until the studies by Sarachek and his colleagues [64,362-365] on factors involved in inactivation of *C. albicans* and other *Candida* spp. by UV-irradiation that a zoopathogen other than a dermatophyte was thoroughly examined. Inactivation of *C. albicans* by UV light was markedly dependent on the cell division stage and on the nutrition and growth temperature both before and after irradiation [64]. *Candida albicans* did not photoreactivate and there was no evidence for a dark-repair of DNA comparable to that in bacteria [363,364]. However, more recent data from Sarachek's laboratory do indicate the existence of DNA repair mechanisms in *C. albicans* [362]. Each of seven pathogenic species of *Candida* exhibited a unique pattern of light and dark recovery responses to UV-irradiation. *Candida guillermondii, C. parapsilosis,* and *C. pseudotropicalis* were photoreactive whereas *C. albicans, C. krusei,* and *C. stellatoides* were not [363,364]. Dark recovery was also observed, but again there were strain variations among species [363,364]. Current work with various mutants of *Saccharomyces cerevisiae* establishes a connection between mutation and faulty repair, but there also seems to be a very large number of genes involved [128]. Similar sorts of UV-sensitive mutants have not been generated with the pathogens. In addition to an error-prone repair pathway, mutations in *C. albicans* are revealed by UV-induced mitotic segregation from heterozygotes. This mechanism may be the most common origin of auxotrophs of *C. albicans*, since most clinical isolates of the fungus appear to be diploids. The ploidy of *C. albicans* would influence greatly conclusions about reactivation (see subsequent discussion in this section).

The largest number of observations on the effects of UV-radiation on zoopathogens has been made as a result of the use of UV light as a mutagen. In addition to those already mentioned, pathogens so handled have included *Aspergillus nidulans* [313], *Emmonsia crescens* [172], *Microsporum gypseum* [438], *Trichophyton sulfureum* [434], *Cryptococcus neoformans* [324], *Coccidioides immitis* [433], among others [78,216,218, and the literature therein cited].

Few topics on the basic biology of zoopathogenic fungi have generated as much debate as has the subject of the ploidy of *Candida albicans*. It has long been recognized that a sexual form of reproduction cannot be displayed with this fungus. This fact coupled with the difficulty encountered in generating certain auxotrophs by UV mutagenesis led Olaiya and Sogen [285] to examine the ploidy of *C. albicans*. From their studies of DNA content, genome sequence complexity, radiation sensitivity, and chemical mutagenesis, they concluded that the strains they studied were diploids. Whelan et al. [442] presented genetic evidence that the auxotrophs of *C. albicans* that arise after UV-irradiation result from induced mitotic segregation from heterozygotes. From such results, these workers inferred that *C. albicans* is diploid and they have gone on to a genetic analysis of *C. albicans* based on this inference [195,195a,441]. Poulter et al. [308] stated that the simplest interpretation of their data meant that *C. albicans* ATCC 10261 was haploid, a conclusion in keeping with that of Sarachek et al. [365] from their studies on hybridization through protoplast fusion. However, more recent data generated in Poulter's group has caused those workers to alter their earlier interpretation and to report that *C. albicans* ATCC 10261 is, after all, diploid [308a]. Although there are a number of complicated possibilities involving various aneuploid arrangements, results of a very recent report show haploid, diploid, and tetraploid examples among isolates of *C. albicans* [412]. This could mean that the disparate results from various laboratories were based on ploidy differences among isolates studied. The majority of the isolates studied by Suzuki et al. [412] were diploid, and this was also noted in a chemical study by Riggsby et al. [327] of some standard laboratory strains. It seems likely that the situation will be further clarified as more comparative genetic studies of various isolates are made. Currently, most of the data [see Refs. 91a,195] support the conclusion that the majority of isolates of *C. albicans* are diploid. Decisions on photoreactivation and study of dark-repair mechanisms will be influenced by the ploidy of the strain of *C. albicans* used. If the predominant effect of UV-irradiation were mitotic recombination in a diploid organism, then a dearth of apparent mutant reversions after light exposure could be misinterpreted as lack of photoactivation when, in point of fact, dimer formation was not the origin of the mutation scored initially.

E. pH and Ionic Strength

Pathogenic fungi are not especially sensitive to pH and grow rather well over a broad range of hydrogen ion concentrations. Advantage of this fact was taken by Sabouraud in the preparation of media with an acid pH of 5.4-5.6 for isolating dermatophytes from the mixed microbial flora of the skin, as was discussed previously in this chapter. Acid tolerance is a property of fungi that has long been recognized [432]. A number of studies on the effects of pH on the growth of zoopathogenic fungi have been published [e.g., 35, 72,154,186,336].

1. pH

The pH of a medium may exercise important control over a given morphogenetic event without influencing remarkably the overall growth of a fungus. A few examples of this sort of control will suffice to emphasize the important monitoring effect of pH:

   a. Conidia Germination: The optimum pH for germination of conidia of *Histoplasma capsulatum* ranges from 6.8 to 7.2 [156]. Germination decreases at acidities grater than 6.5 and does not occur below pH 5.0 [156]. Alkaline conditions are somewhat less inhibitory.

   b. Yeast Cell Germination: Blastoconidial germination of *H. capsulatum* takes place over a range of 4.0 to 7.5; at pH 4.0 and 4.5, the germination event is delayed but eventually takes place to about the same degree as it does at pH 5.0-7.5 (D. H. Howard, unpublished observations). Germination of blastoconidia of *C. albicans* grown under zinc-limiting conditions can be controlled by pH; at pH 4.5, blastoconidia do not germinate in an otherwise conducive environment, whereas similar cells incubated at pH 6.8 germinate in the expected fashion [389].

   c. Acid-Tolerance Yeasts: The yeast *Torulopsis pintolopesii,* which is an indigenous inhabitant of the mouse stomach, initiates growth in media containing various sugars over a pH range of from 2 to 8 [187]. Even among yeasts that do not colonize such acidic environments, growth at acid pH is not uncommon, but sometimes a surprising intolerance of alkaline conditions is found [e.g., 176,261]. This sensitivity was observed in initiating growth from small inocula in peptone media [176] and bears no relation to the sensitivity of creatinine deiminase to ammonia repression discussed earlier.

   d. Sporulation: Amongst entomophthoraceous fungi, vegetative germination predominates at pH 5-8 whereas secondary spore formation is fostered at pH 9-10 [66].

   e. Enzyme Activity: The proteolytic activity of *Candida albicans* was only manifested by cultures grown at a pH 5, whereas growth itself took place in the same medium in a range of pH from 3 to 7 [73,392].

2. Ionic Strength

The ionic strength of a medium as a growth-modifying factor has not been extensively examined. Salt tolerance of some pathogens is clearly indicated by isolation from sea water or sand [10,11,12,34,96,203], and *Coccidioides immitis* is known to survive in highly alkaline desert soils [113]. High salt content intentionally created in nutrient agar does modify the growth rates of zoopathogens [111,202]. Perhaps more interesting is the effect of physiologic saline on certain pathogens. Saline is somewhat toxic to *Candida albicans,* but such an effect is not seen if 0.2% glucose is added to the salt solution [93]. Similarly, saline is not a good diluent for work with the yeast phase of *Histoplasma capsulatum* because of poor survival of the fungus [179,347]. As was seen in *C. albicans,* an additive, in this case 0.1% cysteine, ameliorates the toxic effects [347]. The ionic strength of buffers used in studies with yeast cells of *H. capsulatum* must be quite low (0.01-0.025) to avoid poor survival of suspended cells [179]. Yet survival

Nutrition, Physiology, and Metabolism

of *H. capsulatum* in complete salt solutions (Hanks' balanced salt solution) or in physiological tissue culture media (RPMI 1640) is generally quite good (D. H. Howard, unpublished observations). Thus, balanced salt solutions or complete media do not adversely affect the viability of cell suspensions, but saline and certain buffers may. Clearly, ionic strength per se is not the factor involved but rather direct Na^+ or K^+ toxicity. More work needs to be done on this sort of toxicity and its modification by carbon sources such as glucose or cysteine.

F.   Temperature

In recording the effects of temperature (T) on fungi, it is customary to consider the minimum (min) and maximum (max) temperatures that allow some growth and to identify an optimum (opt) temperature at which growth occurs most abundantly. By such measures, fungi are usually designated as psychrophiles, mesophiles, or thermophiles. The customary definitions [161] given for these categories are:

1. Psychrophiles: Max T, 20°C; min T, 0°C; opt range, 0-17°C
2. Mesophiles: Max T, <50°C; min T, >0°C; opt range, 15-40°C
3. Thermophiles: Max T, >50°C; min T, >20°C; opt range, 20-50°C

There are, of course, a number of fungi that do not fit the classification, e.g., *Aspergillus fumigatus*, which is thermotolerant [89]. An important point is that the temperature tolerances of zoopathogens or potential zoopathogens often allow for colonization of or at least survival in diverse sites in nature [e.g., 1,10,11,96,120,192, 204,256,284,312,369]. Such thermotolerance may also be a basis for identification, especially in difficult groups like the dematiaceous fungi [e.g., 291] or the Mucorales (see Chap. 2, Part A, of this series).

Strains of *Sporothrix schenckii* display a very interesting temperature sensitivity. Kwon-Chung compared isolates from lymphocutaneous and fixed cutaneous disease [217]. Those strains isolated from the lymphocutaneous forms of the disease grew at 37°C, whereas those from fixed cutaneous lesions could not grow above 35°C. This temperature intolerance was also reflected in the sort of disease produced in experimental infections of mice. That strains of *S. schenckii* isolated from nature may vary in the upper limits of temperature at which they will grow has been reported [183], and it is likely that the kind of disease that results from the natural inoculation of these fungi into the tissues reflects the temperature tolerance of the strain.

The effects of temperature on the morphogenesis of zoopathogens has been studied extensively because so many of the pathogens are dimorphic and temperature is decisive in the control mechanisms of that dimorphism. The range of temperature effects extends from instances in which it is the sole controlling factor, e.g., *Blastomyces dermatitidis* and *Paracoccidioides brasiliensis*, to instances in which it is necessary but not sufficient, e.g., *Histoplasma capsulatum*. It is, of course, the metabolic events altered by temperature that are of central interest [19,44,162,271,301,304,331,343, 402; and Chap. 9, Part A, of this series]. A few selected examples that are especially interesting will be mentioned in the section on metabolism to be considered subsequently.

The use of temperature-sensitive (ts) mutants has not yet found wide application to the zoopathogens, perhaps because morphogenetic markers such as spore germination or dimorphism for which ts mutants would be especially useful seem more difficult to select for than small molecule requirements or cell-cycle variants [165,166]. A few instances of the use of ts mutants of zoopathogens are to be noted [viz., 340,360,433]. The appeal of ts mutants in a study of morphogenetic events among zoopathogens seems obvious, but there are technical problems [182,185].

IV. METABOLISM AND METABOLITES

It is customary to consider two general topics under the heading of fungal metabolism: (1) primary metabolism, which includes anabolic and catabolic functions of primary importance to the life of the organism, and (2) secondary metabolism, from which are produced a very large number of compounds whose microbial function is generally unknown, e.g., antibiotics and mycotoxins. The primary metabolism of fungi has been surveyed on a number of occasions [4,130,131,132,170,387] and has been considered in specific chapters on this series (e.g., Chaps. 10, 12, 13, Part A, and Chap. 5, Part B: I of this series; and Chaps. 2 and 3 of this volume). The vast literature on secondary metabolism has been the subject of intense industrial and agricultural interest [e.g., 101, 129; and Chaps. 6, 9, and 10, Part B: I of this series].

Zoopathogens sometimes have been the objects of general metabolic studies [233, 275,294], but more often they have been subjects of special studies to examine some particular aspect of metabolism associated with a certain pathogen, such as the melanin formed by *Cryptococcus neoformans* grown on catecholamines, or some morphogenetic event, such as the dimorphism of systemic pathogens. One of the promises of such studies is that a unique therapeutic approach might be revealed by an understanding of metabolic events in the natural history of the pathogens. Such an expectation is solidly based on the early work regarding the effects of antimetabolites on bacteria and has been pursued vigorously [374,379]. That such studies have not fulfilled their promise has not dampened continuing efforts to generate drugs selectively toxic for pathogens. Another promise in studying metabolic events is that results will yield key information on pathogenesis. In this section, I have selected certain subjects that have been studied in relation to particular pathogens, once again with a view toward describing work that attempts to deal with the unique attribute of pathogens, viz., their ability to cause disease.

Metabolic studies also provide bases for distinguishing among the zoopathogenic fungi. This sort of consideration is contained in a large number of textbooks and manuals [e.g., 27,332].

A. Cysteine Biosynthesis

The sulfur-containing amino acid cysteine has long been recognized as a crucial determinant in the dimorphism of *Histoplasma capsulatum*. Very recently, this amino acid has been shown to play a decisive role in two separate aspects of yeast cell development of the pathogen [245], and this recent work has helped to resolve some uncertainties in the earlier literature.

De Monbreun noted that the mycelial form of *H. capsulatum* was quite stable and thought that the tissue form could *only* be evoked by animal passage after which it could be subcultured quite nicely at 37°C on blood agar media [102]. However, Ciferri and Redaelli [82] and Conant [87] reported that the mycelial form of growth would convert to the parasitic form of growth on sealed blood agar slants at 37°C. Campbell [67] described a medium containing cystine for such conversion, and other media with a high content of sulfur-containing amino acids have been recommended for that purpose [e.g.,

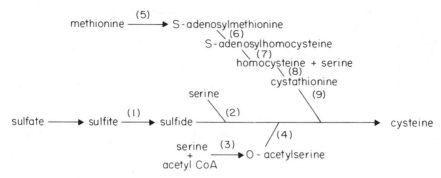

Figure 2 Schematic presentation of cysteine biosynthesis. Reaction in numbered steps mediated by: (1) sulfite reductase; (2) serine sulfhydralase; (3) serine transacetylase; (4) O-acetylserine sulfhydralase; (5) methionine adenosyltransferase; (6) methyl transfer reaction; (7) adenosylhomocysteinase; (8) cystathionine β-synthase; (9) cystathionine γ-lyase. (From Refs. 104,227,400.)

214,251,423]. Salvin studied the nutritional needs of the yeast-like phase of *H. capsulatum* [354,356]. Careful reexamination of his data shows that cysteine or cystine was essential for growth. *Histoplasma capsulatum* has an active cystine reductase which would allow cystine to support yeast-phase growth [243]. Pine [299] and McVeigh and Morton [252] also singled out cysteine or cystine as a required amino acid for the yeast cell growth of *H. capsulatum* in liquid media. More recently, the work of Boguslawski et al. [43,400] and that of Howard et al. [185] reemphasized the cysteine requirement of many laboratory strains of *H. capsulatum* at 37°C. The requirement is based on a defect in inorganic sulfur metabolism at the level of the reduction of sulfite to sulfide [42]. The enzyme sulfite reductase (Fig. 2), which governs this step, is constitutive in mycelial cells but repressible by yeast cells at 37°C [42,43,400].

The early literature contains some contradictory results regarding the substitution of other reduced sulfhydral (-SH) compounds for cysteine. Salvin [354] described a large number of -SH compounds that supported good yeast cell growth. His conclusions were derived from a series of experiments in which one after another amino acid was singly removed from a 17-amino acid medium. Since the medium would have always contained either cysteine, cystine, serine, or methionine, the essential cysteine requirement was not displayed in these experiments. In fact, he concluded, on inadequate grounds as it turns out, that no "single amino acid was necessary for the growth of the mycelial and yeast-like phases of *H. capsulatum*." Furthermore, he stated that "a sulfide or sulfhydral group in a small organic molecule, preferably an amino acid, was essential for the growth of the yeast-like phase." This general conclusion was unsupported by Pine who based his conclusion about the essentiality of cysteine on the fact that glutathione could not substitute for it. McVeigh and Morton also found that neither glutathione nor thio-glycollate could substitute for cysteine (or cystine), though methionine worked to some degree with *some* strains [252]. Interpretation of experiments on the cysteine requirement for yeast form growth by most isolates of *H. capsulatum* was complicated by the fact that cysteine lowers the oxidation-reduction (redox) potential of a medium, a fact that has been judged important to the conversion events [330,331]. In addition, there is some variation among strains with regard to the way they are able to satisfy the cysteine requirement. For example, McVeigh and Morton reported that the growth of some strains was supported by methionine [252], and Boguslawski and Stetler [42,400] report strains that can be grown on serine in the absence of cysteine. Very recently, a prototrophic strain of *H. capsulatum* capable of yeast cell growth on a glucose-salts-biotin medium at 37°C was described [190,191]. The picture that emerges may be summarized as follows (Fig. 2). Most isolates of *H. capsulatum* require cysteine in the yeast cell phase of growth. Some strains can grow in the absence of cysteine if serine is supplied [42]. It is not known whether *H. capsulatum* sulfhydrylates serine directly (serine sulfhydrylase) or through *O*-acetylserine (*O*-acetylserine sulfhydrylase). Both pathways have been described in *Saccharomyces cerevisiae* [104]. From nutritional data, it would appear that *H. capsulatum* yeast cells can also synthesize cysteine from methionine, but no direct information on the pathways is available [252]. Cysteine can arise from methionine in *S. cerevisiae* [104]. In mammalian cells, cysteine is made from methionine, which supplies the sulfur atom, and serine, which provides the carbon chain [227]. Much more work needs to be done to sort out the pathways of cysteine biosynthesis in *H. capsulatum*. Nevertheless, enough is now known to indicate the bases for the contradictory statements on the role of cysteine in the nutrition of *H. capsulatum* that were recorded in the early literature.

In addition to its function in the nutrition of yeast cells of *H. capsulatum*, cysteine also plays a regulatory role in the morphogenesis of the yeast cells from mycelial cells [244,245]. Cysteine stimulates oxygen consumption by yeast cells of *H. capsulatum* [138,139,244]. Recent work by Maresca et al. [245] has suggested that cysteine may be required to activate mitochondrial respiration and that this requirement can be met by other reducing agents, e.g., 2-mercaptoethanol and dithiothreitol. The stimulation of oxygen consumption is due to a cysteine oxidase found in the cytosol of yeast but not in mycelial cells.

In summary, cysteine influences transitional events in *H. capsulatum* by lowering the redox potential of the medium, by stimulating oxygen consumption through a cysteine oxidase, and by fulfilling the auxotrophic requirement of yeast cells at 37°C. Failure to sort out these various effects led to some contradictory assertions in the earlier literature.

B. Enzymes and Pathogenesis

The formation and release of extracellular enzymes by fungi during sporulation or growth is a common occurrence. Some examples of the use made of this fact in fungal identification were given in Table 2. Host penetration by plant pathogens is ascribed to such enzymes [e.g., 17]. Efforts have been made to show that penetration of animal tissue is due to exoenzymes, but results have not been so abundant nor so convincing as with the phytopathogens. There are some recent examples of membrane-bound enzymes that are clearly involved in the attribute of pathogenicity even though they are not active aggressins (e.g., phenoloxidase). A few examples of enzymes studied for their potential role in pathogenesis are gathered in Table 4. It may be that there are several other examples of this sort of association reported in the context of other work, but information is not abundant and it is clear that explanations of pathogenicity will require knowledge on the molecular aspects of tissue invasion.

Another use to which enzymes have been put is a taxonomic one based on isozyme patterns [32,143,194,199,348,372]. The number of examples of this type of work is as yet too few to allow assessment of its ultimate utility.

Table 4 Enzymes That May Play a Pathogenetic Role in Disease

Enzyme[a]	Fungus	Reference
Catalase[b]	*Aspergillus fumigatus*	424
	Histoplasma capsulatum	39
Coagulase	*Candida albicans*	451
Collaginase	*Entomophthora coronata*	134,140
	Trichophyton schoenlienii	329
Elastase	*Allescheria (Petriellidium) boydii*	335
	Blastomyces dermatitidis	335
	Coccidioides immitis	335
	Epidermophyton, Microsporum, and *Trichophyton* spp.	77,328,329
Esterase	*Candida albicans*	31
	Entomophthora coronata	134,140
Hemolysin	*Candida albicans*	213,358
Keratinases[c]	*Candida albicans*	196
	Microsporum canis	417
	Trichophyton mentagrophytes	450
	Trichophyton verrucosum	83,439
Ketoreductase[d]	Mucorales	307
Lipases	*Candida albicans*	309,310,311
	Trichophyton rubrum	98,99
Muscle damage (enzymes unspecified)	*Candida* spp.	279
Peptidase	Dermatophytes	74
Phenoloxidase	*Cryptococcus neoformans*	306
	Phialophora verrucosa	318
Proteinases[e]	*Aspergillus fumigatus*	259
	Blastomyces dermatitidis	28
	Candida albicans[f]	56,75,239,322, 392,393,394
	Candida spp.	56
	Cryptococcus neoformans	263
	Metarhizium anisopliae	209
	Trichophyton mentagrophytes	198
	Trichophyton verrucosum	83

[a]Only hydrolytic enzymes with imaginable pathogenetic activity are included. Other types of enzymatic activities, some of which are useful in identification, have been tabulated in Table 2, q.v.

[b]Catalase activity has been associated with antigenic extracts of *Histoplasma capsulatum* (m antigen) and of *Aspergillus fumigatus*. Current results from my laboratory affirm the close association of *Histoplasma* catalase and m antigen (unpublished observations).

[c]Keratin might also be susceptible to proteinases if it were first denatured by a nonenzymatic sulphitolysis reaction described in cultures of *Microsporum gypseum* [212].

[d]The enzyme allows utilization of ketone bodies.

[e]The role of proteinases in pathogenesis has been considered in a review of proteinases in eucaryotic microorganisms [276].

[f]All of the enzyme activities that have been demonstrated in *Candida* spp. have been tabulated by Odds [280].

C. Macromolecular Synthesis

The major emphasis in the metabolism section of this chapter is on primary catabolic events. Anabolic metabolism has also been studied extensively in the pathogenic fungi. Some of these synthetic activities have been examined in other parts of this series on zoopathogenic fungi. Major topics of macromolecular systems are gathered in Table 5 with key references and will not be considered in detail here.

D. Melanin Production

Cryptococcus neoformans is unique among members of the genus *Cryptococcus* and un-usual among a great many commonly encountered genera of yeasts in producing melanin when grown on media containing di- or polyphenolic compounds. Since Staib's [390] original report of the phenomenon, there have been many publications in which are described modified media designed to test for melanin production by yeast isolates [73, 90,171,277]. The enzyme responsible for pigment formation is a phenoloxidase which is membrane-bound and differs from those of plants and mammals in that tryosine cannot serve as its substrate [306]. A phenoloxidase that forms melanin from catechol has been described in *Phialophora verrucosa* [318]. However, melanin is formed by this fungus on a defined glucose-nitrate-salts [318] medium and other dematiaceous fungi form melanin-like pigments on media unsupplemented with di- or polyphenolic compounds.

The constant association of ability to grow at 37°C and ability to form melanin by *C. neoformans* has led to the suggestion that these two features are important in its pathogenicity [220]. A naturally occurring variant of *C. neoformans* that lacks pheno-loxidase activity has been isolated [326]. With this variant, cosegregation and coreversion of the melanin phenotype and virulence were observed, a fact that suggests that pheno-loxidase is one of the important virulence factors in *C. neoformans* [326]. Further studies on a UV-induced double mutant of *C. neoformans* that lacks the ability to produce melanin on media containing diphenols and fails to grow at 37°C have strengthened this suggestion [220].

The melanin produced by *C. neoformans* is pictured as augmenting its pathogenicity by increasing its resistance to lysis [220]. This is plausible because melanin is a very inert substance for which no hydrolytic enzymes have been discovered [40], and the pigment of the resistant sporangia of *Blastocladiella emersonii* is considered to be melanin [68]. The dematiaceous fungi produce melanins in abundance [133,318], and the suggestion has been made that this contributes to their pathogenicity by increasing resistance to lysis.

E. Mineral Metabolism

The elemental requirements of fungi have been reviewed on a number of occasions [84, 161]. The primary structural elements, e.g., carbon, hydrogen, oxygen, phosphorus, potassium, nitrogen, sulfur, calcium, and magnesium are required in substantial quantity, i.e., about 10^{-3} M, and have thereby been referred to as macronutrients [161]. In contrast, minerals such as iron, copper, manganese, zinc, and molybdenum are required in only very small quantities, i.e., about 10^{-6} M and have been referred to as micro-nutrients [161]. The trace amount of these minerals that will evoke positive responses is a caution in experiments designed to display those responses. Griffin has reviewed the mineral nutrient requirements of fungi. In addition to requiring certain minerals for growth, fungi can reduce certain metallic salts, e.g., tellurite and selenite, and deposit

Table 5 Macromolecular Synthesis Studied in Zoopathogenic Fungi

Synthesis	References[a]
Chitin	14,49,64a,79
Deoxyribonucleic Acid	38,48,104,193,375
Melanin	306,318
Polyamines	248,268
Protein	53,104,141,206,419
Ribonucleic Acid	104,142,206,211,375,401,419

[a]The number of references given is far from comprehensive and each should be consulted for more citations on the subject indicated.

the elemental metals in their cells. If only certain species do so, then the capacity can be used as a test for identification. In keeping with my general approach, only selected examples of mineral metabolism will be discussed. Those chosen are of particular interest in the basic biology of the pathogens or closely related forms.

Minerals are essential to the yeast-like growth of *Mucor rouxii* in cultures incubated under carbon dioxide [20]. In the presence of ethylene diaminetetraacetic acid (EDTA), yeast-like morphogenesis is almost completely suppressed, being replaced by filamentous development. Metal ions added back to EDTA-inhibited cultures antagonize the inhibition and, to varying degrees, allow yeast-like growth to be expressed under carbon dioxide incubation. The transition group metals, Fe^{2+}, Mn^{2+}, Cu^{2+}, Zn^{2+}, Al^{3+}, or Co^{2+} at 10^{-4} M reverse EDTA inhibition of yeast growth; Co^{2+} is the least and Zn^{2+} is the most effective in restoring growth. The alkaline earth metals, Mg^{2+}, Ca^{2+}, and Sr^{2+} do not overcome growth inhibition by EDTA. Cations also reverse the morphogenetic effects of EDTA by restoring pure yeast form growth: Fe^{2+}, Al^{3+}, and Co^{2+} are most active; Mn^{2+} and Cu^{2+} are effective but at higher concentration; and Zn^{2+} only partially reverses morphogenesis in that the cultures to which it is added show both yeast and mycelial growth.

Adequate supplies of Zn^{2+}, Cu^{2+}, Mn^{2+}, and Fe^{2+} are required for the production of phialoconidia of *Phialophora verrucosa* [319]. When Mn^{2+} is omitted from a defined medium, phialoconidia production ceases and is replaced by chlamydoconidia resembling the sclerotic cells of the tissue form of the fungus. This morphogenetic response is specific for Mn^{2+} and is not seen with the other cations [319]. A profound effect of Mn^{2+} on the morphology of *Aspergillus parasiticus* has also been described [105]. In the absence of the cations, spherical yeast-like forms of the fungus appeared, whereas in the presence of Mn^{2+} normal hyphal growth occurred.

The nutritional studies of Pine and Peacock showed that the mycelial phase of *Histoplasma capsulatum* was strongly inhibited at 30°C and 37°C by 1.5% citrate incorporated in a minimal vitamin agar medium, whereas the yeast form of growth was stimulated by the presence of citrate [304]. The ions Ca^{2+} and Mg^{2+} reversed the effect of citric acid on mycelial growth at 30°C, but at 37°C Mg^{2+} stimulated both mycelial and yeast growth and the conversion of the mycelial phase to the yeast phase. In contrast, Ca^{2+} inhibited conversion and stimulated only mycelial growth at 37°C. Conversion to the yeast form of growth was stimulated at 37°C by Zn^{2+}.

The importance of Zn^{2+} in maintaining the yeast form of growth amongst forms capable of mycelial growth observed with *M. rouxii* and *H. capsulatum* has also been recorded for *Candida albicans*. Widra [444] noted that Zn^{2+} deficiency sponsored pseudohyphal formation, and Yamaguchi [448] and Soll et al. [389] have reported on the regulation of yeast cell growth by Zn^{2+} in defined culture media. Interestingly, Cu^{2+} has also been noted to suppress filamentation in *C. albicans* in in vitro cultures [430]. In contrast, a germination-promoting effect of Mn^{2+} has been observed in certain media [76].

Animal serum incorporated into culture media inhibits the growth of many species of fungi [21,65,81,136,184,189,201,267,289,290,320,345,346,378,409,411,440]. Such growth suppression is caused most often by serum transferrin, which binds iron and makes it unavailable for the nutrition of the microorganism [70,99a,114,123,173a,201, 224,378,409,411]. Although factors other than transferrin may account for certain aspects of serum-induced fungistasis in some organisms [81,123,290,321], it is clear that addition of iron to serum-containing media commonly reverses the fungistatis activity of those media [99a,114,201,409]. It is interesting to note that serum from patients with ketoacidotic diabetes and with cirrhosis do not inhibit *Rhizopus* spp. These observations have not been extended to other fungi or correlated with changes in serum transferrin levels [81,290].

The importance of iron has also been documented by the work of Burt and his colleagues on the siderophores of *H. capsulatum* which was described in an earlier section of this chapter (Sec. II.A.2.c).

The reduction of sulfite, tellurite, and selenite by *Candida albicans* has been recorded [241,272,274, and literature cited therein]. This fact has been used in the design of media for detecting species of *Candida*. The effectiveness of selenite and tellurite in modifying form and color of certain yeasts led to an interest in other elements in the same periodic group, viz., molybdenum [241]. The distinctive pigmentation developed by *C. albicans* grown on a medium containing appropriate compounds of molybdenum could be used in clinical identification. However, the usefulness of such relatively protracted culture techniques has been replaced by the more rapid germ tube test.

Phosphate plays an essential role in nucleic acic synthesis, energy transfer, and intermediary metabolism. Among many examples that might be chosen is the one of germ tube formation of blastoconidia of *C. albicans*. Land and co-workers have shown that this event is fostered by conditions of low-phosphate and high-glucose concentrations [207,222]. It is interesting that the glucose-to-phosphate ratio affects both germination [95] and pseudohyphal formation [444].

F. Respiration

Respiration of fungi is fundamentally comprised of the citric acid cycle, electron transport, and oxidative phosphorylation. The overall process is similar among all aerobic organisms and much of the detailed information has been derived from work with fungi. The subject has been reviewed recently [161 and literature therein cited].

Respiratory-deficient mutants called petites have been described in *Saccharomyces cerevisiae* and *Torulopsis glabrata* [128]. A naturally occurring respiratory-deficient strain of *Candida slooffii* has been described [16] and petite mutants of several yeast species might be widespread in environments nonselective for respiratory competence [16]. A few examples include *T. pintolopesii, T. lactis-condensi*, and *Schizosaccharomyces japonicus* var. *versatalis*. The petite mutation is reported to be lethal for *Candida albicans* [9a,57a,57b], but a petite-like variant with an alternate respiratory pathway has been described [208].

Yamaguchi reported that the respiratory activity of yeast cells of *C. albicans* declined when they were placed under germinating conditions [447,448]. Land et al. [222] also reported repression of respiration in germinating blastoconidia of *C. albicans*. However, Shepherd and his colleagues [376] and Aoki and Ito-Kuwa [13] presented data that emphasized that repression of respiration did not play an essential role in yeast cell germination, although there is a difference between yeast and mycelial cells in the ability to induce the cyanide-insensitive respiratory pathway in them.

Respiratory-deficient mutants of *Neurospora crassa* termed "poky" have long been known [52]. A similar phenotype has been described in a mutant of *Arthroderma benhamiae*. The mutant displayed a defective standard cytochrome system and a functional alternate oxidase pathway [182]. A branched electron-transport system consisting of a standard cytochrome system which is inhibited by cyanide and an alternate oxidase system inhibited by salicylhydroxamic acid has been demonstrated in *Histoplasma capsulatum*. This branched system is further augmented by a cysteine oxidase system which is functional during the morphogenesis of yeast phase growth from the mycelium of this dimorphic fungus (see section on cysteine metabolism for a consideration of these matters).

G. Uric Acid Utilization

The association of *Histoplasma capsulatum* and *Cryptococcus neoformans* with avian habitats has led to studies on the ability of these fungi to utilize the prominent nitrogenous components of bird manure [391]. Staib and his colleagues have reported on the growth of *C. neoformans* on various purines and other low molecular weight nitrogenous substances, such as urea and creatinine [398], and have extended their studies to include the formation of basidiospores by *Filobasidiella neoformans* [368,396,398]. The presence of an active urease among species of *Cryptococcus* and *Rhodotorula* and its absence from most species of *Candida* and *Saccharomyces* has long been used as a screening test in the clinical laboratory [370]. The selective occurrence of an urease among other species of pathogens has been chosen as a basis for distinguishing them [e.g., 257, 297,344].

Histoplasma capsulatum var. *capsulatum* and *H. capsulatum* var. *duboisii* have been cultivated on media containing avian manure [384,427]. Throughout the remainder of this discussion, *H. capsulatum* will be used in reference to the *capsulatum* variety for the sake of brevity. Lockwood and Garrison demonstrated the enzymes responsible for the conversion of uric acid to inorganic nitrogen in cell free extracts of *H. capsulatum* [230]. These enzymes included uricase, allantoinase, allantoicase, and urease. The same authors also reported the uricolytic activity of cell-free extracts of *Cryptococcus neoformans*. In fact, it has been known for quite some time that uricase activity is very common among *Candida* spp., dermatophytes, and other zoopathogens [344,422].

The evidence described in the preceding paragraphs suggests that the ability to utilize certain substrates may in part explain the strong association of *H. capsulatum* and *Cryptococcus neoformans* with soils rich in avian fecal matter. There are other interesting suggestions that arise from the uricolytic activities of these two pathogens. Both survive and multiply with murine macrophages cultivated in vitro, and the fate of *H. capsulatum* within such cells has been extensively studied [180]. Soon after the engulfment of a particle by phagocytes, there is a rapid disappearance of cytoplasmic granules which fuse with the intact phagosome [160]. The strategy by which facultative intracellular parasites evade the microbicidal substances to which they might be exposed

Table 6   Key Low Molecular Weight Nitrogenous Ingredients in Serum

Ingredient	Concentration (mg/100 ml)[a]
Urea	20-40
Uric acid	4-8
Creatinine	0.6-1.2
Creatine	0.5-0.9
Ammonia	0.035-0.10
Amino acids (arginine)	3.5-7.0

[a]*Source*: Ref. 169.

after lysosomal fusion is various [160,164], but the mode adopted by *Mycobacterium tuberculosis* is to interfere with or antagonize phagosome-lysosome fusion [160]. Such interference with lysosomal fusion appears to be one method utilized by *Coccidioides immitis* to avoid the antifungal activities of alveolar macrophages [23,24]. In contrast, however, an electron microscopic study of materials from a case of human histoplasmosis by Dumont and Piche [109] showed that phagosomes containing yeast cells of *H. capsulatum* "interacted with lysosome-like granules present in (the) macrophages." Subsequently, Dumont and Robert [110] reported that phagolysosomal fusion took place within peritoneal macrophages from hamsters infected with *H. capsulatum*. Von Behren and Tewari (personal communication) report that phagolysosomes are formed in mouse peritoneal macrophages. Thus, phagosome-lysosome fusion seems to take place in phagocytes and one must look elsewhere for clues as to the intracellular survival of *H. capsulatum* within mammalian macrophages. The question is unresolved and it is interesting to speculate on possible mechanisms that involve intraphagosomal metabolism by the fungus. It is not uncommon to use serum at a level of 20% in the medium used to cultivate the macrophages. *Histoplasma capsulatum* could generate a large amount of ammonia from the nitrogenous compounds included in the nutrient medium surrounding it (Table 6). The pH of the internal milieu of the phagosome could be affected by the ammonia generated. Thus, one could imagine that *H. capsulatum* might affect its own intracellular survival through metabolic events that alter the internal environment of the phagosome [112].

Urea is generally recognized as a utilizable nitrogen source for many fungi [380]. Even organisms, such as *Geotrichum candidum*, that lack urease may nevertheless utilize urea by means of an inducible amidolyase which catalyses the cleavage of urea to carbon dioxide and ammonia [380].

Urea may occur free in fungi and, in the fruiting bodies of some higher basidiomycetes, it comprises a major component of the soluble nitrogen fraction, representing about 6% of the total dry weight [Ref. 380 and literature cited therein]. Presumably under such circumstances, it represents a nitrogen reserve.

ACKNOWLEDGMENTS

The author is grateful to Dr. R. K. Gupta, Department of Surgery, UCLA, who assisted by arranging for an initial review of the literature used in part to construct this chapter and by suggesting alterations after reading a rough draft copy. He also appreciates Dr. June Kwon-Chung's (NIH) critical reading and he thanks Mrs. Bette Y. Tang for her care in preparing the numerous retypings a work of this sort requires.

During the period when this review was composed, the author received grant support from Public Health Service grant AI 16252 from the National Institute of Allergy and Infectious Diseases.

This chapter is publication number 52 of the Collaborative California Universities-Mycology Research Unit (CCU-MRU).

REFERENCES

1. Ahearn, D. G., and W. Kaplan. 1969. Occurrence of *Sporotrichum schenckii* on a cold-stored meat product. Am. J. Epidemiol. *89*:116-124.
2. Ainsworth, G. C. 1952. *Medical Mycology. An Introduction to Its Problems.* Pitman, London.
3. Ainsworth, G. C. 1976. *Introduction to the History of Mycology,* Cambridge University Press, Cambridge.
4. Ainsworth, G. C., and A. S. Sussman (Eds.), *The Fungi. An Advanced Treatise,* Vol. I, Academic, New York, pp. 229-613.
5. Ajello, L. 1956. Soil as a natural reservoir for human pathogenic fungi. Science *123*:876-879.
6. Ajello, L. 1957. Cultural methods for human pathogenic fungi. J. Chronic Dis. *5*:545-551.
7. Ajello, L. 1967. Comparative ecology of respiratory mycotic disease agents. Bacteriol. Rev. *31*:6-24.
8. Ajello, L. 1980. Natural habitats of fungi that cause pulmonary mycoses. Zentralbl. Bakteriol. Parasitenkd. Infektionskr. Hyg., Abt. 1:Orig., Suppl. *8*:31-42.
9. Ajello, L., and L. K. Georg. 1957. *In vitro* hair cultures for differentiating between atypical isolates of *Trichophyton mentagrophytes* and *Trichophyton rubrum*. Mycopathol. Mycol. Appl. *8*:3-17.
9a. Alvarez, A., and J. E. Mackinnon. 1957. Lethal variant of *Candida albicans,* a petite colonie mutant. Science *126*:399-400.
10. Anderson, J. G. 1978. Temperature-induced fungal development. In J. E. Smith and D. R. Berry (Eds.), *The Filamentous Fungi,* Vol. 3, Wiley, New York, pp. 358-375.
11. Anderson, J. H. 1979. *In vitro* survival of human pathogenic fungi in sea water. Sabouraudia *17*:1-12.
12. Anderson, J. H. 1979. *In vitro* survival of human pathogenic fungi in Hawaiian beach sand. Sabouraudia *17*:13-22.
13. Aoki, S., and S. Ito-Kuwa. 1982. Respiration of *Candida albicans* in relation to its morphogenesis. Plant Cell Physiol. *23*:721-726.
14. Archer, D. B. 1977. Chitin biosynthesis in protoplasts and subcellular fractions of *Aspergillus fumigatus*. Biochem. J. *164*:653-658.
15. Area Leão, A. E., and A. Cury. 1950. Deficiencias vitaminecas de cogumelos patogenicos. Mycopathol. Mycol. Appl. *5*:65-90.
16. Arthur, H., K. Watson, C. R. McArthur, and G. D. Clark-Walker. 1978. Naturally occurring respiratory deficient *Candida slooffii* strains resemble *petite* mutants. Nature (Lond.) *271*:750-752.
17. Barash, I. 1968. Liberation of polygalacturonase during spore germination by *Geotrichum candidum*. Phytopathology *58*:1364-1371.
18. Barash, I., M. L. Conway, and D. H. Howard. 1967. Carbon catabolism and synthesis of macromolecules during spore germination of *Microsporum gypseum*. J. Bacteriol. *93*:656-662.

19. Bartnicki-Garcia, S., and I. McMurrough. 1971. Biochemistry of morphogenesis in yeasts. In A. H. Rose and J. S. Harrison (Eds.), *The Yeasts,* Vol. 2, Academic, New York, pp. 441-491.

20. Bartnicki-Garcia, S., and W. J. Nickerson. 1962. Induction of yeast-like development in *Mucor* by carbon dioxide. J. Bacteriol. *84*:829-840.

21. Baum, G. L., and D. Artis. 1961. Growth inhibition of *Cryptococcus neoformans* by cell free serum. Am. J. Med. Sci. *241*:613-616.

22. Bauman, D. S. 1971. Physiology of *Histoplasma capsulatum*. In L. Ajello, E. W. Chick, and M. L. Furcolow (Eds.), *Histoplasmosis,* Proceedings of the Second National Conference, Thomas, Springfield, Ill., pp. 78-84.

23. Beaman, L., and C. A. Holmberg. 1980. In vitro response of alveolar macrophages to infection with *Coccidioides immitis*. Infect. Immun. *28*:594-600.

24. Beaman, L., E. Benjamini, and D. Pappagianis. 1981. Role of lymphocytes in macrophage-induced killing of *Coccidioides immitis in vitro*. Infect. Immun. *34*: 347-353.

25. Beijerinck, M. W. 1889. L'auxanographic ou la methode de l'hydrodiffusion dans la gelatine appliquee aux recherches microbiologiques. Arch. Neerl. Sci. Exactes Natur. *23*:367-372.

26. Beijerinck, M. W. 1901. Anhäufungsversuche mit Ureumbakterien. Centralbl. Bakteriol. Parasitenkd. Abt. II, 7:33-61 (see Ref. 51).

27. Beneke, E. S., and A. L. Rogers. 1980. *Medical Mycology Manual,* Burgess Publishing Co., Minneapolis.

28. Beneke, E. S., R. W. Wilson, and A. L. Rogers. 1969. Extracellular enzymes of *Blastomyces dermatitidis*. Mycopathol. Mycol. Appl. *39*:325-328.

29. Benham, R. W. 1947. Biology of *Pityrosporum ovale*. In W. J. Nickerson (Ed.), *Biology of the Pathogenic Fungi,* Chronica Botanica Co., Waltham, Mass., pp. 63-70.

30. Bennett, J. E., K. J. Kwon-Chung, and T. S. Theodore. 1978. Biochemical differences between serotypes of *Cryptococcus neoformans*. Sabouraudia *16*:167-174.

31. Berchev, K. 1967. Histochemistry of polysaccharides and activity of a group of enzymes in *Candida albicans*. Nauchni Tr. Vissh. Med. Inst. Sofia *46*:1-8.

32. Berchev, K., and I. Izmirov. 1967. Isoenzymes of some oxido-reductases in the *Candida* genus as a basis of species identification after electrophoresis. Experientia *23*:961-962.

33. Berchev, K., and I. Izmirov. 1968. Isoenzymes of G-6-PDH, LDH, and MDH in extracts from *Candida albicans, pseudotropicalis, krusei,* and *utilis* as a basis of species identification after agar electrophoresis. Nauchni Tr. Vissh. Med. Inst. Sofia *47*: 39-46.

34. Bergen, L., and D. T. Wagner-Marner. 1977. Comparative survey of fungi and potential pathogenic fungi from selective beaches in the Tampa Bay area. Mycologia *69*:299-308.

35. Berliner, M. D. 1973. *Histoplasma capsulatum*: effects of pH on the yeast and mycelial phases. Sabouraudia *11*:267-270.

36. Berliner, M. D. 1977. Gelatin hydrolysis for identification of the filamentous phase of *Histoplasma, Blastomyces* and *Chrysosporium* species. Sabouraudia *5*: 274-277.

37. Berliner, M. D., and N. Biundo, Jr. 1973. Effects of continuous light and total darkness on cultures of *Histoplasma capsulatum*. Sabouraudia *11*:48-51.

38. Berry, D. R., and E. A. Berry. 1976. Nucleic acid and protein synthesis in filamentous fungi. In J. E. Smith and D. R. Berry (Eds.), *The Filamentous Fungi,* Vol. 3, Wiley, New York, pp. 238-291.

39. Biguet, J., P. Tran Van Ky, S. Andrieu, and T. Vaucelle. 1967. Premières caractérisations d'activités enzymatiques sur les immunoelectrophorégrammes des extraits antigéniques de *Histoplasma capsulatum*. Conséquences diagnostiques pratiques. Ann. Soc. Belge Med. Trop. *47*:425-434.

40. Bloomfield, B., and M. Alexander. 1967. Melanin and resistance of fungi to lysis. J. Bacteriol. *93*:1276-1280.

41. Blumer, S., and L. Kaufman. 1968. Variation in enzymatic activities among strains of *Histoplasma capsulatum* and *Histoplasma duboisii.* Sabouraudia 6:203-206,

42. Boguslawski, G., and D. A. Stetler. 1979. Aspects of physiology of *Histoplasma capsulatum.* Mycopathologia *67* :17-24.

43. Boguslawski, G., J. M. Akagi, and L. G. Ward. 1976. Possible role for cysteine biosynthesis in conversion from mycelial to yeast form of *Histoplasma capsulatum.* Nature (Lond.) *261*:336-338.

44. Boisseau-Lebreuil, M. T. 1975. Factors influencing the in vitro formation of adiaspores in 10 strains of *Emmonsia crescens* fungal agent of adiasperomycosis. C. R. Acad. Sci. (Paris) *169*:1057-1061.

45. Booth, C. 1971. Fungal culture media. In C. Booth (Ed.), *Methods in Microbiology,* Vol. 4, Academic, New York, pp. 49-94.

46. Bowman, P. I., and D. G. Ahearn. 1975. Evaluation of the Uni-Yeast-Tek kit for the identification of medically important yeasts. J. Clin. Microbiol. *2*:354-358.

47. Bowman, P. I., and D. G. Ahearn. 1976. Evaluation of commercial systems for the identification of clinical yeast isolates. J. Clin. Microbiol. *4*:49-53.

48. Brambl, R., L. D. Dunkle, and J. L. Van Etten. 1978. Nucleic acid and protein synthesis during fungal spore germination. In J. E. Smith and D. R. Berry (Eds.), *The Filamentous Fungi,* Vol. 3, Wiley, New York, pp. 94-118.

49. Braun, P. C., and R. A. Calderone. 1979. Regulation and solubilization of *Candida albicans* chitin synthetase. J. Bacteriol. *140*:666-670.

50. Breslau, A. M., and M. Y. Kubota. 1964. Continuous in vitro cultivation of spherules of *Coccidioides immitis.* J. Bacteriol. *87*:468-472.

51. Brock, T. (Ed.). 1961. *Milestones in Microbiology,* American Society for Microbiology, Washington, D.C.

52. Brody, S. 1981. Genetic and biochemical studies on *Neurospora* conidia germination and formation. In G. Turian and H. R. Hohl (Eds.), *The Fungal Spore: Morphogenetic Controls,* Academic, New York, pp. 605-626.

53. Brummel, M., and D. R. Soll. 1982. The temporal regulation of protein synthesis during synchronous bud or mycelium formation in the dimorphic yeast *Candida albicans.* Dev. Biol. *89*:211-224.

54. Brummer, E., P. A. Morozumi, D. E. Philpott, and D. A. Stevens. 1981. Virulence of fungi: Correlation of virulence of *Blastomyces dermatitidis* in vivo with escape from macrophage inhibition of replication in vitro. Infect. Immun. *32*:864-871.

55. Buchnicek, J. 1976. Light resistance in geophilic dermatophytes. Sabouraudia *14*:75-80.

56. Budtz-Jörgensen, E. 1974. Proteolytic activity of *Candida* spp. as related to the pathogenesis of denture stomatitis. Sabouraudia *12*:266-271.

57. Buesching, W. J., K. Kurch, and G. D. Roberts. 1979. Evaluation of the modified API 20C system for identification of clinically important yeasts. J. Clin. Microbiol. *9*:565-569.

57a. Bulder, C. J. E. A. 1964. Induction of petite mutation and inhibition of synthesis of respiratory enzymes in various yeasts. Antonie Leeuwenhoek J. Microbiol. Serol. *30*: 1-9.

57b. Bulder, C. J. E. A. 1964. Lethality of the petite mutation in petite negative yeasts. Antonie Leeuwenhoek J. Microbiol. Serol. *30*:442-454.

58. Bullen, J. J. 1949. The yeast-like form of *Cryptococcus farciminosus* (Rivalta) : (*Histoplasma farciminosus*). J. Pathol. Bacteriol. *61*:117-120.

59. Buller, A. H. R. 1915. Micheli and the discovery of reproduction in fungi. Trans. R. Soc. Canada, series 3, *9*:1-25.

60. Bulloch, W. 1960. *The History of Bacteriology,* Oxford University Press, London.

61. Burkholder, P. R., and D. Moyer. 1943. Vitamin deficiencies of fifty yeasts and molds. Bull. Torrey Bot. Club *70*:372-377.

62. Burt, W. R. 1982. Identification of coprogen B and its breakdown products from *Histoplasma capsulatum*. Infect. Immun. *35*:990-996.

63. Burt, W. R., A. L. Underwood, and G. L. Appleton. 1981. Hydroxamic acid from *Histoplasma capsulatum* that displays growth factor activity. Appl. Environ. Microbiol. *42*:560-563.

64. Busbee, D. L., and A. Saracheck. 1969. Inactivation of *Candida albicans* by ultraviolet radiation. Arch. Mikrobiol. *64*:289-313.

64a. Cabib, E., and R. Roberts. 1982. Synthesis of the yeast cell wall and its regulation. Annu. Rev. Biochem. *51*:763-793.

65. Caldwell, C. W., and R. F. Sprouse. 1982. Iron and host resistance in histoplasmosis. Am. Rev. Respir. Dis. *125*:674-677.

66. Callaghan, A. A. 1978. Effect of nutrient level, pH, and light on conidial germination in entomophthoraceous fungi. Trans. Br. Mycol. Soc. *70*:271-276.

67. Campbell, C. C. 1947. Reverting *Histoplasma capsulatum* to the yeast phase. J. Bacteriol. *54*:263-264.

68. Cantino, E. C., and E. A. Horenstein. 1955. The role of ketoglutarate and polyphenol oxidase in the synthesis of melanin during morphogenesis in *Blastocladiella emersonii*. Physiol. Plant. *8*:189-221.

69. Carlile, M. J. 1970. The photoreceptors in fungi. In P. Halldal (Ed.), *Photobiology of Microorganisms*, Wiley-Interscience, New York, pp. 309-344.

70. Caroline, L., C. L. Taschdjian, P. J. Kozinn, and A. L. Schade. 1964. Reversal of serum fungistasis by addition of iron. J. Invest. Dermatol. *42*:415-419.

71. Castellani, A. 1928. *Fungi and Fungous Diseases,* American Medical Association, Chicago, Ill.

72. Catchings, B. M., and D. J. Guidry. 1973. Effects of pH and temperature on the in vitro growth of *Sporothrix schenckii*. Sabouraudia *11*:70-76.

73. Chaskes, S., S. C. Edberg, and J. M. Singer. 1981. A D,L-DOPA drop test for the identification of *Cryptococcus neoformans*. Mycopathologia *74*:143-148.

74. Chattaway, F. W., D. A. Ellis, and A. J. E. Barlow. 1963. Peptidases of dermatophytes. J. Invest. Dermatol. *41*:31-37.

75. Chattaway, F. W., F. C. Odds, and A. J. E. Barlow. 1971. An examination of the production of hydrolytic enzymes and toxins by pathogenic strains of *Candida albicans*. J. Gen. Microbiol. *67*:255-263.

76. Chattaway, F. W., P. R. Wheeler, and J. O'Reilly. 1980. Purification and properties of peptides which induce germination of blastospores of *Candida albicans*. J. Gen. Microbiol. *120*:431-437.

77. Cheung, S. C., and J. Maniotis. 1973. A genetic study of an extracellular elastin hydrolysing protease in the ringworm fungus *Arthroderma benhamiae*. J. Gen. Microbiol. *74*:299-304.

78. Chick, E. W., A. B. Hudnell, Jr., and D. G. Sharp. 1963. Ultraviolet sensitivity of fungi associated with mycotic keratitis and other mycoses. Sabouraudia *2*:195-200.

79. Chiew, Y. Y., M. G. Shepherd, and P. A. Sullivan. 1980. Regulation of chitin synthesis during germ-tube formation in *Candida albicans*. Arch. Microbiol. *125*: 97-104.

80. Chin, B., and S. G. Knight. 1957. Growth of *Trichophyton mentagrophytes* and *Trichophyton rubrum* in increased carbon dioxide tensions. J. Gen. Microbiol. *16*: 642-646.

81. Chinn, R. Y. W., and R. D. Diamond. 1982. Generation of chemotactic factor by *Rhizopus oryzae* in the presence and absence of serum : Relationship to hyphal damage mediated by human neutrophils and effects of hyperglycemia and ketoacidosis. Infect. Immun. *38*:1123-1129.

82. Ciferri, R., and P. Redaelli. 1934. *Histoplasma capsulatum* Darling, the agent of "histoplasmosis": systematic position and characteristics. J. Trop. Med. Hyg. *37*: 278-280.

83. Clerivet, A., and J. Ragot. 1974. Keratinolytic and proteolytic activity of *Trichophyton verrucosum* cultured on undenatured Merino wool. C. R. Acad. Sci. (Paris) *278*:3191-3194.

84. Cochrane, V. W. 1958. *Physiology of Fungi*, Wiley, New York.

85. Collard, P. 1976. *The Development of Microbiology*, Cambridge University Press, Cambridge.

86. Conant, N. F. 1936. Studies in the genus *Microsporum*. Arch. Dermatol. Syphilol. *33*:665-683.

87. Conant, N. F. 1941. A cultural study of the life cycle of *Histoplasma capsulatum* Darling 1906. J. Bacteriol. *41*:563-579.

88. Converse, J. L. 1955. Growth of *Coccidioides immitis* in a chemically defined liquid medium. Proc. Soc. Exp. Biol. Med. *90*:709-711.

89. Cooney, D. G., and R. Emerson. 1964. *Thermophilic Fungi*, Freeman, San Francisco.

90. Cooper, B. H. 1980. Clinical laboratory evaluation of a screening medium (CN screen) for *Cryptococcus neoformans*. J. Clin. Microbiol. *11*:672-674.

91. Cooper, B. H., J. B. Johnson, and E. S. Thaxton. 1978. Clinical evaluation of the Uni-Yeast-Tek system for rapid presumptive identification of medically important yeasts. J. Clin. Microbiol. 7:349-355.

91a. Crandall, M. 1983. UV-induced mitotic cosegregation of genetic markers in *Candida albicans*: evidence for linkage. Curr. Genet. 7:167-173.

92. Crellin, J. K. 1966. The problem of heat resistance of microorganisms in the British spontaneous generation controversies of 1860-1880. Med. Hist. *10*:50-59.

93. Dabrowa, N., J. W. Landau, and V. D. Newcomer. 1965. The antifungal activity of physiological saline in serum. J. Invest. Dermatol. *45*:368-377.

94. Dabrowa, N., J. W. Landau, and V. D. Newcomer. 1967. Generation time of *Candida albicans* in synchronized and nonsynchronized cultures. Sabouraudia *6*: 51-56.

95. Dabrowa, N., S. S. S. Taxer, and D. H. Howard. 1976. Germination of *Candida albicans* induced by proline. Infect. Immun. *13*:830-835.

96. Dabrowa, N., J. W. Landau, V. D. Newcomer, and O. A. Plunkett. 1964. A survey of tide-washed coastal areas of southern California for fungi potentially pathogenic to man. Mycopathol. Mycol. Appl. *24*:137-150.

97. Dahlberg, K. R., and J. L. Van Etten. 1982. Physiology and biochemistry of fungal sporulation. Annu. Rev. Phytopathol. *20*:281-301.

98. Das, S. K., and A. B. Banerjee. 1977. Lipolytic enzymes of *Trichophyton rubrum*. Sabouraudia *15*:313-323.

99. Das, S. K., and A. B. Banerjee. 1977. Phospholipid turnover in *Trichophyton rubrum*. Sabouraudia *15*:99-102.

99a. Davis, R. R., and T. J. V. Denning. 1972. Growth and form in *Candida albicans*. Sabouraudia *10*:180-188.

100. De Busk, R. M., and S. Ogilvie-Villa. 1962. Physiological adaptation to the loss of amino acid transport ability. J. Bacteriol. *152*:545-548.

101. Demain, A. L. 1981. Industrial microbiology. Science *214*:987-995.

102. De Monbreun, W. A. 1934. The cultivation and cultural characteristics of Darling's *Histoplasma capsulatum*. J. Trop. Med. *14*:93-125.

103. Denton, J. F., E. S. McDonough, L. Ajello, and R. Ausherman. 1961. Isolation of *Blastomyces dermatitidis* from soil. Science *133*:1126-1127.

104. de Robichon-Szulmajster, H., and Y. Surdin-Kerjan. 1971. Nucleic acid and protein synthesis in yeasts: Regulation of synthesis and activity. In A. H. Rose and J. S. Harrison (Eds.), *The Yeasts*, Vol. 2, Academic, New York, pp. 335-418.

105. Detroy, R. W., and A. Ciegler. 1971. Induction of yeastlike development in *Aspergillus parasiticus*. J. Gen. Microbiol. *65*:259-264.

106. Dodge, C. W. 1935. *Medical Mycology*, Mosby, St. Louis.

107. Doetsch, R. N. 1963. Studies on biogenesis by Sir William Roberts. Med. Hist. 7:232-240.

108. Dubos, R. J. 1950. *Louis Pasteur, Free Lance of Science*, Little, Brown, Boston.

109. Dumont, A., and C. Piche. 1969. Electron microscopic study of human histoplasmosis. Arch. Pathol. *87*:168-178.

110. Dumont, A., and P. Robert. 1970. Electron microscopic study of phagocytosis of *Histoplasma capsulatum* by hamster peritoneal macrophages. Lab. Invest. *23*: 278-286.

111. Dzawachiszwili, N., J. W. Landau, V. D. Newcomer, and O. A. Plunkett. 1964. The effect of sea water and sodium chloride on the growth of fungi pathogenic to man. J. Invest. Dermatol. *43*:103-109.

112. Edwards, M., and D. H. Howard. 1981. The interaction of *Histoplasma capsulatum* with mouse macrophages. Abstr. Annu. Meet. Am. Soc. Microbiol., F4, p. 314.

113. Egeberg, R. O., A. E. Elconin, and M. C. Egeberg. 1964. Effect of salinity and temperature on *Coccidioides immitis* and three antagonistic soil saprophytes. J. Bacteriol. *88*:473-476.

114. Elin, R. J., and S. M. Wolff. 1973. Effect of pH and iron concentration on growth of *Candida albicans* in human serum. J. Infect. Dis. *127*:705-708.

115. Emerson, R., and A. A. Held. 1969. *Aqualinderella fermentans* gen. et sp. nov. II. Isolation, cultural characteristics, and gas relations. Am. J. Bot. *56*:1103-1120.

116. Emerson, R., and W. H. Weston. 1967. *Aqualinderella fermentans* gen. et sp. nov., a phycomycete adapted to stagnant waters. I. Morphology and occurrence in nature. Am. J. Bot. *54*:702-719.

117. Emmons, C. W. 1942. Isolation of *Coccidioides* from soil and rodents. Public Health Rep. *57*:109-111.

118. Emmons, C. W. 1951. The isolation from soil of fungi which cause disease in man. Trans. N.Y. Acad. Sci., Ser. II. *14*:51-54.

119. Emmons, C. W. 1954. Isolation of *Myxotrichum* and *Gymnoascus* from the lungs of animals. Mycologia *46*:334-338.

120. Emmons, C. W. 1962. Nautral occurrence of opportunistic fungi. Lab. Invest., No. 11, Part 2, *11*:1026-1032.

121. Emmons, C. W., and A. Hollaender. 1939. The action of ultraviolet radiation on dermatophytes. II. Mutations induced in cultures of dermatophytes by exposure of spores to monochromatic ultraviolet radiation. Am. J. Bot. *26*:467-475.

122. English, M. P. 1963. The saprophytic growth of keratinophytic fungi in keratin. Sabouraudia *2*:115-130.

123. Esterly, N. B., S. B. Brammer, and R. G. Crounse. 1967. The relationship of transferrin and iron to serum inhibition of *Candida albicans*. J. Invest. Dermatol. *49*:437-442.

124. Faergemann, J., and S. Bernander. 1981. Microacrophilic and anaerobic growth of *Pityrosporum* species. Sabouraudia *19*:117-121.

125. Falcone, G., and W. J. Nickerson. 1963. Reduction of selenite by intact yeast cells and cell-free preparations. J. Bacteriol. *85*:754-762.

126. Farley, J. 1977. *The Spontaneous Generation Controversy from Descartes to Oparin*, Johns Hopkins University Press, Baltimore.

127. Fieldes, P. 1934. Some medical and other aspects of bacterial chemistry. Proc. R. Soc. Med. *28*:79-90.

128. Fincham, J. R. S., P. R. Day, and A. Radford. 1979. *Fungal Genetics*, University of California Press, Berkeley.

129. Flanagan, D. (Ed.). 1981. Industrial microbiology. Sci. Am. *245*(3):226 pp. (N. B. entire issue).

130. Foster, J. W. 1949. *Chemical Activities of Fungi,* Academic, New York.

131. Foster, J. W. 1951. Metabolism of fungi. Annu. Rev. Microbiol. *5*:101-120.

132. Foster, J. W. 1958. An evaluation of the role of molds in the comparative biochemistry of carbohydrate oxidation. Tex. Rep. Biol. Med. *16*:99-100.

133. Freis, J., and P. Ottolenghi. 1969. Pigment formation by the "black yeast" *Phialophora jeanselmei.* Antonie Leeuwenhoek J. Microbiol. Serol. (Suppl.: Yeast Symposium) *35*:H13-H14.

134. Fromentin, H., H. Hurion, and F. Mariat. 1978. Collagenase, esterase, et elastase de pouches pathogene et saprophytes de *Entomophthora coronata*: Cinetique de production. Ann. Microbiol. (Inst. Pasteur) *129A*:425-431.

135. Fuentes, C. A., and Z. E. Bosch. 1960. Biochemical differentiation of the etiologic agents of chromoblastomycosis from non-pathogenic *Cladosporium* species. J. Invest. Dermatol. *34*:419-421.

136. Gale, G. R., and A. M. Welch. 1961. Studies on opportunistic fungi. I. Inhibition of *Rhizopus oryzae* by human serum. Am. J. Med. Sci. *241*:604-612.

137. Garcia, J. P., and D. H. Howard. 1971. Characterization of antigens from the yeast phase of *Histoplasma capsulatum.* Infect. Immun. *4*:116-125.

138. Garrison, R. G. 1961. Studies of the respiratory activity of *Histoplasma capsulatum.* I. Aspects of the aerobic metabolism of the yeast phase. J. Infect. Dis. *108*:120-124.

139. Garrison, R. G., H. T. Dodd, and J. W. Hamilton. 1970. The uptake of low molecular weight sulfur-containing compounds by *Histoplasma capsulatum* and related dimorphic fungi. Mycopathol. Mycol. Appl. *40*:171-180.

140. Garrison, R. G., F. Mariat, K. S. Boyd, and J. F. Tally. 1975. Ultrastructural and electron cytochemical studies of *Entomophthora coronata.* Ann. Microbiol. (Paris) *126B*:149-173.

141. Garvey, M. C., and R. P. Tewari. 1972. A cell-free amino acid incorporating system from yeast-phase cells of *Histoplasma capsulatum.* Sabouraudia *10*:113-121.

142. Gates, D. W., and B. H. Brownstein. 1980. Ribosomal RNA from the yeast and mycelial phases of *Histoplasma capsulatum.* Exp. Mycol. *4*:231-238.

143. Gaur, P. K., R. W. Lichtwardt, and J. L. Hamrick. 1981. Isozyme variation among soil isolates by *Histoplasma capsulatum.* Exp. Mycol. *5*:69-77.

144. Georg, L. K. 1950. The nutritional requirements of the faviform trichophytons. Ann. N.Y. Acad. Sci. *50*:1315-1347.

145. Georg, L. K. 1950. The relation of nutrition to the growth and morphology of *Trichophyton faviforme.* Mycologia *42*:683-692.

146. Georg, L. K. 1952. Cultural and nutritional studies of *Trichophyton gallinae* and *Trichophyton megninii.* Mycologia *44*:470-492.

147. Georg, L. K. 1956. Studies on *Trichophyton tonsurans.* I. The taxonomy of *T. tonsurans.* Mycologia *48*:65-82.

148. Georg, L. K. 1957. *Dermatophytes. New Methods of Classification,* U.S. Dept. Health, Education, and Welfare, Communicable Disease Center, Atlanta.

149. Georg, L. K. 1959. *Animal Ringworm in Public Health. Diagnosis and Nature,* U.S. Dept. Health, Education, and Welfare, Public Health Service, Bureau of State Services, Communicable Disease Center, Atlanta.

150. Georg, L. K., and L. Camp. 1957. Routine nutritional tests for the identification of dermatophytes. J. Bacteriol. *73*:113-121.

151. Georg, L. K., L. Ajello, and C. Papageorge. 1954. Use of cycloheximide in the selective isolation of fungi pathogenic to man. J. Lab. Clin. Med. *44*:422-428.

152. Georg, L. K., W. Kaplan, and L. B. Camp. 1957. *Trichophyton equinum.* A reevaluation of its taxonomic status. J. Invest. Dermatol. *29*:27-37.

153. Germaine, G. R., and L. M. Tellefson. 1981. Effect of pH and human saliva on protease production by *Candida albicans*. Infect. Immun. *31*:313-326.

154. Gilardi, G. L. 1965. Nutrition of systemic and subcutaneous pathogenic fungi. Bacteriol. Rev. *29*:406-424.

155. Gilardi, G. L., and N. C. Laffer. 1962. Nutritional studies of the yeast phase of *Blastomyces dermatitidis* and *B. brasiliensis*. J. Bacteriol. *83*:219-227.

156. Goos, R. D. 1964. Germination of the macroconidium of *Histoplasma capsulatum*. Mycologia *56*:662-671.

157. Gordon, M. A. 1951. Lipophilic yeast-like organisms associated with tinea versicolor. J. Invest. Dermatol. *17*:267-272.

158. Gordon, M. A. 1951. The lipophilic mycoflora of the skin. I. *In vitro* culture of *Pityrosporum obiculare*. Mycologia *43*:525-535.

159. Gordon, R. E., and W. A. Hagan. 1936. A study of some acid-fast actinomycetes from soil with special reference to pathogenicity to animals. J. Infect. Dis. *59*: 200-206.

160. Goren, M. B. 1977. Phagocyte lysosomes: Interactions with infectious agents, phagosomes, and experimental perturbations in function. Annu. Rev. Microbiol. *31*:507-533.

161. Griffin, D. H. 1981. *Fungal Physiology*, Wiley, New York.

162. Haidle, C. W., and R. Storck. 1966. Control of dimorphism in *Mucor rouxii*. J. Bacteriol. *92*:1236-1244.

163. Haley, L. D., J. Trandel, and M. B. Coyle. 1980. *Practical Methods for Culture and Identification of Fungi in the Clinical Microbiology Laboratory*, Cumitech 11 (J. C. Sherris, Coordinating Editor), American Society for Microbiology, Washington, D.C.

163a. Halliday, W. J., and E. Mc Coy. 1955. Biotin as a growth requirement for *Blastomyces dermatitidis*. J. Bacteriol. *70*:464-467.

164. Hart, D'Arcy, P. 1981. Macrophage antimicrobial activity: evidence for participation by lysosomes in the killing of *Saccharomyces cerevisiae* by normal resident macrophages. Infect. Immun. *31*:828-830.

165. Hartwell, L. H. 1974. *Saccharomyces cerevisiae* cell cycle. Bacteriol. Rev. *38*: 164-198.

166. Hartwell, L. H., J. Culotti, and B. J. Reid. 1970. Genetic control of the cell division cycle in yeast. I. Detection of mutants. Proc. Natl. Acad. Sci. U.S.A. *66*:352-359.

167. Hashimoto, T., C. D. R. Wu, and H. J. Blumenthal. 1972. Characterization of L-leucine-induced germination of *Trichophyton mentagrophytes* microconidia. J. Bacteriol. *112*:967-976.

168. Hasyn, J. J., and H. R. Buckley. 1982. Evaluation of the automicrobic system for identification of yeasts. J. Clin. Microbiol. *16*:901-904.

169. Hawk, P. B., B. L. Oser, and W. H. Summerson. 1947. *Practical Physiological Chemistry*, The Blakiston Co., Philadelphia.

170. Hawker, L. E. 1957. *Physiology of Reproduction in Fungi*, Cambridge University Press, Cambridge.

171. Healy, M. E., C. L. Dillavou, and G. E. Taylor. 1977. Diagnostic medium containing inositol, urea, and caffeic acid for selective growth of *Cryptococcus neoformans*. J. Clin. Microbiol. *6*:387-391.

172. Hejtmánek, M., and J. Bártek. 1976. Mutants of *Emmonsia crescens*—their pathogenicity and size of adiaspores in vivo. Folia Microbiol. *21*:297-300.

173. Held, A. A., R. Emerson, M. S. Fuller, and F. H. Gleason. 1969. *Blastocladiella* and *Aqualinderella*: Fermentation water molds with high carbon dioxide optima. Science *165*:706-709.

173a. Hendry, A. T., and A. Bakerspiegel. 1969. Factors affecting serum inhibited growth of *Candida albicans* and *Cryptococcus neoformans*. Sabouraudia 7:219-229.

174. Hilger, A. E., M. J. Lawrie, and D. A. Wilson. 1979. Growth of *Trichophyton mentagrophytes* on individual amino acids. Sabouraudia *17*:299-303.

175. Hopsu-Havu, V. K., S. M. Laiko, and E. R. Lundell. 1967. A colour test for yeasts based on staining of the colonies with aromatic diazonium salts. Mykosen *10*:23-26.

176. Howard, D. H. 1961. Some factors which affect the initiation of growth of *Cryptococcus neoformans*. J. Bacteriol. *82*:430-435.

177. Howard, D. H. 1964. Intracellular behavior of *Histoplasma capsulatum*. J. Bacteriol. *87*:33-38.

178. Howard, D. H. 1973. The commensalism of *Cryptococcus neoformans*. Sabouraudia *11*:171-174.

179. Howard, D. H. 1981. Comparative sensitivity of *Histoplasma capsulatum* conidiospores and blastospores to oxidative antifungal systems. Infect. Immun. *32*: 381-387.

180. Howard, D. H. 1981. Mechanisms of resistance in the systemic mycoses. In A. J. Nahmias and R. O'Reilly (Eds.), *Comprehensive Immunology*, Vol. 8, Plenum, New York, pp. 475-493.

181. Howard, D. H. 1983. The catalase of *Histoplasma capsulatum*. Infect. Immun. *39*:1161-1166.

182. Howard, D. H., and N. Dabrowa. 1979. Mutants of *Arthroderma benhamiae*. Sabouraudia *17*:35-50.

183. Howard, D. H., and G. F. Orr. 1963. Comparison of strians of *Sporotrichum schenckii* isolated from nature. J. Bacteriol. *85*:816-821.

184. Howard, D. H., and V. Otto. 1967. The intracellular behavior of *Torulopsis glabrata*. Sabouraudia *5*:235-239.

185. Howard, D. H., N. Dabrowa, V. Otto, and J. Rhodes. 1980. Cysteine transport and sulfite reductase activity in a germination defective mutant of *Histoplasma capsulatum*. J. Bacteriol. *141*:417-421.

186. Howell, A., Jr. 1941. Studies on *Histoplasma capsulatum* and similar form-species. III. Effect of hydrogen ion concentration. Mycologia *33*:103-117.

187. Huelsmann, C., and D. C. Savage. 1981. pH and growth of *Torulopsis pintolopesii* in media containing various sugars as carbon and energy sources. Appl. Environ. Microbiol. *43*:554-555.

188. Huppert, M., G. Harper, S. H. Sun, and V. Delanerolle. 1975. Rapid methods for identification of yeasts. J. Clin. Microbiol. *2*:21-34.

189. Igel, H. J., and R. P. Bolande. 1966. Humoral defense mechanisms in cryptococcosis: substances in normal human serum, saliva, and cerebrospinal fluid affecting the growth of *Cryptococcus neoformans*. J. Infect. Dis. *116*:75-83.

190. Jacobson, E. S., and A. C. Harrell. 1982. A prototrophic yeast-strain of *Histoplasma capsulatum*. Mycopathologia *77*:65-68.

191. Jacobson, E. S., and A. C. Harrell. 1982. Cysteine-independent and cysteine-requiring yeast strains of *Histoplasma capsulatum*. Mycopathologia *77*:69-73.

192. Jaitly, A. K., and J. N. Rai. 1982. Thermophilic and thermotolerant fungi isolated from mangrove swamps. Mycologia *74*:1021-1022.

193. Jaso-Friedmann, L., and G. Boguslawski. 1981. DNA polymerases from a dimorphic fungus, *Histoplasma capsulatum*. Exp. Mycol. *5*:89-100.

194. Jones, M. G., and W. C. Noble. 1982. An electrophoretic study of enzymes as a tool in the taxonomy of the dermatophytes. J. Gen. Microbiol. *128*:1101-1107.

195. Kakar, S. N., and P. T. Magee. 1982. Genetic analysis of *Candida albicans*:

identification of different isoleucine-valine, methionine, and arginine alleles by complementation. J. Bacteriol. *151*:1247-1252.

195a. Kakar, S. N., R. M. Partridge, and P. T. Magee. 1983. A genetic analysis of *Candida albicans*: isolation of a wide variety of auxotrophs and demonstration of linkage and complementation. Genetics *104*:241-255.

196. Kapica, L., and F. Blank. 1957. Growth of *Candida albicans* on keratin as sole sources of nitrogen. Dermatologia *115*:81-105.

197. Karling, J. S. 1946. Keratinophilic chytrids. Am. J. Bot. *33*:751-757.

198. Kashkin, A. P., and Y. N. Voevidin. 1976. Proteolytic enzymes of *Trichophyton mentagrophytes* (Robin) Blanchard Str. 69. Mikol. Fitopatol. *10*:179-185.

199. Kashkin, K. P. 1980. Dimorphism and antigens. Zentralbl. Bakteriol. Parasitenkd. Infektionskr., Hyg., Abt. 1, Suppl. *8*:3-15.

200. Kim, Y. P., K. Adachi, and D. Chow. 1962. Leucine aminopeptidase in *Candida albicans*. J. Invest. Dermatol. *38*:115-116.

201. King, R. D., H. A. Khan, J. C. Faye, J. H. Greenberg, and H. E. Jones. 1975. Transferrin, iron and dermatophytes. I. Serum dermatophyte inhibitory component definitively identified as unsaturated transferrin. J. Lab. Clin. Med. *86*:204-212.

202. Kirk, P. W., Jr. 1967. A comparison of saline tolerance and sporulation in marine and clinical isolates of *Allescheria boydii* Shear. Mycopathol. Mycol. Appl. *33*:65-75.

203. Kishimoto, R. A., and G. E. Baker. 1969. Pathogenic and potentially pathogenic fungi isolated from beach sands and selected soils of Oahu, Hawaii. Mycologia *61*:537-548.

204. Kitz, D. J., R. W. Embree, and J. Cazin, Jr. 1980. *Radiomyces* a genus in the Mucorales pathogenic for mice. Sabouraudia *18*:115-121.

205. Knight, B. C. J. G. 1938. *Bacterial Nutrition,* Medical Research Council Special Report Series, No. 2101, London.

206. Knight, R. H., B. A. Body, G. S. Kobayashi, and G. Medoff. 1980. Balanced growth and morphogenesis of *Histoplasma capsulatum* in a defined synthetic medium. Sabouraudia *18*:39-50.

207. Koobs, D. H. 1972. Phosphate mediation of the Crabtree and Pasteur effects. Science *178*:127-133.

208. Kot, E. J., V. L. Olson, L. J. Rolewic, and D. O. McClary. 1976. An alternate respiratory pathway in *Candida albicans*. Antonie Leeuwenhoek. J. Microbiol. Serol. *42*:33-48.

209. Kucera, M. 1981. The production of toxic protease by the entomopathogenic fungus *Metarhizium anisopliae* in submerged culture. J. Invertebr. Pathol. *38*:33-38.

210. Kuehn, H. H., and G. F. Orr. 1962. Tolerance of certain fungi to actidione and its use in isolation of *Gymnoascaceae*. Sabouraudia *1*:220-229.

211. Kumar, B. V., R. A. McMillian, G. Medoff, M. Gutwein, and G. Kobayashi. 1980. Comparison of the ribonucleic acid polymerases from both phases of *Histoplasma capsulatum*. Biochemistry *19*:1080-1087.

212. Kunert, J. 1972. Keratin decomposition by dermatophytes. Evidence of the sulphitolysis of the protein. Experientia *28*:1025-1026.

213. Kuprowski, M. 1966. The influence of the quality of agar in the occurrence of haemolysis in cultures of *Candida albicans*. Zentralbl. Veterinaermed, Ser. B, *13*:364-368.

214. Kurung, J. M., and D. Yegian. 1954. Medium for maintenance and conversion of *Histoplasma capsulatum* to yeastlike phase. Am. J. Clin. Pathol. *24*:505-508.

215. Kwon-Chung, K. J. 1969. Studies on the sexuality of *Nannizzia*. II. Morphogenesis of gametangia of *N. incurvata*. Mycologia *61*:593-605.

216. Kwon-Chung, K. J. 1974. Genetics of fungi pathogenic for man. CRC Crit. Rev. Microbiol., February: 115-133.

217. Kwon-Chung, K. J. 1979. Comparison of isolates of *Sporothrix schenckii* obtained from fixed cutaneous lesions with isolates from other types of lesions. J. Infect. Dis. *139*:424-431.

218. Kwon-Chung, K. J., and W. B. Hill. 1970. Studies on the pink, adenine-deficient strains of *Candida albicans*. I. Cultural and morphological characteristics. Sabouraudia *8*:48-59.

219. Kwon-Chung, K. J., I. Polacheck, and J. E. Bennett. 1982. Improved diagnostic medium for separation of *Cryptococcus neoformans* var. *neoformans* (serotypes A and D) and *Cryptococcus neoformans* var. *gattii* (serotypes B and C). J. Clin. Microbiol. *15*:535-537.

220. Kwon-Chung, K. J., I. Polacheck, and T. J. Popkin. 1982. Melanin-lacking mutants of *Cryptococcus neoformans* and their virulence for mice. J. Bacteriol. *150*:1414-1421.

221. Land, G. A., W. H. Fleming III, T. A. Beadles, and J. H. Foxworth. 1979. Rapid identification of medically important yeasts. Lab. Med. *10*:533-541.

222. Land, G. A., W. C. McDonald, R. L. Stjernholm, and L. Friedman. 1975. Factors affecting filamentation in *Candida albicans*: Relationship of the uptake and distribution of proline to morphogenesis. Infect. Immun. *11*:1014-1023.

223. Land, G. A., B. A. Harrison, K. L. Hulme, B. H. Cooper, and J. C. Byrd. 1979. Evaluation of the new API 20C strip for yeast identification against a conventional method. J. Clin. Microbiol. *10*:357-364.

224. Landau, J. W., N. Dabrowa, V. D. Newcomer, and J. Rowe. 1964. The relationship of serum transferrin and iron to the rapid formation of germ tubes by *Candida albicans*. J. Invest. Dermatol. *43*:473-482.

225. Leach, C. M. 1971. A practical guide to the effects of visible and ultraviolet light on fungi. In C. Booth (Ed.), *Methods in Microbiology*, Vol. 4, Academic, New York, pp. 609-664.

226. Lee, K. L., M. E. Reca, R. R. Watson, and C. C. Campbell. 1975. Identification of yeast phase of pathogenic fungi by the specificity of their aminopeptidases. Sabouraudia *13*:132-141.

227. Lehninger, A. L. 1982. *Principles of Biochemistry*, Worth Publishers, Inc., New York.

228. Levine, S., and Z. J. Ordal. 1946. Factors influencing the morphology of *Blastomyces dermatitidis*. J. Bacteriol. *52*:687-694.

229. Lewis, D. H. 1973. Concepts in fungal nutrition and the origin of biotrophy. Biol. Rev. *48*:261-278.

230. Lockwood, G. F., and R. G. Garrison. 1968. The possible role of uric acid in the ecology of *Histoplasma capsulatum*. Mycopathol. Mycol. Appl. *35*:377-388.

231. Lodder, J. (Ed.). 1970. *The Yeasts. A Taxomic Study*, North-Holland, Amsterdam.

232. Loeffler, F. 1887. *Vorlesungen über die geschichtliche Entwickelung der Lehre von den Bacterien*, F. C. W. Vogel, Leipzig.

233. Lones, G. W. 1967. Studies of intermediary metabolism of *Coccidioides immitis*. In L. Ajello (Ed.), *Coccidioidomycosis*, Papers from the Second Symposium on Coccidioidomycosis, University of Arizona Press, Tucson, pp. 349-353.

234. Lones, G. W., and C. L. Peacock. 1960. Role of carbon dioxide in the dimorphism of *Coccidioides immitis*. J. Bacteriol. *79*:308-309.

235. Lones, G. W., and C. L. Peacock. 1960. Studies on the growth and metabolism of *Coccidioides immitis*. Ann. N.Y. Acad. Sci. *89*:102-108.

236. Lubarsky, R., and O. A. Plunkett. 1955. In vitro production of the spherule phase of *Coccidioides immitis*. J. Bacteriol. *70*:182-186.

237. Lund, A. 1958. Ecology of yeasts. In A. H. Cook (Ed.), *The Chemistry and Biology of Yeasts,* Academic, New York, pp. 63-91.

238. Macdonald, F., and F. C. Odds. 1980. Purified *Candida albicans* proteinases in the serological diagnosis of systemic candidosis. JAMA *243*:2409-2411.

239. Macdonald, F., and F. C. Odds. 1983. Virulence for mice of a proteinase-secreting strain of *Candida albicans* and a proteinase-deficient mutant. J. Gen. Microbiol. *129*:431-438.

240. Macfayden, A. 1896. A contribution to the biology of the ringworm organism. J. Pathol. Bacteriol. *3*:176-183.

241. MacLaren, J. A., and D. Armen. 1958. Pigmentation of *Candida albicans* by molybdenum. Am. J. Clin. Pathol. *30*:411-422.

242. Mandels, G. R. 1965. Kinetics of fungal growth. In G. C. Ainsworth and A. S. Sussman (Eds.), *The Fungi. An Advanced Treatise,* Academic, New York, pp. 599-623.

243. Maresca, B., E. Jacobson, G. Medoff, and G. Kobayashi. 1978. Cystine reductase in the dimorphic fungus *Histoplasma capsulatum.* J. Bacteriol. *135*:987-992.

244. Maresca, B., A. M. Lambowitz, G. S. Kobayashi, and G. Medoff. 1979. Respiration in the yeast and mycelial phases of *Histoplasma capsulatum.* J. Bacteriol. *138*:647-649.

245. Maresca, B., A. M. Lambowitz, V. B. Kumar, G. A. Grant, G. S. Kobayashi, and G. Medoff. 1981. Role of cysteine in regulating morphogenesis and mitochondrial activity in the dimorphic fungus *Histoplasma capsulatum.* Proc. Natl. Acad. Sci. U.S.A. *78*:4596-4600.

246. Mariat, F. 1960. Action de l'anhydride carbonique sur la croissance de *Sporotrichum schenckii.* C. R. Acad. Sci. (Paris) *250*:3503-3505.

247. Mariat, F., and E. Drouhet. 1952. Étude des facteurs déterminant le développement de la phase levure de *Sporotrichum schenckii.* Ann. Inst. Pasteur (Paris) *83*:506-515.

248. Marshall, M., G. Russo, J. Van Etten, and K. Nickerson. 1979. Polyamines in dimorphic fungi. Curr. Microbiol. *2*:187-190.

249. McDonough, E. S., L. K. Georg, L. Ajello, and S. Brinkman. 1960. Growth of dimorphic human pathogenic fungi on media containing cycloheximide and chloramphenicol. Mycopathol. Mycol. Appl. *13*:113-120.

250. McGinnis, M. R. 1980. *Laboratory Handbook of Medical Mycology,* Academic, New York.

251. McMillan, S. 1958. A simple fluid medium for diphasic fungi. J. Lab. Clin. Med. *51*:141-142.

252. McVeigh, I., and K. Morton. 1965. Nutritional studies of *Histoplasma capsulatum.* Mycopathol. Mycol. Appl. *25*:294-309.

253. McVickar, D. L. 1951. Factors important for the growth of *Histoplasma capsulatum* in the yeast cell phase on peptone media. J. Bacteriol. *62*:137-143.

254. Meevootisom, V., and D. J. Niederpruem. 1979. Control of exocellular proteases in dermatophytes and especially *Trichophyton rubrum.* Sabouraudia *17*:85-170.

255. Meinhof, W., C. Scherwitz, and K. Pupaibul. 1973. Comparative study of physiological properties for identification of *Trichophyton rubrum* and *Trichophyton mentagrophytes* pigment production, urease, and lipase activity, growth in peptone solution, and by hair performation test. Arch. Dermatol. Forsch. *248*:247-256.

256. Menges, R. W., M. L. Furcolow, H. W. Larsh, and A. Hinton. 1952. Laboratory studies on histoplasmosis. I. The effect of humidity and temperature on the growth of *Histoplasma capsulatum.* J. Infect. Dis. *90*:67-70.

257. Merz, W. G., I. Weitzman, and M. Silva-Hutner. 1974. Characterization and

mating reactions of clinical isolates of *Trichophyton mentagrophytes* and *T. rubrum* which produce a diffusible brownish pigment. Sabouraudia *12*:7-11.

257a. Main, K. H., and K. J. Kwon-Chung. 1983. Glycine utilization by *C. neoformans* species. Abstr. Annu. Meet. ASM, F10, p. 384.

258. Minocha, Y., J. S. Pasricha, L. N. Mohapatra, and K. C. Kandhari. 1972. Proteolytic activities of dermatophytes and its role in the pathogenesis of skin lesions. Sabouraudia *10*:79-85.

259. Miyaji, M., and K. Nishimura. 1977. Relationship between proteolytic activity of *Aspergillus fumigatus* and the fungus invasiveness of mouse brain. Mycopathologia *62*:161-166.

260. Montes, L. F., and V. S. Constantine. 1968. Cytochemical demonstration of aminopeptidase in *Candida albicans*. J. Invest. Dermatol. *51*:1-3.

261. Mosberg, W. H., Jr., and J. A. Alvarez-de Chaudens. 1951. Torulosis of the central nervous system; effect of change in pH and temperature on growth of causal organism. Lancet *260*:1259-1260.

262. Mosher, W. A., D. H. Saunders, L. B. Kingery, and R. J. Williams. 1936. Nutritional requirements of the pathogenic mold *Trichophyton interdigitale*. Plant Physiol. *11*:795-806.

263. Mueller, H. E., and K. K. Sethi. 1972. Proteolytic activity of *Cryptococcus neoformans* against human plasma proteins. Med. Microbiol. Immunol. *158*:129-134.

264. Murphy, J. W., and D. O. McDaniel. 1982. In vitro reactivity of natural killer cells against *Cryptococcus neoformans*. J. Immunol. *128*:1577-1583.

265. Murray, P. R., R. E. Van Scoy, and G. D. Roberts. 1977. Should yeasts in respiratory secretions be identified? Mayo Clinic Proc. *52*:42-45.

266. Nazzaro Porro, M., S. Passi, F. Caprilli, P. Nazzaro, and G. Morpurgo. 1976. Growth requirements and lipid metabolism of *Pityrosporum orbiculare*. J. Invest. Dermatol. *66*:178-182.

267. Newcomer, V. D., J. W. Landau, N. Dabrowa, and M. L. Fenster. 1968. Effects of human body fluids on *Candida albicans*. In *Proceedings of the XIIIth International Congress of Dermatology*, Munich, Springer-Verlag, Berlin, pp. 813-817.

268. Nickerson, K. W., B. K. McCune, and J. L. Van Etten. 1977. Polyamine and macromolecule levels during spore germination in *Rhizopus stolonifer* and *Botryodiplodia theobromae*. Exp. Mycol. *1*:317-322.

269. Nickerson, W. J. (Ed.). 1947. *Biology of Pathogenic Fungi*, Chronica Botanica, Waltham, Mass.

270. Nickerson, W. J. 1953. Reduction of inorganic substances by yeasts. I. Extracellular reduction of sulfite by species of *Candida*. J. Infect. Dis. *93*:43-56.

271. Nickerson, W. J., and S. Bartnicki-Garcia. 1964. Biochemical aspects of morphogenesis in algae and fungi. Annu. Rev. Plant Physiol. *15*:327-344.

272. Nickerson, W. J., and G. Falcone. 1963. Enzymatic reduction of selenite. J. Bacteriol. *85*:763-771.

273. Nickerson, W. J., and J. W. Williams. 1947. Nutrition and metabolism of pathogenic fungi. In W. J. Nickerson (Ed.), *Biology of the Pathogenic Fungi*, Chronica Botanica, Waltham, Mass., pp. 130-156.

274. Nickerson, W. J., W. A. Taber, and G. Falcone. 1956. Physiological bases of morphogenesis in fungi. 5. Effect of selenite and tellurite on cellular division of yeastlike fungi. Can. J. Microbiol. *2*:575-584.

275. Niederpruem, D. J. 1965. Carbohydrate metabolism. 2. Tricarboxylic acid cycle. In G. C. Ainsworth and A. S. Sussman (Eds.), *The Fungi. An Advanced Treatise*, Vol. 1, Academic, New York, pp. 269-300.

276. North, M. J. 1982. Comparative biochemistry of the proteinases of eucaryotic microorganisms. Microbiol. Rev. *46*:308-340.

277. Nurudeen, T. A., and D. G. Ahearn. 1979. Regulation of melanin production by *Cryptococcus neoformans*. J. Clin. Microbiol. *10*:724-729.

278. Oblack, D. L., J. C. Rhodes, and W. J. Martin. 1981. Clinical evaluation of the Automicrobic system yeast biochemical card for rapid identification of medically important yeasts. J. Clin. Microbiol. *13*:351-355.

279. Oblack, D., J. Schwarz, and I. A. Holder. 1980. In vivo muscle damage during *Candida* infection. Sabouraudia *18*:21-31.

280. Odds, F. C. 1979. *Candida and Candidosis*, University Park Press, Baltimore.

281. Odds, F. C., and A. B. Abbott. 1980. A simple system for the presumptive identification of *Candida albicans* and differentiation of strains within the species. Sabouraudia *18*:301-317.

282. Odds, F. C., and A. Trujillo-Gonzales. 1974. Acid phosphatase levels in the genus *Candida* and their application to the taxonomy and identification of pathogenic *Candida* species. Sabouradia *12*:287-294.

283. Odds, F. C., C. A. Hall, and A. B. Abbott. 1978. Peptones and mycological reproducibility. Sabouraudia *16*:237-246.

284. Ogundero, V. W. 1981. Nutritional physiology of pathogenic species of thermophilic *Mucor*. Sabouraudia *12*:287-294.

285. Olaiya, A. F., and S. J. Sogen. 1979. Ploidy determination of *Candida albicans*. J. Bacteriol. *140*:1043-1049.

286. Onions, A. H. S. 1971. Preservation of fungi. In C. Booth (Ed.), *Methods in Microbiology,* Vol. 4, Academic, New York, pp. 113-151.

287. Onions, A. H. S., H. O. W. Eggins, and D. Allsopp. 1982. *Smith's Introduction to Industrial Mycology,* 7th ed., Wiley, New York.

288. Orr, G. F. 1969. Keratinophilic fungi isolated from soil by a modified hair bait technique. Sabouraudia *7*:129-134.

289. Otto, V., and D. H. Howard. 1976. Further studies on the intracellular behavior of *Torulopsis glabrata*. Infect. Immun. *14*:433-438.

290. Owens, A. W., M. H. Shacklette, and R. D. Baker. 1965. An antifungal factor in human serum. I. Studies on *Rhizopus rhizopodiformis*. Sabouraudia *4*:179-186.

291. Padhye, A. A., M. R. McGinnis, and L. Ajello. 1978. Thermotolerance of *Wangiella dermatitidis*. J. Clin. Microbiol. *8*:424-426.

292. Padhye, A. A., C. N. Young, and L. Ajello. 1980. Hair performation as a diagnostic criterion in the identification of *Epidermophyton, Microsporum,* and *Trichophyton* species. In *Proceedings of the Fifth International Conference on the Mycoses,* Pan Am. Health Organ. Sci. Publ. No. 396, Washington, D.C., pp. 115-120.

293. Pagano, J., J. D. Levin, and W. Trejo. 1958. Diagnostic medium for differentiation of species of *Candida*. Antibiot. Annu. *1957-58*:137-143.

294. Pappagianis, D., and G. S. Kobayashi. 1960. Approaches to the physiology of *Coccidioides immitis*. Ann. N.Y. Acad. Sci. *89*:109-121.

295. Petri, R. J. 1887. Eine kleine Modification des Koch'schen Plattenverfahrens. Centralbl. Bakteriol. Parasitenkd. *1*:279-280. (see Ref. 51).

296. Phaff, H. J., and D. G. Ahearn. 1970. *Rhodotorula* (Harrison). In J. Lodder (Ed.), *The Yeasts. A Taxonomic Study,* North-Holland, Amsterdam, pp. 1187-1223.

297. Philpot, C. M. 1967. The differentiation of *Trichophyton mentagrophytes* from *T. rubrum* by a simple urease test. Sabouraudia *5*:189-193.

298. Philpot, C. M. 1977. The use of nutritional tests for the differentiation of dermatophytes. Sabouraudia *15*:141-150.

299. Pine, L. 1954. Studies on the growth of *Histoplasma capsulatum*. I. Growth of the yeast phase in liquid media. J. Bacteriol. *68*:671-679.

300. Pine, L. 1955. Studies on the growth of *Histoplasma capsulatum*. II. Growth of the yeast phase on agar media. J. Bacteriol. *70*:375-381.

301. Pine, L. 1962. Nutritional determinants of fungous morphology. In G. Dalldorf (Ed.), *Fungi and Fungous Diseases*, Thomas, Springfield, Ill., pp. 84-101.

302. Pine, L. 1972. Growth on amino acids, cell wall proteins, and hydrolysis of yeast phase cell walls of *Histoplasma capsulatum* and *Histoplasma duboisii*. Sabouraudia *10*:244-255.

303. Pine, L., and E. Drouhet. 1963. Sur l'obtention et la conservation de la phase levure d'*Histoplasma capsulatum* et d'*H. duboisii* en millieu chemiquement define. Ann. Inst. Pasteur (Paris) *105*:798-804.

304. Pine, L., and C. L. Peacock. 1958. Studies on the growth of *Histoplasma capsulatum*. IV. Factors influencing conversion of the mycelial phase to the yeast phase. J. Bacteriol. *75*:167-174.

305. Polacheck, I., and K. J. Kwon-Chung. 1980. Creatinine metabolism and *Cryptococcus neoformans* and *Cryptococcus bacillisporus*. J. Bacteriol. *142*:15-20.

306. Polacheck, I., V. J. Hearing, and K. J. Kwon-Chung. 1982. Biochemical studies of phenoloxidase and utilization of catecholamines in *Cryptococcus neoformans*. J. Bacteriol. *150*:1212-1220.

307. Polli, V. C., H. Diekmann, Z. Kis, and L. Ettlinger. 1965. Über das Vorkommen von keton reduktase bei Mikroorganismen. Pathol. Microbiol. *28*:93-98.

308. Poulter, R., K. Jeffery, M. J. Hubbard, M. G. Shepherd, and P. A. Sullivan. 1981. Parasexual genetic analysis of *Candida albicans* by spheroplast fusion. J. Bacteriol. *146*:833-840.

308a. Poulter, R., V. Hanrahan, K. Jeffery, D. Markie, M. G. Shepherd, and P. A. Sullivan. 1982. Recombination analysis of naturally diploid *Candida albicans*. J. Bacteriol. *152*:969-975.

309. Price, M. F., and R. A. Cawson. 1977. Phospholipase activity in *Candida albicans*. Sabouraudia *15*:179-186.

310. Pugh, D., and R. A. Cawson. 1975. The cytochemical localization of phospholipase a and lysophospholipase in *Candida albicans*. Sabouraudia *13*:110-115.

311. Pugh, D., and R. A. Cawson. 1977. The cytochemical localization of phospholipase in *Candida albicans* infecting the chick chorio-allantoic membrane. Sabouraudia *15*:29-35.

312. Purchio, A., C. R. Paula, and W. Gambale. 1979. Isolation of *Sporothrix schenckii*. Rev. Microbiol. *10*:69-71.

313. Purnell, D. M. 1973. The effect of specific auxotrophic mutations on the virulence of *Aspergillus nidulans* for mice. Mycopathol. Mycol. Appl. *50*:195-203.

314. Ramirez-Martinez, J. R. 1972. Growth and physiological characteristics of *Paracoccidioides brasiliensis*. In *Paracoccidioidomycosis*, Proceedings of the First Pan American Symposium, Pan Am. Health Organ. Sci. Publ. No. 254, Washington, D.C., pp. 13-20.

315. Raulin, J. 1869. Étude chemiques sur la végétation. Ann. Sci. Nat. Paris, Ser. 5, *11*:93-299. (as thesis in 1870).

316. Reca, M. E., and C. C. Campbell. 1967. Growth curves with the yeast phase of *Histoplasma capsulatum*. Sabouraudia *5*:267-277.

317. Redline, R. W., and B. B. Dahms. 1981. *Malessezia* pulmonary vasculitis in an infant on long-term intralipid therapy. N. Engl. J. Med. *305*:1395-1398.

318. Reiss, E., and W. J. Nickerson. 1974. Characterization of 2 melanins produced by *Phialophora verrucosa*. Sabouraudia *12*:193-201.

319. Reiss, E., and W. J. Nickerson. 1974. Control of dimorphism in *Phialophora verrucosa*. Sabouraudia *12*:202-213.

320. Reiss, F., and G. Szilagyi. 1967. The effect of mammalian and avian sera on the growth of *Cryptococcus neoformans*. J. Invest. Dermatol. *48*:264-265.

321. Reiss, F., G. Szilagyi, and F. Mayer. 1975. Immunological studies of the anti-cryptococcal factor of normal human serum. Mycopathologia *55*:175-178.

322. Remold, H., H. Fasold, and F. Staib. 1968. Purification and characterization of a proteolytic enzyme from *Candida albicans*. Biochim. Biophys. Acta *167*: 399-406.

323. Restrepo, A., B. E. Jiménez, and C. de Bedout. 1981. Survival of *Paracoccidioides brasiliensis* yeast cells under microacrophilic conditions. Sabouraudia *19*: 301-305.

324. Rhodes, J. C., and D. H. Howard. 1980. Isolation and characterization of arginine auxotrophs of *Cryptococcus neoformans*. Infect. Immun. *27*:910-914.

325. Rhodes, J. C., and G. D. Roberts. 1975. Comparison of four methods for determining nitrate utilization by cryptococci. J. Clin. Microbiol. *1*:9-10.

326. Rhodes, J. C., I. Polacheck, and K. J. Kwon-Chung. 1982. Polyphenol oxidase activity and virulence in isogenic strains of *Cryptococcus neoformans*. Infect. Immun. *36*:1175-1184.

327. Riggsby, W. S., L. J. Torres-Bauza, J. W. Wills, and T. M. Townes. 1982. DNA content, kinetic complexity, and the ploidy question in *Candida albicans*. Mol. Cell. Biol. *2*:853-862.

328. Rippon, J. W. 1967. Elastase: production by ringworm fungi. Science *157*: 947.

329. Rippon, J. W. 1968. Extracellular collagenases from *Trichophyton schoenleinii*. J. Bacteriol. *95*:43-46.

330. Rippon, J. W. 1968. Monitored environment system to control cell growth, morphology, and metabolic rates in fungi by oxidation-reduction potential. Appl. Microbiol. *16*:114-121.

331. Rippon, J. W. 1980. Dimorphism in pathogenic fungi. CRC Crit. Rev. Microbiol. *8*:49-97.

332. Rippon, J. W. 1982. *Medical Mycology,* Saunders, Philadelphia.

333. Rippon, J. W., and D. N. Anderson. 1970. Metabolic rate of fungi as a function of temperature and oxidation-reduction potential (EH). Mycopathol. Mycol. Appl. *40*:349-352.

334. Rippon, J. W., and L. J. LeBeau. 1965. Germination and initial growth of *Microsporon audouinii* from infected hairs. Mycopathol. Mycol. Appl. *26*:273-287.

335. Rippon, J. W., and D. P. Varadi. 1968. The elastases of pathogenic fungi and actinomycetes. J. Invest. Dermatol. *50*:54-58.

336. Robbins, W. J., and R. Ma. 1945. Growth factors of *Trichophyton mentagrophytes*. Am. J. Bot. *32*:509-523.

337. Robbins, W. J., J. E. Mackinnon, and R. Ma. 1942. Vitamin deficiencies of *Trichophyton discoides*. Bull. Torrey Bot. Club *69*:509-521.

338. Roberts, G. D., H. S. Wang, and G. E. Hollick. 1976. Evaluation of the API 20C microtube system for the identification of clinically important yeasts. J. Clin. Microbiol. *3*:302-305.

339. Roberts, J. A., J. M. Counts, and H. G. Crecelius. 1970. Production in vitro of *Coccidioides immitis* spherules and endospores as a diagnostic aid. Am. Rev. Respir. Dis. *102*:811-813.

340. Roberts, R. L., and P. J. Szaniszlo. 1980. Temperature-sensitive multicellular mutants of *Wangiella dermatitidis*. J. Bacteriol. *135*:622-632.

341. Roberts, R. L., and P. J. Szaniszlo. 1980. Yeast-phase cell cycle of the polymorphic fungus *Wangiella dermatitidis*. J. Bacteriol. *144*:721-731.

342. Roessler, W. G., E. J. Herbst, W. G. McCullough, R. C. Mills, and C. R. Brewer. 1946. Studies with *Coccidioides immitis*. I. Submerged growth in liquid mediums. J. Infect. Dis. *79*:12-26.

343. Romano, A. H. 1966. Dimorphism. In G. C. Ainsworth and A. S. Sussman (Eds.), *The Fungi. An Advanced Treatise*, Vol. 2, Academic, New York, pp. 181-209.

344. Rosenthal, S. A., and H. Sokolsky. 1965. Enzymatic studies with pathogenic fungi. Dermatol. Int. *4*:72-79.

345. Roth, F. J., Jr., and M. I. Goldstein. 1961. Inhibition of growth of pathogenic yeasts by human serum. J. Invest. Dermatol. *36*:383-387.

346. Roth, F. J., Jr., C. C. Boyd, S. Sagami, and H. Blank. 1959. An evaluation of the fungistatic activity of serum. J. Invest. Dermatol. *32*:549-555.

347. Rowley, D. A., and M. Huber. 1955. Pathogenesis of experimental histoplasmosis in mice. I. Measurement of infecting dosages of the yeast phase of *Histoplasma capsulatum*. J. Infect. Dis. *96*:174-183.

348. Roy, I., and J. W. Landau. 1971. Polymorphism of malate dehydrogenase in cytoplasmic and mitochondrial fractions of *Blastomyces dermatitidis*. Sabouraudia *9*:39-42.

349. Rüchel, R., R. Tegeler, and M. Trost. 1982. A comparison of secretory proteinases from different strains of *Candida albicans*. Sabouraudia *20*:233-244.

350. Sabouraud, R. 1908. Milieux de culture des champignons dermatophytes (Technique de fabrication des géloses sucries dites: Milieux d'épreuve). Ann. Dermatol. Syphiligr. IV, *9*:99-101.

351. Salkin, I. F. 1975. Adaptation to cycloheximide: *In vitro* studies with filamentous fungi. Can. J. Microbiol. *21*:1413-1419.

352. Salkin, I. F., and N. J. Hurd. 1982. New medium for differentiation of *Cryptococcus neoformans* serotype pairs. J. Clin. Microbiol. *15*:169-171.

353. Salomonsen, C. J. 1876. Zur Isolation differenter Bacterienformen. Bot. Ztg. *34*:609-622.

354. Salvin, S. B. 1947. Cultural studies on the yeastlike phase of *Histoplasma capsulatum* Darling. J. Bacteriol. *54*:655-660.

355. Salvin, S. B. 1947. Multiple budding in *Sporotrichum schenckii* Matruchot. J. Invest. Dermatol. *9*:315-320.

356. Salvin, S. B. 1949. Cysteine and related compounds in the growth of the yeastlike phase of *Histoplasma capsulatum*. J. Infect. Dis. *84*:275-283.

357. Salvin, S. B. 1949. Phase determining factors in *Blastomyces dermatitidis*. Mycologia *43*:311-319.

358. Salvin, S. B. 1962. Hemolysin from the yeastlike phases of some pathogenic fungi. Proc. Soc. Exp. Biol. Med. *76*:852-854.

359. San-Blas, F., and L. J. Cova. 1975. Growth curves of the yeast-like form of *Paracoccidioides brasiliensis*. Sabouraudia *13*:22-29.

360. San-Blas, F., G. San-Blas, and L. Yarzàbal. 1981. A mycelial mutant of *Paracoccidioides brasiliensis* defective in dimorphism: chemical and immunological characterization. Exp. Mycol. *5*:23-34.

361. Sanger, V. K., J. M. Cortes, and L. W. Self. 1975. Acid phosphatase production as an aid in rapid characterization of *Candida* species. Am. J. Med. Technol. *41*:327-332.

362. Sarachek, A. 1977. Ergosterol-enhanced recovery of mutagen treated *Candida albicans*. Z. Allg. Mikrobiol. *17*:481-485.

363. Sarachek, A., and J. T. Bish. 1976. Effects of growth, temperature, and caffeine on genetic responses of *Candida albicans* to ethyl methanesulfonate, nitrous acid and ultraviolet radiation. Mycopathologia *60*:51-56.

364. Sarachek, A., and J. A. Brammer. 1976. Differentiation of pathogenic species of *Candida* by their recovery characteristics following UV-irradiation. Antonie Leeuwenhoek J. Microbiol. Serol. *42*:165-180.

365. Sarachek, A., D. D. Rhoads, and R. H. Schwarzhoff. 1981. Hybridization of *Candida albicans* through fusion of protoplasts. Arch. Microbiol. *129*:1-8.

366. Scherr, G. H. 1957. Studies on the dimorphism of *Histoplasma capsulatum*. Exp. Cell Res. *12*:92-107.

367. Schønheyder, H., and A. Stenderup. 1982. Isolation of *Cryptococcus neoformans* from pigeon manure on two media inducing pigment formation. Sabouraudia *20*:193-197.

368. Schwartz, D., and F. Staib. 1980. Effect of purines on the formation of the perfect state of *Cryptococcus neoformans, Filobasidiella neoformans*. Zentralbl. Bakteriol. Parasitenkd. Infektionskr. Hyg., Abt. I: Orig. *248*:274-280.

369. Scott, W. W., and C. O. Warren, Jr. 1964. *Studies on the Host Range and Chemical Control of Fungi Associated With Diseased Tropical Fish*, Technical Bulletin No. 171, Virginia Agricultural Experimental Station, Blacksburg, Virginia.

370. Seeliger, H. P. R. 1956. Use of a urease test for the screening and identification of cryptococci. J. Bacteriol. *72*:127-131.

371. Segal, E., and L. Ajello. 1976. Evaluation of a new system for the rapid identification of clinically important fungi. J. Clin. Microbiol. *4*:157-159.

372. Sekhon, A. S., A. A. Padhye, and J. W. Carmichael. 1974. Disc-gel electrophoresis of + and − strains and of gymnothecial cultures of *Arthroderma tuberculatum*. Sabouraudia *12*:12-17.

373. Shadomy, H. J., and C. M. Philpot. 1979. Utilization of standard laboratory methods in the laboratory diagnosis of problem dermatophytes. Am. J. Clin. Pathol. *74*:197-201.

374. Shaw, E. 1953. Antimetabolites. A review. Metabolism *2*:103-119.

375. Shearer, G., J. C. Hubbard, and H. W. Larsh. 1980. Non-specific incorporation of nucleic acid precursors in *Blastomyces dermatitidis* and *Histoplasma capsulatum*. Mycopathologia *72*:111-119.

376. Shepherd, M. G., C. M. Chin, and P. A. Sullivan. 1978. The alternate respiratory pathway of *Candida albicans*. Arch. Microbiol. *116*:61-67.

377. Shields, A. B., and L. Ajello. 1966. Medium for selective isolation of *Cryptococcus neoformans*. Science *151*:208-209.

378. Shiraishi, A., and T. Arai. 1979. Antifungal activity of transferrin. Sabouraudia *17*:79-83.

379. Shive, W. 1952. Biological activities of metabolite analogues. Annu. Rev. Microbiol. *6*:437-466.

380. Shorer, J., I. Zelmanowicz, and I. Barash. 1972. Utilization and metabolism of urea during spore germination by *Geotrichum candidum*. Phytochemistry *11*:595-605.

381. Silva, M. 1958. The effect of amino acids on the growth and sporulation of *Trichophyton rubrum*: Possible application to diagnosis and therapy. J. Invest. Dermatol. *30*:69-76.

382. Skinner, C. E., C. W. Emmons, and H. M. Tsuchiya. 1947. *Henrici's Molds, Yeasts, and Actinomycetes*, 2nd ed., Wiley, New York.

383. Smith, C. D. 1971. Nutritional factors that are required for growth and sporulation of *Histoplasma capsulatum*. In L. Ajello, E. W. Chick, and M. L. Furcolow (Eds.), *Histoplasmosis*, Proceedings of the Second National Conference, Thomas, Springfield, Ill., pp. 64-77.

384. Smith, C. D., and M. L. Furcolow. 1964. The demonstration of growth stimulating substances for *Histoplasma capsulatum* and *Blastomyces dermatitidis* in infusions of Starlings's (*Sturnis vulgaris*) manure. Mycopathol. Mycol. Appl. *22*:73-80.

385. Smith, C. E., E. G. Whiting, E. E. Baker, H. G. Rosenberger, R. R. Beard, and M. T. Saito. 1948. The use of coccidioidin. Am. Rev. Tuberc. *57*:330-360.

386. Smith, G. 1938. *An Introduction to Industrial Mycology*, Edward Arnold & Co., London.

387. Smith, J. E., and D. R. Berry (Eds.). 1975, 1976, and 1978. *The Filamentous Fungi*, Vol. 1, 2, 3, Wiley, New York.

388. Smith, R. F., D. Blasi, and S. L. Dayton. 1973. Phosphatase activity among *Candida* species and other yeasts isolated from clinical material. Appl. Microbiol. *26*:364-367.

389. Soll, D. R., G. W. Bedell, and M. Brummel. 1981. Zinc and the regulation of growth and phenotype in the infectious yeast *Candida albicans*. Infect. Immun. *32*:1139-1147.

390. Staib, F. 1962. *Cryptococcus neoformans* and *Guizotia abyssinica* (syn. *G. oleifera* D.C.) Farbenreaktion für *Cryptococcus neoformans*. Z. Hyg. Infektionskr. *148*:466-475.

391. Staib, F. 1962. Vogelkot, ein Nähsubstrate für die Gattung *Cryptococcus*. Zentralbl. Bakteriol. Parasitenkd. Infektionskr. Hyg., Abt. 1:Orig. *186*:233-247.

392. Staib, F. 1964. Das Serum-Reststickstoff-Auxanogramm (mit Sprossund Schimmelpilzen). Zentralbl. Bakteriol. Parasitenkd. Infektionskr. Hyg., Abt. 1: Orig. *194*:379-406.

393. Staib, F. 1965. Serum-proteins as nitrogen source for yeastlike fungi. Sabouraudia *4*:187-193.

394. Staib, F. 1969. Proteolysis and pathogenicity of *Candida albicans* strains. Mycopathol. Mycol. Appl. *37*:345-348.

395. Staib, F., and A. Blisse. 1974. Stellungnahme zu *Sporothrix schenckii* var. *luriei*. Ein Beitrag zum diagnostischen Wert der Assimilation von Kreatinin, Kreatin und Guanidinoessigsäure durch *Sporothrix schenckii*. Zentralbl. Bakteriol. Parasitenkd. Infektionskr. Hyg., Abt. I: Orig. *229*:261-263.

396. Staib, F., and A. Blisse. 1982. Bird manure filtrate agar for the formation of the perfect state of *Cryptococcus neoformans*, *Filobasidiella neoformans*. Zentralbl. Bakteriol. Parasitenkd. Infektionskr. Hyg., Abt. I: Orig. *251*:554-562.

397. Staib, F., A. Blisse, and H. S. Randhawa. 1972. Creatine and creatinine assimilation by *Sporothrix schenckii*. Zentralbl. Bakteriol. Parasitenkd. Infektionskr. Hyg., Abt. I: Orig. *221*:94-99.

398. Staib, F., S. K. Mishra, T. Abel, and A. Blisse. 1976. Growth of *Cryptococcus neoformans* on uric acid agar. Zentralbl. Bakteriol. Parasitenkd. Infektionskr. Hyg., Abt. I: Orig. *236*:374-385.

399. Stanier, R. Y., M. Doudoroff, and E. A. Adelberg. 1970. *The Microbial World*, Prentice-Hall, Englewood Cliffs, New Jersey.

400. Stetler, D. A., and G. Boguslawski. 1979. Cysteine biosynthesis in a fungus *Histoplasma capsulatum*. Sabouraudia *17*:23-34.

401. Stetler, D. A., G. Boguslawski, and C. J. Decedue. 1978. Effect of elevated temperature on growth and ribonucleic acid synthesis in *Cryptococcus albidus*. J. Gen. Microbiol. *106*:67-72.

402. Stewart, P. R., and P. J. Rogers. 1978. Fungal dimorphism: a particular expression of cell wall morphogenesis. In J. E. Smith and D. R. Berry (Eds.), *The Filamentous Fungi*, Vol. 3, Wiley, New York, pp. 164-196.

403. Stewart, R. A., and K. F. Meyer. 1932. Isolation of *Coccidioides immitis* (Stiles) from soil. Proc. Soc. Exp. Biol. Med. *29*:937-938.

404. Stewart, R. A., and K. F. Meyer. 1938. Studies in the metabolism of *Coccidioides immitis*. J. Infect. Dis. *63*:196-205.

405. Stier, T. J. B., R. C. Scalf, and M. C. Brockman. 1950. An all-glass apparatus for the continuous cultivation of yeasts under anaerobic conditions. J. Bacteriol. *59*:45-49.

406. Stockdale, P. M. 1968. Sexual stimulation between *Arthroderma simii* Stockd., Mackenzie & Austwick and related species. Sabouraudia *6*:176-181.

407. Stockdale, P. M. 1981. Sexual stimulation between *Arthroderma simii* and other dermatophytes. In R. Vanbreuseghem and C. DeVroey (Eds.), *Sexuality and Pathogenicity of Fungi,* Masson, Paris.

408. Stotsky, G., and R. D. Goos. 1965. Effect of high CO_2 and low O_2 tensions on the soil microbiota. Can. J. Microbiol. *11*:853-868.

409. Summers, D. F., and H. F. Hasenclever. 1964. In vitro inhibition of yeast growth by mouse ascites fluid and serum. J. Bacteriol. *87*:1-7.

410. Sun, S. H., and M. Huppert. 1976. A cytological study of morphogenesis in *Coccidioides immitis.* Sabouraudia *14*:185-198.

411. Sutcliffe, M. C., A. M. Savage, and R. H. Alford. 1980. Transferrin-dependent growth inhibition of yeast-phase *Histoplasma capsulatum* by human serum and lymph. J. Infect. Dis. *142*:209-219.

412. Suzuki, T., S. Nishibayashi, T. Kuroiwa, T. Kanbe, and K. Tanaka. Variance of ploidy in *Candida albicans.* J. Bacteriol. *152*:893-896.

413. Swartz, H. E., and L. K. Georg. 1955. The nutrition of *Trichophyton tonsurans.* Mycologia *47*:475-493.

414. Szawatkowski, M., and J. M. T. Hamilton. 1977. Anaerobic growth and sensitivity of *Candida albicans.* Microbios Lett. *5*:61-66.

415. Szilvingi, A., and U. Rosenkrantz. 1961. Radiation effects on yeast of the genus *Candida* Berkhout. Nature (Lond.) *190*:1212-1213.

416. Tabak, H. H., and W. B. Cooke. 1968. Growth and metabolism of fungi in an atmosphere of nitrogen. Mycologia *60*:115-140.

417. Takiuchi, I., D. Higuchi, Y. Sei, and M. Koga. 1982. Isolation of an extracellular proteinase (keratinase) from *Microsporum canis.* Sabouraudia *20*:281-288.

418. Tan, K. K. 1976. Light-induced fungal development. In J. E. Smith and D. R. Berry (Eds.), *The Filamentous Fungi,* Vol. 3, Wiley, New York, pp. 334-357.

419. Tang, S. L., and D. H. Howard. 1973. Metabolism macromolecular synthesis and nuclear behavior of *Cryptococcus albidus* at 37°C. J. Bacteriol. *115*:574-581.

420. Tanner, F. W., and E. Ryder. 1923. Action of ultraviolet light on yeast like fungi. Bot. Gaz. *75*:309-317.

421. Tate, P. 1929. On enzymes of certain dermatophyte or ringworm fungi. Parasitology *21*:31-54.

422. Taylor, J. J. 1962. Demonstration and possible significance of uricase in human pathogenic fungi. Nature (Lond.) *194*:403-404.

423. Titsworth, E. H., and E. Grunberg. 1950. A medium for the growth and maintenance of the yeast-like phase of *Histoplasma capsulatum.* Mycologia *42*:298-300.

424. Tran Van Ky, P., J. Biguet, and T. Vaucelle. 1968. Étude d'une fraction antigénique d'*Aspergillus fumigatus* support d'une activité catalasique. Consequence sur le diagnostic immunologique de l'Aspergillose. Rev. Immunol. (Paris) *32*:37-52.

425. Vanbreuseghem, R. 1952. Keratin digestion by dermatophytes: A specific diagnostic method. Mycologia *44*:176-182.

426. Vanbreuseghem, R. 1952. Technique biologique pour l'isolement des dermatophytes der sol. Ann. Soc. Belge Med. Trop. *32*:173-178.

427. Vanbreuseghem, R., and J. Eugene. 1958. Culture d'*Histoplasma capsulatum* et d'*Histoplasma duboisii* sur un milieu à base de terre et de matières fécales provenant de divers animaux. C. R. Soc. Biol. *152*:1602-1605.

428. Vandervliet, G. 1971. *Microbiology and the Spontaneous Generation Debate During the 1870's,* Coronado Press, Lawrence, Kans.

429. Vandevelde, A. G., A. A. Mauceri, and J. E. Johnson, III. 1972. 5-fluorocytos-ine in the treatment of mycotic infections. Ann. Intern. Med. *77*:43-53.

430. Vaughn, V. J., and E. D. Weinberg. 1978. *Candida albicans* dimorphism and virulence: Role of copper. Mycopathologia *64*:39-42.

431. Verujsky, D. 1887. Recherches sur la morphologie et la biologie du *Trich-ophyton tonsurans* et de'l'*Achorion schoenlienii.* Ann. Inst. Pasteur *1*:369-391.

432. Waksman, S. A. 1922. A method for counting the number of fungi in the soil. J. Bacteriol. *7*:339-341.

433. Walch, H. A., Jr., and R. K. Walch. 1967. Studies with induced mutants of *Coccidioides immitis.* In L. Ajello (Ed.), *Coccidioidomycosis,* Papers from the Second Symposium on Coccidioidomycosis, University of Arizona Press, Tucson, pp. 339-347.

434. Walker, J. 1958. Effect of ultraviolet irradiation on the spores of *Trichophyton sulfureum.* Arch. Dermatol. *78*:153-156.

435. Weidman, F. D. 1928. Comparison of ringworm culture ingredients. II. The nitrogen factor. Arch. Dermatol. Syphilol. *18*:829-837.

436. Weidman, F. D., and T. M. Macmillan. 1921. A comparison of ingredients of ringworm culture mediums with special reference to American and French crude maltose. Arch. Dermatol. Syphilol. *4*:451-468.

437. Weidman, F. D., and D. Spring. 1928. Comparison of ringworm culture ingred-ients. III. Grütz, Goldschmitt, Sabouraud (honey modification), Sabouraud's glycerin and certain synthetic mediums. Arch. Dermatol. Syphilol. *18*:837-850.

438. Weigl, E. 1980. Conditioned pathogenicity of *Microsporum gypseum* bio-chemical mutants. Mycopathologia *70*:3-8.

439. Weigl, E., M. Hejtmánek, N. Hejtmankova, J. Kunnert, and K. Lenhart. 1975. Biochemical mutants of *Trichophyton mentagrophytes.* Acta Univ. Palacki Olomuc. Fac. Med. *74*:69-82.

440. Weinberg, E. D. 1974. Iron and susceptibility to infectious diseases. Science *184*:952-956.

441. Whelan, W. L., and P. T. Magee. 1981. Natural heterozygosity in *Candida albicans.* J. Bacteriol. *145*:896-903.

442. Whelan, W. L., R. M. Partridge, and P. T. Magee. 1980. Heterozygosity and segregation in *Candida albicans.* Mol. Gen. Genet. *180*:107-113.

443. Wickerham, L. J. 1981. *Taxonomy of Yeasts,* Tech. Bull. No. 1029, U.S. Dept. Agriculture, Washington, D.C.

444. Widra, A. 1964. Phosphate directed Y-M variation in *Candida albicans.* Myco-pathol. Mycol. Appl. *23*:197-202.

445. Wildiers, E. 1901. Nouvelle substance indispensable au développement de la levure. La Cellule *18*:313-332.

446. Winogradsky, S. 1890. Sur les organismes de la nitrification. C. R. Acad. Sci. (Paris). *110*:1013-1016.

447. Yamaguchi, H. 1974. Dimorphism in *Candida albicans.* I. Morphology-dependent changes in cellular content of macromolecules and respiratory activity. J. Gen. Appl. Microbiol. *20*:87-99.

448. Yamaguchi, H. 1975. Control of dimorphism in *Candida albicans* by zinc: Effect on cell morphology and composition. J. Gen. Microbiol. *86*:370-372.

449. Yarzàbal, L. A., S. Andrieu, D. Bout, and F. Naquira. 1976. Isolation of a specific antigen with alkaline phosphatase activity from soluble extracts of *Paracoccidioides brasiliensis.* Sabouraudia *14*:275-280.

450. Yu, R. J., S. R. Harmon, S. F. Grappel, and F. Blank. 1971. Two cell-bound keratinases of *Trichophyton mentagrophytes.* J. Invest. Dermatol. *56*:27-32.

451. Zaikina, N. A., and N. P. Elinov. 1968. Fungal plasmocoagulase. Mycopathol. Mycol. Appl. *35*:10-16.

452. Zellner, J. 1907. Chemie der höreren Pilze. Eine Monographie, Leipzig.
453. Zopf, W. 1890. *Die Pilze in morphologischer, physiologischer, und systematischer Beziehung,* Breslau.
454. Zwadyk, P., Jr., R. A. Tarlton, and A. Proctor. 1977. Evaluation of the AP1 20C for identification of yeasts. Am. J. Clin. Pathol. *67:*269-271.

2

Cell Wall Composition

Errol Reiss / Centers for Disease Control, Atlanta, Georgia

I. INTRODUCTION

The protoplasts of filamentous and yeast-like fungi are encased in a rigid, laminated, largely polysaccharide protective covering that reinforces the cylindrical or ellipsoidal shape of the cells. This cell wall is plasticized at the tips of growing hyphae and at the radius of maximum curvature in yeasts that undergo multipolar budding. Thus, fungi demonstrate the phenomenon of apical growth. Changes in the cell shape are often reflected in changes in the cell wall composition. The fundamental observations of (1) apical growth, (2) the wall as a determinant of shape, and (3) the corollary that morphogenesis is reflected in the mural composition of the cell wall were introduced to me in the laboratory of Walter J. Nickerson, and continue to influence current thought about the fungal cell wall [122].

The perspective conveyed in this chapter is to view the structure of the wall as a surface that the host recognizes as a foreign antigenic complex. If the wall is sufficiently porous, it can be penetrated by oxidative and nonoxidative fungicidal mechanisms which then act on the plasmalemma. On the other hand, it may be necessary for the host phagocytes to grapple with the wall itself, in an attempt to degrade the slimy outer coat and the inner fibrillar and more chemically inert mural layers. We are still far from understanding the host-fungus interaction, but knowledge of the molecular organization of the cell wall can help to attain this goal.

Reviews of various aspects of the fungal cell wall appear with increasing frequency. The important subject of mannan has been addressed both structurally [8] and in terms of its genetics [9]. Frequent revisions of our concept of the antigenic structure of yeast mannans have been necessary [128,166]. The diversity of mannose-based heteroglycans is recognized as a general property of them [58], and specific examples of that diversity are seen among the pathogenic fungi [154] and in the intricate complexity of a model lipopeptidophosphogalactomannan [59,60]. The structure and localization of yeast glucans and chitin are becoming well-understood [6,30,112]. Chitin is of particular interest because of its role in conferring strength, in assisting in orderly cell division [17,78,79,84], and as a potential target for specific drugs [62]. An array of glycanases has been classified and their action patterns discussed in relation to enzymatic cell wall degradation [133]. The compendium of analyses of carbohydrate and amino acid composition of fungal cell walls has reached a considerable size [14]. More general approaches are evident in monographs directed toward cell wall biosynthesis [54], morphogenesis [163], and composition [150].

The fundamental differences between bacterial and fungal cell walls are important in understanding the phagocyte-fungus interaction, in developing chemotherapeutic strategy, and in delineating the antigenic mosaic. Fungi lack peptidoglycan (muramic acid-glucosaminyl polymer cross-linked by peptide bridges), glycerol or ribitol teichoic acids, and the lipopolysaccharide endotoxin class of macromolecules. As a result, fungi are resistant to antibacterial agents like penicillin that interfere with bacterial cell wall synthesis. In place of these procaryotic wall structures, fungi have outer layers of readily soluble peptidomannans embedded in a matrix of α- and β-glucans. Structural rigidity is increased by crystalline chitin fibrils arrayed as rings or disks in the bud scars of yeast forms and as a thin microcrystalline sleeve, interwoven with glucan fibrils, that covers the lateral walls of mycelial forms. Chitin antagonists like polyoxin D can exert a static or cidal effect on fungi. Chitin is important in the budding process because it provides a channel for the nucleus to migrate into the daughter cell. Not all genera of zoopathogenic fungi have an identical macromolecular construction and such taxonomic considerations are discussed below.

II. PEPTIDOMANNANS

The peptidomannans are a family of mannose-based polymers that form the readily soluble outer layers of the cell wall. They are either homopolymers of mannose or heteroglycans with α-D-mannan backbones. Peptidomannans are the major mural antigens that determine serotypes. Serological cross-reactions occur to a moderate extent among pathogenic fungi, but in many genera there are substituents that confer a good degree of specificity. Three general plans for fungal mannan can be recognized: mural, capsular, and secreted.

A. Mural

Most mannans are embedded in the glucan-chitin wall matrix and are major structural elements. In this type, α-1,6-linked mannan backbones predominate with side chains 2-5 sugar residues in length. Structural analyses by Ballou's group on the mannans of *Saccharomyces cerevisiae* have resulted in the structure proposed in Fig. 1 [8,9] which serves as a model for the mannan of *Candida* species. Sequences of α-1,6-mannan are joined by glycopeptide bonds to structural protein. The mannan is organized into an inner core, outer chain, and base-labile oligomannosides. Antigenic specificity is determined by the outer-chain region consisting of three or four repeating blocks of linear α-1,6-mannan substituted with oligomannosides having a degree of polymerization (d.p.) of one to four. *Candida albicans* mannan has longer side chains; mannopentaose and mannohexaose are encountered. The predominant linkage in the side chains is α-1,2- with α-1,3- residues disposed as nonreducing termini. Other substituents have been described in the outer-chain region, e.g., phosphodiester-mannose and *N*-acetylglucosamine (GlcNAc) [8]. The inner-core region connects the α-1,6-mannan to protein via an *N,N'*-diacetylchitobiosyl-asparagine glycopeptide bond. Yeast mannan shares this initiation sequence with mammalian glycoproteins [175]. Alkali-labile oligomannosides are joined to the structural protein via hydroxyamino-acid ester bonds between mannose residues and serine or threonine of the peptide moiety. The observed molecular weight of mannans depends on the method of preparation. The use of Fehling solution [132] results in some alkaline degradation and a molecular weight of about 40,000, whereas complexing with borate-cetyltrimethylammonium bromide (CTAB) preserves a higher molecular weight species of 133,000 [121]. Mannan prepared by the method of Peat et al. [132] is serologically active and the serotype specificity of *C. albicans* mannan is preserved [164], but it is not immunogenic in depot injections with complete Freund's adjuvant [106]. Anti-mannan IgG can be induced more easily by injection of soluble peptidoglucomannan, which is extracted with cold alkali from isolated cell walls [106,143]. The higher antibody-precipitating activity of bakers' yeast mannan prepared by the CTAB method as compared with that obtained by Fehling precipitation has been attributed to β-1,3-mannobiosyl and mannosyl phosphodiesters [129]. The mannan isolated with Fehling solution in which acid is used to dissociate the Cu(II)-mannan complex is therefore a degradation product that has lost alkali-labile and acid-labile oligomannosyl residues. The same interpretation may hold for the mannan of *C. albicans*, which is more highly phosphorylated than bakers' yeast [68].

B. Capsular

This type of mannan is restricted to a single genus of the pathogenic fungi, *Cryptococcus*, representing the genetically compatible A and D serotypes (*C. neoformans* var.

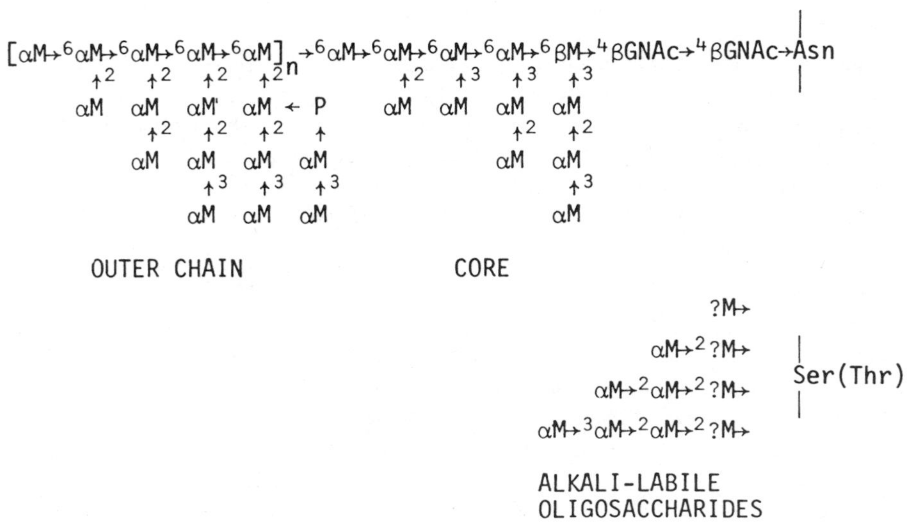

$$[\alpha M \xrightarrow{6} \alpha M \xrightarrow{6} \alpha M \xrightarrow{6} \alpha M \xrightarrow{6} \alpha M]_n \xrightarrow{6} \alpha M \xrightarrow{6} \alpha M \xrightarrow{6} \alpha M \xrightarrow{6} \alpha M \xrightarrow{6} \beta M \xrightarrow{4} \beta GNAc \xrightarrow{4} \beta GNAc \rightarrow Asn$$

Structure continued (outer chain and core branches):

OUTER CHAIN   CORE

Alkali-labile oligosaccharides:

?M→
αM→²?M→
αM→²αM→²?M→   Ser(Thr)
αM→³αM→²αM→²?M→

ALKALI-LABILE
OLIGOSACCHARIDES

Figure 1 Structure of bakers' yeast mannan (*Saccharomyces cerevisiae* X2180) according to Ballou (From Ref. 9).

neoformans) and the B and C serotypes (*C. neoformans* var. *gattii*) [102]. The serotypes are based on agglutinin adsorption [53,180] and by immunofluorescent cross-staining and adsorptions [91]. There has been concern about the serotyping of *C. neoformans*, especially of serotypes A and D. Bennett has serotyped some clinical isolates as "AD," and Bhattacharjee et al. [21] reported the isolation of D clones from a culture originally thought to represent only A. Serotypic determinants are considered to reside in the capsular polysaccharide, but thus far structural analyses have not yielded definitive information about type-specific epitopes. Capsule diameters vary, depending on the isolate, from barely detectable to greater than 4 μm. The capsular polysaccharide is a viscous glucuronoxylomannan of high molecular weight, measured by gel permeation chromatography as 7×10^5 to 8×10^5 [18,20]. The heteroglycan consists of linear α-1,3-mannan backbone singly substituted with β-1,2-glucuronosyl or β-1,4-xylosyl residues. The ratio of xylose:mannose:glucuronic acid varies according to the serotype (Table 1). In serotypes B and C, the mannose residues in the backbone are all trisubstituted and some are tetrasubstituted with xylosyl at O-2, O-4, and glucuronosyl at O-2 [19]. Serotypes A and D have some unbranched mannosyl residues and no tetrasubstituted ones. A significant O-acetyl content occurs in these mannans that contributes to their antigenicity [35,63], but the sites of the O-acetylation have not been identified. The presence of galactose in preparations of the major viscous acidic glucuronoxylomannan is an artifact resulting from contamination with another secreted heteroglycan, galactoxylomannan [36].

C. Secreted

Some mannans appear to occur in equilibrium between the plasma membrane and the extracellular milieu. Such a polysaccharide is not considered a major structural com-

Table 1   Composition of the Glucuronoxylomannans of the Four Serotypes of
Cryptococcus neoformans

| Serotype | Carbohydrates[a] | | | O-Acetyl (%) | Reference |
	Xyl	Man (Molar ratios)	GlcUA		
A	2	3	1	n.d.[b]	114
A	2	5	1	6.5	35
B	3	3	1	10.5	20
C	4	3	1	3.0	19
D	1	3	1	10.3	18

[a]Xyl, xylose; Man, mannose; GlcUA, glucuronic acid.
[b]n.d., not determined.

ponent of the wall. An example of this type is the peptidophosphogalactomannan
(PPGM) of *Penicillium charlesii* [59]. The galactoxylomannan of *C. neoformans* may
also belong in this category [36]. The PPGM secreted into the growth medium is at
first of high molecular weight (68,000) and has a high galactose content (69.9%).
Later, as the culture ages, the weight of the PPGM declines by two-thirds and only 12%
galactose is present. The decline is due to the action of exo-β-galactofuranosidase on
the polymer. The heteroglycan is composed of linear 1,6-linked mannose residues
with linear 1,2-mannosyl side chains and major side chains of 1,4-linked galactofuranosides. The proposed functions for this mannan are: (1) the carbohydrate is a portion
of a glycoenzyme that fastens the enzyme to the cell wall; (2) the carbohydrate
component is amphipathic containing ethanolamine and it reacts with charged groups
in the plasma membrane anchoring enzymes in the region between the plasma membrane and the cell wall [59]; and (3) the carbohydrate serves as a safe-conduct pass
by protecting mural enzymes from premature proteolysis while they travel from the
ribosome to the plasmalemma [59]. This protection may continue once the enzyme
is situated in the periplasmic space. These polymers are reminiscent of the lightly and
heavily galactosylated mannans that have been characterized for *Trichophyton
mentagrophytes* [23,24].

III. GLUCANS

Glucans are a major mural constituent of fungi. Among the zoopathogenic species, the
glucans are α-1,3-, β-1,3-, or β-1,6-glucosyl polymers. To the extent that they occur
as linear sequences, the 1,3-glucans associate to form fibrils that increase the strength of
the wall. But none of these glucans is completely unbranched, and as the percent of
branching increases, opportunities for helical formations are reduced. There is a close
association of glucan and chitin as an insoluble matrix in the mycelial forms [117, 162].
Linkages between insoluble glucan and chitin are known in the basidiomycete *Schizo-
phyllum commune* [160]. The glucan becomes soluble after digestion of the associated

chitin with chitinase from *Streptomyces tatsumaensis*. The residue after chitinase digestion is enriched in lysine and citrulline, accounting for 80% of the total amino acid content. These same amino acids are detected after the glucan-chitin matrix is digested with β-1,3-glucanase. Bridges between glucan chains and chitin contain lysine and citrulline connected to the chitin moiety by glycosylamine bonds. Much of the structural analysis of glucans has been accomplished with the saprophytes and these serve as models until more definitive work on the pathogens is available.

Glucan cannot be released from whole *Saccharomyces cerevisiae* with hot dilute alkali because alkali-resistant β-1,6-glucan is a superficial layer that acts as a filter to block passage of the β-1,3-glucan. Preparation of isolated cell walls is thus justified not only to account for the mural constituents, but is required for the extraction of β-1,3-glucan. A three-stage extraction is used for β-glucan preparation. Isolated walls are extracted with hot dilute alkali to solubilize the major β-1,3-glucan, then the alkali-resistant residue is treated with hot dilute acetic acid to liberate a mainly β-1,6-glucan, which is a minor component of the wall dry weight [6,30]. Exposure of the acid-resistant residue to alkali results in a further release of β-1,3-glucan. The β-1,3-glucan of *S. cerevisiae* contains 3-4% of branching through C-6 [6]. This is a point that is important in understanding the extent to which this glucan can associate into fibrils. Known standards of linear β-1,3-glucan, i.e., paramylon of Euglenophytes, are fibrillar and the long, unbranched β-1,3-sequences associate in a hydrated triple helix [112]. X-ray diffraction patterns that are very similar to the one observed with paramylon are found with acid-treated cell walls of *S. cerevisiae* and of the basidiomycete *Armillaria mellea* [81]. In spite of the branching that occurs in *S. cerevisiae*, glucan microfibrils are distributed over the surface of yeast walls in (1) shadowed wall fragments, (2) next to the plasmalemma in freeze-etched samples, and (3) during regeneration of protoplasts [6]. The sharpening of X-ray diffraction patterns that is obtained after hot dilute acid treatment is explained by the unmasking of β-1,3-glucan fibrils by solubilization of β-1,6-glucan, but more important, acid treatment cleaves branching points by hydrolysis, resulting in freedom of β-1,3-glucan chains to crystallize [81]. Glucan fibrils in native walls are thin, densely woven, and have a low order of crystallinity [6].

A. *Saccharomyces cerevisiae* and *Candida albicans*

Glucan accounts for 47% of the dry weight of *C. albicans* yeast-form cell walls [32]. Structural analysis of glucan solubilized from whole *C. albicans* serotype-B yeast with boiling dilute alkali indicated a majority of β-1,6-linkages (67.4 mol %) and 6 mol % 1,3-linkages [183]. In light of subsequent work on *S. cerevisiae* mentioned above, the choice of whole yeast cells as the starting material, instead of isolated walls, probably inhibited release of β-1,3-glucan. Further investigations of *C. albicans* glucans will thus be necessary, using either the three-stage extraction method and/or cell walls. Three distinct glucans were characterized from *S. cerevisiae* according to solubility properties, molecular size, and linkage-sequence analysis: alkali-insoluble β-1,3-glucan; alkali-insoluble acetic acid-soluble, highly branched β-1,6-glucan; and alkali-soluble, water-insoluble β-1,3-glucan [56]. The difference in alkali solubility of the two β-1,3-glucans is related to the presence in the soluble glucan of 8-12% β-1,6- linkages occurring in repeat sequences of at least three such bonds, and at branch points [56]. The β-1,6-glucan has a lower molecular weight than alkali-soluble β-1,3-glucan. Linkages between glucan and protein or between mannan and glucan in the intact wall are suspected but

not proven. Soluble glucan-mannan complexes have been extracted from defatted
C. albicans cell walls with dilute alkali, but further characterization and linkage-
sequence analysis of these fractions have not appeared [94,117].

B. *Aspergillus niger*

A crystalline glucan, nigeran, composed of alternating α-1,3- and α-1,4- linkages is extracted from *A. niger* with hot water [25]. This polymer does not occur in *A. fumigatus*.
A highly dextrorotatory α-1,3-glucan which is alkali-soluble and acid-precipitable is
isolated from *A. niger* [83]. About 54% of the cell walls of *A. niger* is not soluble in
alkali and consists of a chitin-associated β-1,3-glucan [162]. The alkali-insoluble wall
fraction contained 52.4% glucan and 29.8% chitin. This fraction was solubilized in
dimethylsulfoxide after nitrous acid treatment. Nitrous acid does not deaminate
acetylated amino groups, so that sufficient depolymerization occurred to enhance
solubility without destruction of chitin. The methylation-fragmentation gas chroma-
tography-mass spectrometry (GC-MS) analysis of this fraction showed that the major
glucosyl linkage was 1,3- with a minority (up to 15%) of 1,4- linkages.

C. Dimorphic Systemic Fungi

Two types of glucans are encountered in walls of *Histoplasma capsulatum*. A β-1,3-
glucan has been detected on the basis of enzymatic digestion by β-1,3-glucanase purified
from snail (*Helix pomatia*) digestive juice [89] or from *Cladosporium resinae* [141].
About 22% of the glucans in *H. capsulatum* G-184B yeast form cell walls (chemotype 2)
and 52% of the alkali-resistant residues were solubilized by β-1,3-glucanase. Chemotype 2
of *H. capsulatum* contains large amounts of alkali-soluble α-1,3-glucan. This polymer is
absent in the walls of chemotype 1 [134,141,155]. The α-1,3-glucan is considered to
occupy an exterior position in the wall as short, thick fibrils; once these are removed by
alkali extraction, a network of fine fibrils remains. These are considered to be composed
of chitin [89], but a role for a fibrillar β-1,3-glucan is conceivable in view of its occurrence
as fibrils in bakers' yeast walls. Structural analysis of the β-1,3-glucan of *H. capsulatum*
remains to be performed.

The main glucosyl polymer of *Paracoccidioides brasiliensis* yeast-form cell walls is
an α-1,3-glucan that can account for 45% of the mural dry weight [31,86,88,156].
The α-1,3-glucan was characterized by its specific rotation, $[\alpha]_D^{25}$ = +233 (1 M NaOH)
and susceptibility to α-1,3-glucanase of *Trichoderma viride*. It is resistant to β-1,3-glucanases
present in digestive juice of *Helix pomatia* and that from the Basidiomycete QM806.
Methylation-fragmentation GC-MS showed the major linkage was 1,3- with a small number
of branch points through C-6. The large α-1,3-glucan component of yeast forms contributes
to a wall thickness of 200-600 nm compared with the 80-150-nm wall thickness of
mycelial forms. Yeast-form cell walls contain about 4% β-glucan.

When the temperature of growth is shifted from 37°C to 20°C, conversion to the
mycelial form occurs and α-1,3-glucan synthesis is repressed. There is a corresponding
increase in long, thin, interwoven β-1,3-glucan fibrils. Ultrastructural evidence has
shown that α-1,3-glucan occurs as short, thick fibrils in an outer wall layer and is
covered by a thin coat of galactomannan. The α-1,3-glucan is solubilized with alkali
and precipitates upon acidification. Mutants deficient in α-1,3-glucan can convert to
the yeast form, but they have diminished virulence for mice [156] and they are more
readily killed by human polymorphonuclear neutrophils [61]. Thus, α-1,3-glucan is
itself a determinant of virulence or is genetically linked to a virulence factor.

D. Dermatophytes

Glycogen-like glucans have been characterized from surface mats of *Trichophyton rubrum* [74,75]. The glucans are extracted from acetone powders of mycelia with ethylene glycol and purified by gel permeation and ion exchange chromatography. Enzymic digestions with pullulanase (specific for α-1,6-glucosyl-flanking α-1,4-glucosyl residues), alpha-amylase, and beta-amylase, contributed to the view that at least 80% of the glucan consists of linear sequences of α-1,4-glucosyl units joined by α-1,6-branch points. The glucans could evoke immediate cutaneous hypersensitivity and passive cutaneous anaphylaxis when donor guinea pigs were sensitized with whole, killed *T. rubrum* mycelia.

IV. CHITIN

Chitin exists as insoluble sheets or fibrils composed of long, unbranched chains of poly β-1,4-*N*-acetylglucosamine (GlcNAc). It is more inert and rigid than cellulose because the acetamido group at C-2 limits rotation around the glycosidic bond [181]. The rigidity of chitin chains is further enhanced by intramolecular H-bonding through 0-3 and 0-5 of neighboring GlcNAc residues and by intermolecular H-bonding with the amide groups. Chitin chains stack on top of each other by hydrophobic contacts. Stacks of chains may be packed in antiparallel form, α-chitin, which probably results from chain folding, or in the parallel β-chitin form [181]. The crystallinity of deproteinized chitin is reflected in characteristic X-ray diffraction patterns. When α-chitin from crab shell (*Cancer magister*) was used as a standard, the X-ray diffraction pattern agreed with chitin from *Mucor rouxii* [153]. This finding is consistent with other studies on fungal cell walls [13,137]. Chitin is a major constituent of the cell walls of filamentous fungi [14,17] (Table 2). At the other extreme is *Saccharomyces cerevisiae,* where the chitin content is 1% of the mural dry weight [30]. Despite being a minor component, it serves a crucial role in cell division [26]. The yeast forms of the primary systemic fungal pathogens have a high chitin content comparable to that of filamentous fungi.

A. Chitin Detection in Fungi

X-ray diffraction patterns consistent with α-chitin have been detected in several genera of fungi and were well studied in fibrillar cell wall residues of *Neurospora crassa* after cycles of alkali and acid extraction [79,137]. Isolated fungal cell walls demonstrate X-ray diffraction bands with the same *d* values as purified crustacean chitin [174]. The diffuse pattern obtained with walls is sharpened after digestion with glucanases. Microbial chitinases and *N*-acetylglucosaminidases from *Streptomyces griseus* [16,17] and *Serratia marcescens* [17,118] act on chitin-containing fungal cell walls, releasing chito-oligosaccharides and GlcNAc [50,77,141,161]. Molano et al. [117] localized chitin in the wall of *Saccharomyces cerevisiae* with fluorescein-labeled chitinase. The lectin wheat germ agglutinin, having specificity for GlcNAc, is also a suitable probe for chitin. Colloidal gold- and fluorescein-labeled wheat germ agglutinin bind to chitin in bakers' yeast walls [73,117]. A significant protion of [^{14}C] glucosamine taken up by *S. cerevisiae* is deposited in the cell wall [117] and is released from cell ghosts by chitinase. Cell-free synthesis of chitin microfibrils was reported with extracts of *Mucor rouxii* [153], and chitin synthetase is known to occur in many genera of fungi [54].

Table 2 Chitin in the Cell Walls of Some Pathogenic Fungi

| | Chitin (% of dry weight of cell wall) | | |
Fungus	Yeast form	Mycelial form	Reference
Candida albicans	1.7	7.6	32
Sporothrix schenckii	7.0	7.0	138
Phialophora verrucosa	n.a.[a]	5.9	168
Fonsecaea pedrosoi	n.a.	5.7	168
Cladosporium carrionii	n.a.	7.6	168
Trichophyton mentagrophytes	n.a.	30.4	123
Aspergillus fumigatus	n.a.	22.0	69
Coccidioides immitis			
Silveira	32.5 spherules	n.d.	38
M 11	28.0 spherules	33.0	177,178
Histoplasma capsulatum			
chem 1 SwA	37.6	20.1	50
chem 2 G184B	11.5	25.8	89
Blastomyces dermatitidis			
F,Mc	32.1	24.9-30.4	50
Ga-1, KL-1	22.7, 34.9	n.d.	41
BD 64	48.0	13.9	88
Paracoccidioides brasiliensis			
7193	32.2	18.0	88
Pb 73	29.8	5.9	157

[a]n.a., not applicable; n.d., not determined.

1. Filamentous Fungi

The wall at the hyphal tips in *Neurospora crassa* has an inner layer of chitin fibrils covered by a thin, amorphous layer. The growing point is where chitin synthetase is most active, as shown by autoradiography with tritiated GlcNAc-labeled hyphae [62]. The apical dome shows bright fluorescence when stained with the optical brightener Calcofluor White M2R, which is also considered a probe for chitin [79]. As growth occurs, the wall increases in thickness and the microcrystalline sleeve of chitin is embedded with glucan and proteins giving a laminated reinforced resin quality and high tensile strength to the intact wall [79,181]. The location of chitin in *N. crassa* walls was studied after either chitinase digestion or cycles of acid and alkali extractions [111]. A chitinase released only GlcNAc from the walls, but digestion proceeded to a limited extent. The additional presence of β1,3-glucanase potentiated the attack of chitinase. These findings are evidence that chitin occurs as a skeletal core protected by an external glucan layer. Cycles of acidic and alkaline extraction reveal a fibrillar chitin layer distributed uniformly along the lateral walls of the hyphae. The cross walls seem especially resistant to chitinase unless steps are taken to dissolve glucan-peptide with alkali, whereupon rings of chitin-rich undigested cross walls are released.

Septa of *N. crassa* have been isolated by mechanical disruption of the cells [78]. The inner layer of the hyphal wall, known to contain chitin, is contiguous with the septum. An outer amorphous layer of the septum is removed with pronase, revealing microfibrils that are oriented tangentially and, to an extent, radially. The fibrillar structure resists drastic chemical treatment with alkali, permanganate, and acid. It is readily dissolved by chitinase but not by β-1,3-glucanase. Autoradiography of the incorporation of tritiated GlcNAc shows that silver grains occur in a highly ordered distribution, consistent with the microfibrillar arrangement. These observations agree with the hypothesis that septa arise as a rim of chitin which develops centripetally leaving a small, central pore.

2. Yeasts

Chitin is a minor component of the *S. cerevisiae* wall, comprising less than 1% of the mural dry weight [29]. Greater than 90% of this chitin forms the primary septum between the mother cell and bud, providing a channel through which the nucleus can pass [30]. The chitin ring that forms around the neck of the mother cell is further developed as a disk of chitin formed by centripetal growth to give a cross wall that is the primary septum of the bud scar [117]. Chitin in the bud scars of *S. cerevisiae* was investigated by electron microscopy before and after glucanase or chitinase treatment. The chitin content of cell ghosts made by cyclic alkaline and acetic acid extractions was enriched to 14.5% compared with 0.8% in cell walls [29]. The ghosts consisted of bud scars held together by a thin matrix that retained the ellipsoid cell shape. When ghosts were digested with glucanase, most of the matrix was solubilized, releasing intact bud scars. Treatment with chitinase, on the other hand, left the ghosts intact but the thick ridges of the bud scars disappeared.

Wheat germ agglutinin (WGA) is a probe for β-1,4-GlcNAc polymers that has been used to identify chitin in *S. cerevisiae*. Horisberger and Rosset [73] prepared bud scars by extraction of cell walls with β-1,3-glucanase and showed that colloidal gold-labeled WGA bound to rings that delimit the bud scars. The binding of fluorescein-WGA to yeast cell ghosts was localized in the bud scars but also occurred to a weaker extent along the whole contour of the wall. Chitinase-digested ghosts retained considerable fluorescence in the bud scars and this was removed either by repeated digestion with the same enzyme or with β-1,6-glucanase [117]. *Saccharomyces cerevisiae* cells were grown with [^{14}C]GlcNAc under conditions where the label was incorporated into chitin and not into other wall polymers. Enzymolysis of the corresponding radiolabeled cell ghosts showed that a minority (about 8%) of the chitin is in the lateral walls and the remainder is in the bud scars. Chitin not present in bud scars forms a thin layer uniformly distributed over the lateral walls in *S. cerevisiae* and also in *Candida albicans* [173]. This layer can be demonstrated in chemically produced cell wall ghosts or in pronase-digested thin sections of whole yeast cells. The reaction of labeled WGA with chitin in the lateral walls was ablated by chitinase digestion. A mutually supportive role for β-1,6-glucan and chitin in the inner layers of the *S. cerevisiae* cell wall was proposed because digestion with β-1,6-glucanase from *Bacillus circulans* could also remove [^{14}C]chitin from cell wall ghosts [117]. The occurrence of a thin, uniform chitin layer in *S. cerevisiae* may represent the remnant of an evolutionary link between yeasts and the filamentous fungi. In the latter, chitin exists not only in the septa but as a substantial microcrystalline sleeve for the growing hypha.

The critical role that chitin plays in yeast morphogenesis is illustrated by the effect of the inhibitor of chitin synthesis, polyoxin D, a structural analog of UDP-GlcNAc [62]. Budding occurs and the daughter cell is fully grown when the cell cycle is interrupted just before separation. Extrusion of the cytoplasm occurs at the neck between the two cells, giving an exploded pair configuration [26]. This is the effect of failure to form the primary septum because of inhibition of chitin synthesis.

3. Pathogenic Genera

The chitin content of some principal genera of zoopathogenic fungi is shown in Table 2. These estimates are based either on acid hydrolyzates of cell walls or on chitinase digests. Rarely has more than one isolate of each species been compared in a single study [50]. These data should thus be regarded as pending confirmation by other definitive studies. The chitin content of the tissue form of the systemic dimorphic fungi is approximately one-third of the mural dry weight.

The two yeast-form chemotypes of *Histoplasma capsulatum* differ markedly in their cell wall composition. Yeast forms of chemotype 1 have a high chitin content ranging from 31% to 53.7% of the dry weight [141,155]. Chemotype-2 walls have a reduced amount of chitin, 12.3-20.1%, [50,155], and instead there is a major amount of α-1,3-glucan which is absent in walls of chemotype 1. The chitin content of yeast-form walls is higher than that from mycelial walls. Chitinases from two sources differed in the ability to digest yeast-form walls of chemotype 1 [45]. The chitinase-β-1,3-glucanase complex of *Streptomyces* sp. released 25-38% of the cell wall as GlcNAc and a minor amount of glucose, but the chitinase-chitobiase of *Serratia marcescens* which does not co-produce a glucanase, only hydrolyzed 12-15% of the cell wall to GlcNAc. This finding argues for an occluding effect or linkage between β-1,3-glucan and chitin in the *H. capsulatum* cell wall.

The wall of the mature spherule form of *Coccidioides immitis* is highly susceptible to the chitinase of *Streptomyces antibioticus*, which contains β-1,3-glucanase as a minor component [38]. Dissolution of the wall occurs, leaving a resistant residue of less than 10% of the mass of the mature spherule. GlcNAc and glucose, equivalent to 32.5% and 19% of the mural dry weight, respectively, are liberated in the process. Egg white lysozyme has a significant but limited ability to release GlcNAc from spherule walls, opening the question of whether lysozyme in polymorphonuclear neutrophils may contribute to host defense against *C. immitis*. Spherules incubated in buffer alone undergo moderate autolysis within 48 h, releasing glucose, but not GlcNAc, into the supernatant. The effects of chitinase-glucanase complex on the ultrastructure of immature spherules was assessed [71]. This chitinase complex removed an inner layer along the entire perimeter of the lateral wall and a contiguous layer within the cleavage planes. The further effect of α-1,3-glucanase from *Bacillus circulans* W-12 was partially or completely to lyse the remaining outer mural layer.

Differences in the chitin content of the yeast form cell walls from two isolates of *Blastomyces dermatitidis* have been noted [41]. The avirulent Ga-1 isolate has a chitin content of 24%, whereas 43% was detected in walls of the KL-1 isolate. The trypsin-digested and alkali-insoluble portion of these cell walls evoked tissue necrosis in mice [44]. The intact walls of the virulent strain, in addition, could promote granuloma formation; an observation related to the occurrence of an alkali-soluble antigen. The role of chitin as a factor that makes killing by polymorphonuclear neutrophils, or by macrophages, more difficult seems a tempting possibility but one for which no proof is available.

Hen egg white lysozyme (EC 3.2.1.17) and human leukocyte lysozyme are effective muramidases with only weak chitinase activity. The enzymes attack chitopentaoses resulting in 54% digestion in 1 h, and 88% digestion after 16 h; but colloidal chitin is a relatively poor substrate [84]. Colloidal crustacean chitin is probably not a suitable substrate to judge the efficacy of lysozyme against fungi, particularly in view of the lytic effect of lysozyme on dividing cells of *Candida albicans* [85]. Although chitin is a minor constituent by weight, its critical role in providing a channel for nuclear migration during budding suggests that even minor interruption of chitin synthesis at this stage may cause a sufficient derangement to arrest cell division or even lyse the yeast. Further investigation of lysozyme interactions with growing fungi is indicated.

V. FUNCTIONS OF THE CELL WALL

The primary role of the cell wall of fungi is protective. The wall provides a supporting superstructure for the growing protoplast and assists in orderly cell division. The abundance of murolytic enzymes secreted by bacteria, actinomycetes, and fungi suggests the existence of antagonism among competing soil microflora [133]. It has been pointed out repeatedly that outer wall layers act as filters to block aqueous extraction of more deeply situated glucans and, moreover, that the fibrillar β-glucan-chitin matrix in the inner wall layer limits the activity of chitinase. The same protective devices that fungi have evolved for survival in the soil serve them well in the host-fungus interaction. Primary systemic, dimorphic fungal pathogens, perhaps because of the high chitin content in their walls, resist lysis in the host and evoke a granulomatous reaction. This is end-stage cell-mediated immunity, the classic form of hypersensitivity of infection. A vivid illustration of persistence in tissue are the multiple calcified foci in both lung fields that are the hallmarks of healed acute histoplasmosis resulting from exposure to heavily spore-laden dusts [58]. *Histoplasma capsulatum* yeast forms survive and multiply within macrophages. Discussion of this aspect is outside the scope of this review, but it appears that the oxidative and nonoxidative fungicidal mechanisms are not sufficient for killing the yeast forms, or that the fungus can turn off the lysosomal processes [52,76]. It is held by some that the cell wall is a highly porous structure and does not present a barrier to lysosomal factors that produce lethal hits in the fungal plasmalemma. For reasons that are unclear, lethal hits do not occur efficiently for yeast forms phagocytosed by macrophages. Lysis of the *H. capsulatum* cell wall also is inefficient, perhaps because the correct assortment of enzymes is not present. Indirect evidence of this is the limited success with which lysozyme can degrade chitin in the spherules of *Coccidioides immitis* [38]. In the extreme where a zoopathogen like *Cryptococcus neoformans* has evolved a viscous, acidic, polysaccharide capsule, opportunities are increased to evade phagocytosis, penetrate the blood-brain barrier, and establish meningitis. Although *C. neoformans* may be the gastronomic delight of a soil ameba [28], the capsule in experimental murine models has been characterized as antiphagocytic and tolerogenic [100,120].

The description of phagocytic lysosomal enzymes capable of acting on fungal cell walls is an active area of research. Pseudohyphal forms of *Candida albicans*, too large for endophagocytosis, are subject to damage by polymorphonuclear neutrophils. Adherence is followed by the discharge of granules, loss of integrity of cytoplasmic organelles, and eventual dissolution of the cell wall [47-49].

Another aspect of protection is the locus that the wall provides for periplasmic enzymes. Acid phosphatase has been identified in seven pathogenic *Candida* species, in *Cryptococcus neoformans,* and in *Torulopsis glabrata* [127]. In *Candida albicans,* this enzyme is a mannoprotein with a hexose:protein ratio of 7:1. *N*-acetylglucosaminidase was identified in a superficial wall layer of *C. albicans* [139]. Acidic carboxyl proteinase is a glycoprotein that is secreted by most *C. albicans* isolates [152]. Although its location has not been cytochemically confirmed, it probably occupies a periplasmic niche. Gander and Fang [60] have proposed that the peptidophosphogalactomannan of *Penicillium charlesii* functions to protect mural enzymes from proteolytic cleavage during transport between the ribosome and the wall, and second, to anchor enzymes in the periplasmic space. These speculations may have broad implications for the pathogenic genera in which galactomannans are well represented.

Other physicochemical properties of the fungal cell wall have implications for protection. Mannose-based glycans occur almost universally in the outer mural layers. As readily soluble polymers, these mannans probably exist in a hydrated form and serve as a gel in the cell microenvironment giving some protection against desiccation. Charged wall polymers have the potential to act as ion exchangers. Glucuronosyl groups in cryptococcal polysaccharides can bind cations, and the chitosan of *Mucor* species can act as an anion exchanger [15].

The fungal cell wall is sometimes regarded as a highly porous structure that does not pose a serious barrier to the oxidative and cationic protein-mediated fungicidal mechanisms of granulocytes. The porosity of *C. albicans* cell walls was surveyed with polyethylene glycols as model compounds [40]. When the molecular weight of the solute exceeded 600, corresponding to an Einstein-Stokes radius of 0.8 nm, the polymer was effectively excluded by the cell wall.

Adherence to buccal and vaginal epithelial cells is displayed by *C. albicans* and to a much lesser extent by other *Candida* species [97]. Adherence is inhibited by digestion of yeast with proteinase, suggesting that the outer coat protein or glycoprotein of the cell wall has a functional role in mediating adherence; this may explain how *C. albicans* has become well-adapted to life on the mucosae of warm-blooded animals and humans.

The wall should also be considered as the source of antigen most accessible to the host. The weight of evidence favors peptidomannans as the principal mural antigens. The proteins that occur in the periplasmic space and those that are being secreted into the external milieu are also capable of providing potent antigenic stimuli, as shown in the instances of acid phosphatase and acidic carboxyl proteinase of *C. albicans* [109,127], and the H and M factors of histoplasmin [52,136].

Antigen-processing that involves collaboration among T-lymphocytes, B-lymphocytes, and macrophages is the major circuit of specific immune recognition, but in the instance of the fungi, another less specific type of recognition serves as an accessory host defense mechanism during the latent period of the primary immune response. The direct activation of complement via the alternative pathway was first described using *zymosan,* an alkali-extracted bakers' yeast [72]. Since then, other fungal polysaccharides have been described as alternative pathway activators including the cell wall of *Cryptococcus neoformans* [104] and the mannan of *Candida albicans* [96]. Acute-phase reactants such as the C-reactive protein found in plasma also have an affinity for fungal polysaccharides. This observation was made by Longbottom and Pepys [108] who described C-substance activity in polysaccharides of *Aspergillus fumigatus.* Peptidomannan from *Epidermophyton floccosum* was characterized as containing phosphorylcholine and was precipitated by human serum containing C-reactive protein [7].

The functions of the cell wall can be summarized as follows: (1) maintenance of shape and orderly cell division; (2) resistance to lysis by competing microflora and host phagocytes; (3) locale of periplasmic enzymes; (4) prevention of desiccation and action as a filter and ion exchanger; (5) mediation of adherence; and (6) immune recognition at the level of antibody responses, direct complement activation, and C-reactive protein.

VI. PREPARATION AND CRITERIA FOR PURITY

Cell walls are typically prepared by the mechanical disruption of cells and removal of cytoplasmic membranes by repeated washing. A consideration in manipulating batches of pathogenic fungi for cell wall preparation is to kill them before processing. This can be accomplished by immersion in 0.2% neutral, buffered formaldehyde. After a suitable time of standing in the cold, about 48 hr, a sample should be centrifuged and checked for sterility on enriched medium.

The phenomenon of cell wall autohydrolysis has been described. Washed cells of *Schizosaccharomyces pombe* incubated in buffer release proteins, β-1,3-glucose oligosaccharides, and soluble glycans [133]. Endogenous glucanases have also been characterized in *Histoplasma capsulatum* [45]. The culture fluid from 5-day-old *Aspergillus nidulans* contained enzymes that could partially digest the alkali-resistant fraction of the *A. nidulans* cell walls [185]. Inhibition of glucanases is desirable to prevent autohydrolysis during the multiple washings used in cell wall purification. Glucono-δ-lactone is a potent inhibitor of glucanase reactions. Some glucanases, e.g., zymolyase, are rapidly inactivated at 60°C [133]. Boiling cell walls for brief periods (5 min) has been used to inactivate glucanases [55], but controls to determine the presence of heat-labile determinants would be necessary if the antigenic structure of the walls is to be investigated.

A. Isolation and Purification

Yeast-form cells can be directly disrupted but mycelial mats or the balls of mycelia that form in liquid shake cultures may need pretreatment to break up large aggregates. This is conveniently done in a Waring Blendor or Virtis homogenizer. Experience in this laboratory favors the use of the Braun MSK cell homogenizer as the method of choice for disrupting fungi to produce cell walls. Less efficient methods of fungal cell disruption such as sonication, French pressure cell, or Ribi cell fractionator also have a place, especially if the goal is to strip mural outer layers without substantial cytoplasmic contamination. The Ribi fractionator has been used to strip the outer layer of the *Coccidioides immitis* endospores, after which the remaining inner layer was disrupted with the Braun cell homogenizer [37]. Under different conditions, the Ribi fractionator was used to disrupt *C. immitis* spherules releasing intact endospores that were separated from large pieces of spherule wall by differential centrifugation [176]. The MSE microblender (a device similar to the Waring Blendor, but made in England) has been used effectively to prepare detached septa of *Neurospora crassa* [78] and to macerate *A. fumigatus* mycelia before Braun homogenization [69]. Cell walls prepared by disrupting bakers' yeast in a Braun cell homogenizer followed by multiple washings in buffer still contained trapped membrane vesicles [149]. These could be removed by repeated treatments with a Lourdes multimix and washings.

The conditions for successful homogenization require close attention to the duration and to temperature control [130].

A washed, killed, yeast cell suspension, or analogous preparation of disaggregated mycelia is resuspended in 0.1 M Tris, tris(hydroxymethyl) aminomethane-HCl buffer, pH 7.5-8.0, giving a packed cell-to-buffer ratio of 1:2 or 1:2.5. Then 32.5 ml of this suspension is added to 42.5 g of 0.5-mm diameter glass beads in a 60-ml screw cap serum bottle. The bottles are packed in ice and subsequent steps are carried out at ice bath temperature. The bottle is lubricated with glycerol and seated in the chamber of the Braun cell homogenizer. The chamber is cooled with liquid CO_2 from a cylinder with a siphon tube. A spare cylinder is kept in reserve because there is no easy way to determine the residual liquid CO_2 level of the tank. The operator gauges the effectiveness of the flaked CO_2 flow rate and should wear a plastic visor against the small possibility of a broken flask. The instrument is operated from about 3 ft away with a remote switch. The flask in the chamber is cooled with CO_2 for about 30 s before beginning the first 30 s cycle of homogenization. The CO_2 is allowed to flow over the flask in a constant stream that is metered by the operator to prevent either warming of the contents or freezing to a solid plug. After the first 30 s cycle, the machine is stopped and the flask is removed from the chamber using an ordinary laboratory clamp as an extracting tool. Excess glycerol is removed and the contents are examined for indication of proper temperature which should not rise about 10°C. A thin layer of frozen material should coat the base and the adjacent few millimeters of the flask walls. This layer is dislodged and thawed by wrist-action shaking and, if necessary, brief immersion in warm water. Contents are sampled for the extent of breakage by phase-contrast microscopy. A compromise is made between too little breakage and excessive fragmentation. Samples are taken after each 30 s cycle of homogenization until there is ⩾80% breakage, but while most of the yeast cells still retain their ellipsoidal shape. Three minutes of homogenization is usually sufficient. The flasks are replaced in ice and twirled to encourage separation of the upper homogenate layer from the lower bead layer. The upper layer is aspirated with a syringe fitted with polyethylene or similar tubing that is wide enough in diameter so that it is not blocked by entrapment of a few beads that frequently carry over. About 25 ml of buffer washings are used to transfer quantitatively the homogenate to a 250-ml polycarbonate centrifuge bottle. The walls and unbroken cells are washed 3× at 4000 g in Tris buffer plus 0.1% of a nonionic detergent such as Triton X-100, then resuspended in a packed cell:buffer ratio of 1:1 and subjected to additional disruption with glass beads in two 30 s cycles. We and others have previously used sodium dodecyl sulfate (SDS) as a detergent [110,130,147], but its incompatibility with antigen-antibody reactions and difficulty with its complete removal prompted a change to nonionic detergents. Among these, Tween 80 [174] and Triton X-100 [69,70] have been used to purify cell walls. The walls are resuspended and washed in Tris-Triton-10% sucrose, 2× at 5500 g; and then allowed to stand in an ice bath overnight with stirring in Tris-Triton-10% sucrose. Walls are then transferred for convenience to 50-ml polycarbonate Oak Ridge tubes, washed 3× with Tris-Triton-10% sucrose at 5500 g. At this point, nonhomogenous areas on the top and bottom of the pellet are discarded after each washing. Three washes in 0.14 M NaCl are used to chase the detergent and sucrose. After six washes in distilled water, a thin slurry of walls is made, shell-frozen, and lyophilized. Cell walls are stored at $-40°C$ in 1-oz plastic bottles inside of "zip-lock" polyethylene bags with blue indicating silica gel as desiccant.

B. Further Purification of Isolated Cell Walls

The Gram reaction and phase-contrast microscopy are used to determine the extent of breakage. Intact cells are gram-positive and refractile and lose these properties once they are broken. Electron microscopy of negatively stained or cross-sectioned walls will indicate the relative absence of gross debris and the extent of fragmentation. Sedimentation of a whole-cell homogenate, or partially purified walls, through a density gradient removes intact cells and provides a more uniform wall fraction. A 9-21% dextran gradient has been used for bakers' yeast walls [126] and a discontinuous 0.4-1.6 M sucrose gradient aided in purifying walls of *Trichophyton mentagrophytes* [123]. Cell walls accumulate at the interface between the two sucrose solutions.

Digestion of walls with enzymes is another means of ridding them of cytoplasmic contamination. Walls of *Blastomyces dermatitidis* were digested with trypsin [41]. Trypsin and pepsin reduced the mural weight of *Histoplasma capsulatum* walls 27-69%, depending on the isolate [134]. Both trypsin and chymotrypsin were used on mycelial walls of *Neurospora crassa* [137]. A sequence of proteinase treatments with papain, nagarse, and trypsin was applied to *T. mentagrophytes* walls [123,124]. It is difficult to compare the effects of proteinase treatments among different studies because of variation in the choice of enzymes and conditions for their use. One can only suggest criteria for the proteinase digestions. Measurements should be made of the release of ninhydrin-positive material so that the extent of digestion can be determined. Antimicrobial agents should be added to inhibit contamination. A combination of cycloheximide and chloramphenicol has been adequate for this purpose [141]. The removal of extraneous nucleic acid with RNase is recommended by Taylor and Cameron [169], who advise that tests to exclude the presence of nucleic acid should rely on measurement of nucleotide bases rather than on pentoses, because the latter may be part of the mural heteroglycans.

Reports of the lipid content of the walls in excess of 8-10% should be regarded critically to see if the purification procedure was rigorous enough to exclude cytoplasmic contamination. If the objective is antigenic analysis, organic solvents are best avoided as a means of defatting in favor of nonionic detergents. The third stage of the lipid extraction procedure that consists of (1) ethanol-diethyl ether, (2) chloroform, and (3) acidified ethanol-ether [15] is risky for the preservation of acid-labile antigenic determinants such as phosphodiester-linked mannan.

C. Summary of Criteria For Cell Wall Preparation and Purity

Selection of a method to prepare cell wall fractions is obviously influenced by the objective of the investigation. If antigenic structure is to be studied, then denaturing conditions must be avoided to preserve antigenic determinants. On the other hand, if composition analysis of the cell wall matrix is the object of the studies, then all noncovalent lipid and protein must be excluded, and this requires more rigorous purification procedures which involve denaturing conditions. The isolation of outer mural layers and periplasmic enzymes is only indirectly concerned with the cell wall composition. Complete breakage of fungal cells is usually necessary, but rupture of the cells is an obvious disadvantage leading to cytoplasmic contamination. Activation of autolysis may aid in the release of outer mural layers and enzymes. The following guides are intended to accomplish the three different objectives mentioned:

1. Antigenic Structure

1. The use of nonviable fungal cells is necessary for safety considerations.
2. Provide for inactivation of autolytic enzymes.
3. Break cells, but avoid excessive fragmentation.
4. Remove intact cells and subcellular organelles by differential centrifugation. This step most likely requires a dense osmoticum or a density gradient.
5. Remove lipid and protein with a nonionic detergent.
6. Divide walls into portions and extract one sample with a proteinase of relatively narrow specificity, e.g., trypsin. Digestion with an RNase is optional.
7. Monitor the purification by release of $A_{260\ nm}$-$A_{280\ nm}$ material and by the total nitrogen content of the walls.

2. Compositional Analysis

The steps taken are the same as in Sec. VI.B.1, except that lipid and noncovalent protein are removed with SDS and proteinases of broader specificity may be used on samples of the walls. Digestion with RNase is desirable. Monitoring of purification should measure the removal of nucleic acid and the amino acid content of walls at different stages of purification.

3. Outer Layers and Periplasmic Enzymes

The choice of agents for killing cells is limited because formaldehyde may fix and inactivate periplasmic enzymes. Activation of autolytic enzymes is a desirable means of releasing mural outer layers and increasing the access to enzymes. Mild sonication provides the maximum tolerable force to remove outer layers while avoiding fungal cell breakage. Reducing compounds, especially dithiothreitol, and chelating agents like EDTA can loosen the mural outer layers with the aid of added proteinases [170] or perhaps even without proteinases.

It is conceivable that the objectives of recovering readily soluble outer mural layers and periplasmic enzymes and studying the antigenic structure and chemical composition of cell walls could all be met by applying the above methods in series. In that event, soluble outer layers and mural enzymes are isolated first since they would otherwise be lost during the cell disruption and multiple washing steps. Next, disruption of the cells and removal of cytoplasm would be accomplished with nonionic detergents. Finally a portion of the wall preparation would be exposed to stronger detergents and enzymes to remove traces of noncovalent polymers.

The criteria for purity of cell walls are summarized as follows:

1. Absence of intact cells is indicated by phase-contrast microscopy and staining reactions.

2. The retention of cell shape and the absence of cytoplasmic debris is verified by electron microscopy.

3. Total nitrogen and amino acid nitrogen are reduced to constant levels usually less than 15% protein in the wall. This reduction may require the use of a proteinase-like trypsin.

4. The absence or reduction of lipids to constant amounts that are less than 10% of the dry weight. The lipid content of the material can be ascertained by extraction of a sample with chloroform-methanol and subsequent thin-layer chromatography.

5. The absence of nucleic acids measured as nucleotide bases instead of as pentoses. Supplementary criteria that increase confidence in the purity of the cell wall preparation are:

6. If walls are prepared by methods that do not lead to enzyme inactivation, then cytoplasmic contamination may be assayed by the presence of the membrane marker enzyme, adenosine triphosphatase [1].

7. The infrared (IR) spectra of fungal cell walls provide a means of inferring the presence of cellulose, β-1,3-glucan, and chitin [116]. Moreover, the IR spectra of isolated cell walls show a marked decrease in absorption at most wavelengths during purification, especially at an 8.1-μm absorption band corresponding to P=O of nucleic acids and polyphosphate. Thus, spectral analyses also aid in determining cell wall purity [140].

8. The purity of bakers' yeast cell walls has been assessed at various stages by two-dimensional polyacrylamide gel electrophoresis (PAGE) consisting of isoelectric focusing followed by SDS-PAGE [149]. Approximately 170 proteins were present in crude cell walls. After several washings the number of proteins was reduced to 107, and they were weaker in intensity except for component 16w, which was the only wall-associated protein that co-purified with the wall. It was a glycoprotein with an isoelectric pH of 5.0 and a molecular weight of 25,000. Two-dimensional PAGE in conjunction with electron microscopy is a useful way of assessing the occurrence of proteins firmly bound to the cell wall and those that are there due to contamination with cytoplasm.

9. The ^{13}C-nuclear magnetic resonance (NMR) spectra of intact cells and cell walls are markedly different. This observation was adapted to monitor cell walls of *Penicillium ochrochloron* during purification [113]. The disappearance of resonances attributable to triglycerides and mannitol occurred during purification but the polysaccharide resonances persisted. The major polysaccharide resonances were due to β-galactofuranosides present in a galactan. Chitin and β-1,3-glucan because of their highly ordered, rigid structures do not yield resonances.

VII. COMPARATIVE ANALYSIS OF PEPTIDOMANNANS

The peptidomannans are the principal surface antigens of fungi; the fibrillar glucans and chitin are not known to be antigenic. Knowledge about peptidomannans has thus far been restricted by the extremes of pH that are used to isolate them, resulting in the probable destruction of antigenic determinants. Linkage and sequence analysis of mannans has proceeded to a considerable degree in some genera of pathogenic fungi, and information on the fine structure has been reviewed [154]. This section focuses attention on the isolation and characterization of peptidomannans of the principal genera of zoopathogenic fungi. The common theme and generic variations that help to explain antigenic diversity are reviewed.

A. *Histoplasma capsulatum*

Galactomannan (GM) forms an outer amorphous wall layer that accounts for a small percentage of the yeast form mural dry weight (1.5-11.5%, [50]), and is the only known antigenic polysaccharide of *H. capsulatum*. It appears in the soluble fraction after treatment of cell walls with ethylenediamine [50] or dilute alkali. GM has most often been extracted from mycelial forms where it occurs in greater abundance

(9.8-16.9%, [50]). Polysaccharide is also shed into the medium during growth, and its persistence in histoplasmin remains the greatest obstacle to purification of individual protein factors H and M [136]. Anderson [2] extracted GM with hot neutral buffer and precipitated it as the Cu(II) complex with Fehling solution. Acetolysis was carried out and the oligosaccharide fragments were separated by gel permeation. A tetrasaccharide was obtained, containing mannose, galactose, and glucosamine, that could efficiently inhibit immune precipitation in the reaction between the parent GM and antiserum. The GM extracted from defatted mycelia with dilute alkali could be fractionated by anion exchange chromatography into a GM-polysaccharide and a GM-protein, both of which contained galactose and mannose in a molar ratio of 2:5 [143]. The GM and GM-protein had similar serological activity; in addition, the GM-protein was a potent elicitor of macrophage migration inhibition factor (MIF) in the peritoneal exudate cells of guinea pigs primed with the antigen in adjuvant. Azuma et al. [5] also characterized a GM that was extracted with hot alkali from mycelial forms and then precipitated with Fehling solution. Methylation-fragmentation analyses indicated a 1,6-linear backbone with 1,2-mannosyl oligosaccharides and galactofuranosyl nonreducing termini. The GMs of three genera, *Histoplasma*, *Blastomyces*, and *Paracoccidioides* cross-react extensively in quantitative precipitin and immunodiffusion tests. Because of that finding, it is suspected that serotypic factors 1 and 4, which are shared between *B. dermatitidis* and *H. capsulatum*, reside in the GM [92,93]. The remaining factors 2 and 3 specific for *H. capsulatum* yeast forms have not been characterized.

B. *Blastomyces dermatitidis*

An alkali-soluble fraction (B-ASWS) was prepared from *B. dermatitidis* yeast-form cell walls [42,43]. It contains 31.3% carbohydrate composed of mannose, glucose, and galactose [42]. Analysis by SDS-PAGE showed that B-ASWS contains three to four proteins and a periodic acid-Schiff (PAS)-positive component that does not correspond to a protein. The B-ASWS can stimulate peritoneal exudate cells of infected guinea pigs to produce MIF [46]. Peripheral blood lymphocytes from infected guinea pigs undergo blastogenesis when stimulated by B-ASWS to a greater extent than when stimulated by blastomycin [66]. GM has been extracted from *B. dermatitidis* mycelia with dilute alkali and precipitated with Fehling solution [5]. The GM is less abundant in the yeast forms. The molar ratio of galactose:mannose is 1:2.9. All of the galactose occurs as single nonreducing terminal galactofuranosides. The mannan is 1,6-linked in the linear portion and heavily substituted with short 1,2-linked side chains. Extensive cross-reactions are observed among the GMs of *H. capsulatum*, *H. capsulatum* *P. brasiliensis*, and *B. dermatitidis*.

C. *Coccidioides immitis*

Alkaline extraction of *C. immitis* mycelial cell walls results in a mixture of glucan and GM, whereas hot aqueous phenol selectively removes a 3-*O*-methylmannose polysaccharide or glycoprotein from defatted mycelia [176,178]. The phenol-soluble material is 68% protein and 15% neutral sugar. Analysis of the carbohydrates present shows 3-*O*-methylmannose (20%), mannose (74%) with traces of galactose and glucose. The 3-*O*-methylmannose-containing fraction is active in detecting delayed cutaneous hypersensitivity but less so than coccidioidin.

D. *Paracoccidioides brasiliensis*

GM comprises 5% of the wild-type yeast-form cell walls but 16.6% of that from the mycelial form. A mutant deficient in α-1,3-glucan has an increased amount of GM in yeast-form walls [156]. The serological cross-reactions of this GM with that from other genera of primary systemic fungal pathogens is mentioned above. A 1,6-linked mannan from *Alternaria kikuchiana* having 1,2- and 1,3-mannosyl side chains did not cross-react, giving indirect evidence that galactose is an antigenic determinant. *Alternaria zinniae* GM has a 1,6-linear mannan backbone with galactofuranose linked to C-3 in the main chain, and it cross-reacted with antiserum to heat-killed *P. brasiliensis* [5]. This indicated the importance of galactofuranose as an antigenic determinant. Methylation-fragmentation analysis of the GM showed that the major linkage was linear 1,6-mannosyl residues (24.3 mol %) with 8.7 mol % mannosyl nonreducing termini, and 27.5% terminal galactofuranosides. The linear backbone is punctuated with frequent branches (38.3 mol %) linked through C-1, C-3, C-6 or C-1, C-2, C-6 [5]. The major difference between GMs from *P. brasiliensis* and those from *H. capsulatum* is that in the latter there is relatively more galactose and fewer branch points.

E. *Sporothrix schenckii*

Peptidorhamnomannan complexes occur as the readily soluble surface coat of this fungus. Different ratios of L-Rhamnose (Rha):Mannose (Man) are found, depending on the form of this dimorphic fungus. Yeast forms contain monorhamnosyl side chains whereas dirhamnosyl units are displayed in mycelial forms [172]. The peptido-rhamnomannans can be isolated directly from supernatants of mature cultures or by autoclaving *S. schenckii* cells at neutral pH. The polysaccharide portion of the extract is concentrated by ethanol precipitation during which a GM is co-precipitated. Selective precipitation of peptidorhamnomannan is accomplished with Fehling solution. The major mannan component contains linear α-1,6-sequences heavily substituted at C-3 with L-Rha. When present, the second L-Rha residue is 1,2-linked. Proof of the trisaccharide α-L-Rha-1→2- α-L-Rha-1→ 3-Man was obtained because the α-1,6-linkages in the backbone are susceptible to acetolysis. The trisaccharide fragment was isolated as an acetolysis product from mycelia and identified by methylation-fragmentation GC-MS.

F. *Cryptococcus neoformans*

The major capsular polysaccharide of *C. neoformans* is a glucuronoxylomannan (GXM). Proof that serotype specificity resides in the capsule depends on the observed loss of serotype in acapsular mutants [80,101]. The GXMs are viscous, high molecular weight, essentially N-free polysaccharides (Table 1). The main structural feature is a linear α-1,3-mannan backbone heavily substituted with xylosyl or glucuronosyl residues. O-acetylation occurs, but the site of this substituent has not been clarified. The GXM of *C. neoformans* differs from the majority of mannans of pathogenic fungi in which the major linkage in the linear sequences is 1,6-. In serotypes B and C, the GXMs are completely substituted and every third mannosyl is doubly substituted at C-4 with xylosyl and at C-2 with glucuronic acid [19,20]. Serotypes A and D have some unbranched mannosyl residues in the backbone but no tetra-substituted ones [18,21,35,36,114]. The *C. neoformans* of serotype A was grown on semisynthetic medium and the GXM was isolated by CTAB complexation [35]. The material solubilized into the medium during growth is assumed to be identical to the capsule that remains adherent to the yeast cells. Galactoxylomannan is a soluble peptidomannan that is co-produced by *C. neoformans,* grown on chemically defined medium [36]. It is chemically and antigenically distinct from the major GXM, having a significant peptido-component as well as phosphate. The galactoxylomannan is not capable of organizing a capsule, and it is not known whether its appearance in culture supernatants is a result of active secretion or merely sloughing off of a readily soluble outer mural layer. Acapsular mutants that are no longer typable continue to produce galactoxylomannan, so it is not likely to direct serotype specificity. Recent investigations (unpublished observations) suggest the galactoxylomannan is itself heterogeneous and is separable by Concanavalin A (Con A) affinity into a heavily galactosylated polymer that does not bind, and a mannan that binds to the lectin.

G. *Candida* species

The general plan for yeast peptidomannans is a valid model for *Candida* species. To reiterate, the plan consists of an outer chain carrying determinant groups, an inner core linked to structural protein, and base-labile oligomannosides linked directly via hydroxyamino acid esters to the peptide moiety. The method of preparation influences the molecular weight of mannan [121]. Mannan isolated by CTAB complexation, avoiding high pH, has a molecular weight of 133,000, and further exposure of this mannan to dilute alkali at ambient temperature reduces the size to 40,000. More drastic basic conditions, i.e., boiling in 0.4 M KOH, are sometimes used to extract mannan from yeast cells [64]. This can lead to cleavage of *O*-phosphonomannan, *O*-mannosyl hydroxyamino acid esters, and glycosylamine glycopeptide bonds.

The A and B serotypes that allow discrimination between *C. albicans* isolates were found to reside in mannan [164]. Adsorption of type A antiserum with type-B yeast cells leaves A-specific globulins that can be used as a typing reagent [67]. Antiserum to *Saccharomyces cerevisiae* does not cross-react with type-A mannan but does with that of type B [164]. Quantitative precipitin reactions [164,165] show that *C. tropicalis* mannan is related to type A. Reciprocal adsorptions between *C. stellatoidea* and *C. albicans* B mannans revealed no differences, but these mannans are not identical because in the quantitative precipitin reaction *C. stellatoidea* mannan precipitates less globulin from anti-*C. albicans* B than does the homologous mannan. Controlled partial acetolysis is a fragmentation method that provides fingerprints of the oligomannoside chain removed from the mannan [99]. These are the antigenic oligosaccharides from the outer-chain region. The longest oligosaccharides isolated from *C. albicans* serotype-A mannan are heptasaccharides, whereas those from *C. albicans* B are hexasaccharides [167]. Oligomannosides that are sized on Biogel P-2 gel or equivalent columns inhibit the quantitative precipitin reaction of mannan with antibody. In the homologous mannan-A-anti-A reaction, the order of inhibitory power was heptasaccharides > hexasaccharides [165], but in the reaction of serotype-B mannan with globulins of serotype A, the order of inhibitory power was hexasaccharides of serotype A > heptasaccharides. It was concluded that serotype specificity is related to the length of the oligomannoside chains. Oligomannosides were analyzed by proton magnetic resonance, methylation-fragmentation, and quantitative precipitins [57]. Serotype-A mannohexaose gave rise to four anomeric proton signals including one referrable to a terminal α-1,3-linkage, whereas only three such signals appeared in the spectrum for serotype B, indicating the absence of a 1,3-terminal. Methylation-fragmentation further indicated that serotype-B mannohexaose has a 1,3-linkage occurring as an internal branch point. Results with exo-α-mannan hydrolase [146] showed that mannan of serotype A was resistant to the enzyme whereas mannan of serotype B was susceptible. Considering the available data, serotype specificity appears to reside in the mannohexaose, which is a straight-chain 1,2-linked oligosaccharide in serotype A, with a 1,3- terminal. The corresponding hapten of serotype B is more complex, lacking a terminal 1,3- linkage but having instead a single C-1, C-2, C-3 branch point and an additional internal 1,3- linkage.

Fractionation of bulk *S. cerevisiae* mannan on diethylaminoethyl (DEAE) anion exchanger results in neutral mannan in the effluent and acidic mannan subfractions eluted according to phosphate content with a salt gradient [39]. Such heterogeneity of charged species also occurs in *C. albicans* [128], even though the total phosphate content is less than 1% of the weight of mannan [*C. albicans* B792 (serotype B), 0.86% and *C. albicans* B311 (serotype A), 0.25%] [68]. Serological activity appeared to concentrate in fractions enriched in phosphate [128]. The nature of *O*-phosphonomannan in *C. albicans* is not yet determined, but in bakers' yeast, phosphodiesters in the outer-chain region link Man-(1→ 3)-α-Man to a mannotetraose at the C-6 position of the mannose next to the reducing end of the oligosaccharide [8].

H. *Aspergillus fumigatus*

The surface coat of *A. fumigatus* is an alkali-soluble GM [4,144]. The GMs of *A. fumigatus* and *A. niger* resist extraction with hot neutral buffer [10,144] but *A. fumigatus* GM and a glucan are extracted from the hot buffer residue with cold dilute alkaline borohydride [144]. Both the glucan and GM are retained by Con A agarose columns, and further chromatography on Sephacryl S-200 was necessary to separate the higher molecular weight glucan from the GM. The GM isolated from *A. fumigatus* by Azuma et al. [4] had a galactose (Gal):Man ratio of 1:1.5, total N, 1%, and $[\alpha]_D^{25} = +7.6$. A structure was proposed of a -1,2-linked backbone with side chains of galactofuranose residues joined by -1,6-bonds and other side chains of -1,6-mannosyl residues. Reiss and Lehmann [144] reported a Gal:Man ratio of 1:1.2 and a molecular weight of 25,000-75,000 for *A. fumigatus* 2085 GM. Methylation-fragmentation analysis was consistent with 1,6-linked mannan and oligogalactosides three units long terminating in galactofuranose. The affinity for Con A, in this instance, implies the existence of mannosyl nonreducing termini. These different analyses need to be reconciled by GC-MS. Earlier studies [108] described C-substance activity in a hot aqueous phenol extract of *A. fumigatus*. This extract contained a specific antigen as well as C substance. The relation of *A. fumigatus* GM to C-substance activity is not known.

I. Dermatophytes

Glycopeptide antigens of *Trichophyton mentagrophytes* have been solubilized from mycelia with ethylene glycol and precipitated with CTAB in borate buffer [11]. Three GM peptides were resolved on DEAE-Sephadex columns, including GM peptide II having a Gal:Man = 1:9.2 and a protein content of 11.3%. Galactosyl residues were labile to mild acid hydrolysis indicative of galactofuranosyl termini. Methylation-fragmentation analysis has been interpreted as follows: Linkages in the main chain are 1,2- and 1,4- and 39% of the mannosyl residues occur as branch points [12]. GM peptide II is soluble in Fehling solution probably because galactose is in higher abundance than in GM peptide I, e.g., for *Trichophyton mentagrophytes* var. *interdigitale* the Gal:Man of GM II is 33:67 [65]. GM peptide I, a lightly galactosylated mannan, is precipitated with Fehling solution. Polysaccharides extracted from dermatophytes with hot alkali have also been characterized as lightly galactosylated GM I and heavily galactosylated GM II [23,24]. Methylation-fragmentation analysis of GM I from *Trichophyton granulosum* [23] revealed linear 1,6-linked mannosyl residues with single galactofuranosyl substituents. The structure of GM II is more complex with relatively more 1,2-linked mannose and branch points linked through C-1, C-2, and C-6. The authors proposed a linear sequence of alternating 1,2- and 1,6- bonds. It is probable that the dermatophyte glycopeptides and polysaccharides, although isolated by different means, are the same mixture of two GMs. The GM I is a lightly galactosylated polymer with a Gal:Man of 1:11-12 [23,24,119] which does not bind to ion exchangers but precipitates with Fehling solution. The GM II is a heavily galactosylated, lower molecular weight species with a Gal:Man of 1:2.4-3.1, which can bind to DEAE-Sephadex in borate buffer. Discrepancies in the methylation fragmentation patterns observed by Barker et al. [11] and Bishop et al. [23] should be reconciled with more current GC-MS and ^{13}C-NMR spectroscopy.

Young and Roth [182] extracted trichophytin glycopeptides from cultures of *Trichophyton mentagrophytes* using the ethylene glycol procedure [11,131]. In this instance, the material contained 80% carbohydrate, 65% as neutral sugar, and 35% as amino sugar. The neutral sugar fraction was composed of equimolar amounts of Gal: Man, and the amino sugar component had both GlcNAc and GalNAc in a ratio of 1.5:1. Amino sugars have not been detected in trichophytin glycopeptides before [11,12] and the Gal:Man ratios are different from those previously reported. Galactosamine was not found in the wall of *T. mentagrophytes* [123]. The presence of GalNAc in trichophytin glycopeptides seems important to verify in view of the report that antibodies to the glycopeptides cross-react with the A-blood group substance in which GalNAc is an immunodominant epitope [182]. Although a chemically defined medium for the production of trichophytin glycopeptides has been recommended [131], in a recent study [182] peptones and yeast extract were added to the medium. Blood group substance A can be isolated directly from peptone. Nevertheless, a sample of trichophytin glycopeptide grown on chemically defined medium also precipitated with blood group substance A in agar gel. The use of chemically defined medium for production of trichophytin glycopeptides is recommended because the standard protocol [11,12] uses the entire culture including the mycelia and the supernatant as the material for extraction.

J. *Exophiala werneckii*

A peptidophosphogalactomannan has been extracted from whole cells with hot neutral buffer and selectively precipitated as the borate complex with CTAB. Quantitative analysis showed Gal, 14%; Man, 78%; phosphate, 3.2%; and protein, 11.3% [107]. Galactomannan sequences were joined in the main chain by phosphodiesters so that a reduction in molecular weight occurred as a result of mild acid hydrolysis. The glycosidic portion of the molecule (phosphogalactomannan) was β-eliminated from the protein by alkaline borohydride, and the carbohydrate-containing portion was sized on a G100 column giving a nominal molecular weight of 50,000-60,000. This component contained Gal:Man:PO$_4$ in molar ratios of 1:3.7:0.55. Further studies have shown that one of every five mannosyl residues is O-acetylated [105]. The parent peptidophosphogalactomannan was bound to Con A but after β-elimination, the galactose-enriched phosphogalactomannan did not have affinity for the lectin.

K. *Mucoraceae*

Peptidofucomannan is a minor component (less than 5%) of the cell walls of *Absidia cylindrospora* but a major antigen of that fungus and is common to other genera in the *Mucoraceae*. The fucose (Fuc) content of these fungi varies, being higher in *Mucor* species and *Absidia* species than in *Rhizopus* species [115]. In *A. cylindrospora* the molar ratio of Fuc:Man = 1:2.5. Hot aqueous phenol treatment of *A. cylindrospora* mycelia or cell walls results in partition of the peptidofucomannan into the aqueous phase. The peptidofucomannan is purified by affinity for Con A. Oligomannosides have been produced from peptidofucomannan by partial acid hydrolysis; these were composed of 1,6- linkages, a major structural feature of the linear sequences in the main chain of the molecule.

L. Summary of Peptidomannan Structure

This class of macromolecules is comprised of branched mannose-based polymers that are the readily soluble outer coating of the fungal cell wall. They are the principal, if not only, cell wall glycans capable of producing an antigenic stimulus. In the main chain, they are linked to structural protein via glycosylamine or hydroxyamino acid ester linkages. The occurrence of a small (about 10%) protein component influences the way in which the antigens are processed, so it is not safe to assume that, like pure polysaccharides, they are independent of T-lymphocyte help. A notable exception is the major viscous, acidic glucuronoxylomannan of *Cryptococcus neoformans,* which appears to be a pure polysaccharide. Specificity in peptidomannans resides in the short or single substituents disposed along the linear mannan sequences. The major linkage in the linear portions is α-1,6-, although α-1,3- linkages occur in cryptococcal polysaccharides. If, as in the case of *Candida* species, the mannan is a homopolymer, specificity is provided by the glycosidic bond arrangements in the oligomannosides of the outer-chain region. Otherwise, substituents of xylose, rhamnose, fucose, 3-O-methylmannose and, possibly, glucosamine function as determinants, and these have been discussed in relation to their occurrence in individual genera. Galactose is a constituent of mannans from several genera including all the primary systemic fungi, the dermatophytes, and the aspergilli. The role of galactosyl residues as a cross-reactive determinant seems major, but more fine structural analysis will be required to see how this substituent could contribute to specificity. Noncarbohydrate determinants, particularly O-acetyl and O-phosphonomannan, also affect antigenic specificity.

Two properties of mannans that aid in their purification are the formation of Cu(II) complexes with Fehling solution and affinity for the lectin Con A. Both of these properties are dependent on the presence of nonreducing terminal mannosyl residues. Thus heavily galactosylated mannans, for example, the GM II of the dermatophytes and the phosphogalactomannan of *Exophiala werneckii,* neither bind to Con A nor form Cu(II) complexes.

The use of hot alkali should be discouraged as a means of extracting mannans from fungi if the goal is maximum preservation of antigenic determinants. Alkaline degradation is a peeling reaction which releases sugars from reducing termini. Fragmentation occurs under more drastic alkaline conditions as, for example, the conversion of glucose to D,L-lactate by intramolecular oxidation-reduction [179]. Dilute alkali can effect de-*O*-acetylation and β-elimination of hydroxyamino acid ester glycopeptide bonds, whereas boiling in 1 M alkali will destroy relatively stable glycosylamine bonds.

VIII. PROTEIN IN THE CELL WALL

The sources of protein reported to be in the cell wall vary. Certainly some of it may be cytoplasmic in origin and find its way into cell wall preparations as a result of insufficient purification [133]. However, walls of fungi subjected to extensive washings still contain 10-15% protein which is considered to be a structural component [176]. Harsh disruption and washing procedures may remove readily soluble mural outer layers with accidental loss of native protein. Reports of either high protein content or none at all [174] are open to question. Model studies on bakers' yeast [8] have elucidated the peptido or protein content of mannan that is linked to the polysaccharide via *N,N'*-diacetylchitobiosyl glycosylamine bonds to asparagine, and by alkali-labile hydroxyamino acid ester linkages to mannosyl-reducing termini. Recent studies indicate the occurrence in *Schizosaccharomyces pombe* of glycopeptide bonds between β-1,3-glucan ("R"-glucan) and chitin in which the amino acids involved are lysine and citrulline [160]. It is probable that other glycopeptide bonds will be discovered, for example, those that may link glucan to mannan.

Proteins associated with cell wall preparations have received attention in *Blastomyces dermatitidis* [151] and *Aspergillus fumigatus*. Cell walls of both dimorphic states of *B. dermatitidis* have been prepared by disruption in the Braun cell homogenizer; the walls were then washed in buffer and defatted by the three-stage extraction procedure mentioned above [15]. The walls were partially solubilized with 1 M alkali, and the extract was partitioned by adding ammonium sulfate. Two proteins were located in the supernatant and also in the precipitated material by SDS-PAGE; each of the four proteins had distinctive mobility [151]. Cell walls of *B. dermatitidis* yeast forms were digested with trypsin and exposed to 1 M alkali [42,43]. The soluble portion was dialyzed which precipitated an α-1,3-glucan. The protein content of the alkali-soluble water-soluble (ASWS) fraction was 44-70% of the total weight. SDS-PAGE revealed the presence of three to four proteins of between 30,000-50,000 daltons. The ASWS fraction is antigenically potent.

Cell walls have been produced from 3-day-old mycelia of *Aspergillus fumigatus* [69, 70]. The walls were prepared by shaking the mycelia with glass ballotini and multiple washings with hot water. Next, the detergent, Triton X-100, was used to release five or more proteins that were found to be serologically active against sera from aspergillosis patients. The antigens were resolved by two-dimensional, crossed rocket immunoelectrophoresis and their immunological activity was ablated by pronase digestion or by placing Con A or wheat germ agglutinin in the intermediate gel. These observations are evidence for the glycoprotein nature of the Triton-extracted mural antigens of *A. fumigatus*.

Beyond the structural and other wall-associated proteins are the mural enzymes, or glycoenzymes that reside in the periplasmic space (Table 3). These enzymes are important from the viewpoint of antigenic structure, because of their potential of providing an antigenic stimulus in the host. As attention is focused on the host-fungus interaction, factors mediating adherence are becoming known, such as the protein microfibrils that provide the means of adherence of *C. albicans* to vaginal epithelia [98].

Table 3 Mural Enzymes of Zoopathogenic Fungi and Related Genera

Enzymes	Species	Reference
(a) Mural location proven		
Acidic carboxyl proteinase	*Candida albicans*	109,148,152
Acid phosphatase	*Candida albicans*	33,34,127
β-1,4-xylanase	*Cryptococcus albidus* var. *aerius*	125
(b) Mural location suspected		
Chymotrypsin-like proteinase	*Aspergillus fumigatus*	171
H and M[a] proteins of histoplasmins	*Histoplasma capsulatum*	135, 21a
Keratinase II and III	*Trichophyton mentagrophytes*	184

[a]Catalase activity has been shown to be associated with the M but not the H protein (21a), but it is uncertain whether the enzyme is the M antigen or closely associated with it (D. H. Howard, personal communication).

Different and even mutually exclusive approaches are needed to study these sources of protein in the cell wall. Mild sonication may suffice to shear off outer wall layers containing surface microfibrils. The detection of mural enzymes first requires that the yeast or mold is grown under the correct induction conditions. The proteinase of *Candida albicans* is induced by serum albumin [148], and acid phosphatase is repressed by high levels of inorganic phosphate [3]. Some enzymes are directly assayable in intact cells including the acid phosphatase and the β-1,4-xylanase of *Cryptococcus albidus* [125]. Sometimes "permeabilizing" fungal cells by exposure to toluene [126] or ethyl acetate [3] improves the conditions for enzyme assays by activating the autolytic enzyme system. Trapping of mural enzymes behind disulfide-bridged wall components has been proposed for the invertase of bakers' yeast [95]. In that event, sulfhydryl reagents like dithiothreitol aid in the release of invertase and acid phosphatase [3,33].

IX. COMPARATIVE CELL WALL COMPOSITION

The objectives of cell wall analysis of zoopathogenic fungi are (1) to delineate the antigenic structure, (2) to understand the role of the cell wall in resistance to lysis by host phagocytes and, (3) to discover molecular consequences of dimorphism according to the dictum that changes in shape are reflected by changes in the cell wall composition. Despite a significant body of accumulated literature, these problems are still largely unsolved and remain a challenge for further investigations.

It is obvious that before the cell wall analysis of a yeast or mold can be accepted with confidence the culture must be grown under standard conditions, preferably on chemically defined medium to facilitate reproducibility of results among laboratories. Certain objective criteria for cell wall purity, discussed above, ought to be observed. If general conclusions are to be drawn, then more than one isolate of a species should be examined. Results of different laboratories should be in reasonable agreement. There are few if any species c ⁞ medically important yeasts or molds where these conditions have been fulfilled. The approach taken in this section is to collate the data for each species and to rearrange them, where necessary, to express the wall composition in terms of the percentage by dry weight of each component. It should be borne in mind that some authors have been more

Table 4 Composition of the Cell Walls of *Aspergillus* Species

Component[a]	*Aspergillus niger* 17454[b]	*Aspergillus fumigatus* NCPF2109[c]	*Aspergillus nidulans* 13.1. OL[d]
Glucose	65.4	17.0	28.9
Mannose	3.1	11.0	2.8
Galactose	12.1	30.0	3.8
Hexosamine	12.5	22.0	25.1[e]
Protein	1.1	10.0	9.2
Lipid	2.0	7.2	9.0
Phosphorus	0.03	0.4	0.9
Acetyl	3.2	n.d.[f]	n.d.
Glucuronic acid	n.d	n.d.	3.5
Melanin	n.d.	n.d.	0[g]
Recovery (%)	99.4	97.6	83.2

[a]Results recorded as percent of dry weight of walls.
[b]*Source*: Ref. 82.
[c]*Source*: Ref. 69.
[d]*Source*: Ref. 27. This strain is a pigmentless mutant.
[e]Glucosamine + *N*-acetylglucosamine = 14.3%; galactosamine = 10.8%.
[f]n.d., not determined.
[g]Wild type = 17.3%.

interested in fractionating the cell wall based on its alkali solubility and then analyzing the composition of the fractions, instead of the whole wall. In those instances the data are recalculated from the original reports. The process of exposing the isolated wall to extremes of pH tends to fragment the more reactive moieties, especially the mannans. Thus, in some analyses the percentage accounted for as mannan is lower than expected.

Among the aspergilli (Table 4), the cell wall analyses reported are so distinct as to suggest that wall composition may have taxonomic implications. The black molds (Table 5) present a cell wall profile that is relatively low in amino sugar, regarded as

Table 5 Chemical Compositions of the Hyphal Walls of Three Chromomycosis Agents

Component[a]	*Phialophora verrucosa* 204	*Fonsecaea pedrosoi* SA-14	*Cladosporium carrionii* 8620
Glucose	30.9	27.7	16.6
Mannose	8.3	9.2	13.7
N-acetylglucosamine	5.9	5.7	7.6
Protein (amino acid)	36.0	29.5	42.4
Recovery (%)	81.1[b]	72.1	80.3

[a]Results given as percent of dry weight of walls. *Source*: Ref. 168.
[b]Melanin content (18.6%) of *P. verrucosa* P&S 639 cell walls determined independently. *Source*: Ref. 145.

Table 6 Cell Wall Composition of *Candida albicans*

Component[a]	Hyphae[b]	Blastoconidia[b]	Blastoconidia[c] (806)
Glucose	23.2	29.5	56.5
Mannose	18.0	15.2	22.9
N-acetylglucosamine	7.6	1.7	1.4
Protein	19.8	35.4	5.2
Lipid	5.5	0.6	1.1
Phosphate	1.4	2.4	n.d.[d]
Recovery (%)	75.5	84.8	87.1

[a]Results recorded as percent of dry weight of walls. Data are recalculated from original reports.
[b]Fresh clinical isolate; hyphae grown on 100% ox serum at 37°C; blastoconidia grown on yeast extract-peptone-glucose. *Source*: Ref. 32.
[c]Grown on defined medium. Results within one percentage point of those for isolate 582. *Source*: Ref. 94.
[d]n.d., not determined.

the chitin component. The protein contents reported are among the highest for the fungal cell walls reviewed. Melanins of these fungi have only been studied in a preliminary way [145]. The composition of *Candida albicans* (Table 6) walls that is often cited, partly because of the paucity of other reports, is also subject to verification. This may be especially worthwhile for the mycelial forms because the recovery of components was relatively low and the medium for growth (ox serum) may not have been optimal for normal expression of the cell wall mosaic.

Table 7 Cell Wall Composition of *Trichophyton mentagrophytes* and *Epidermophyton floccosum*

Component[a]	T. mentagrophytes[b]	E. floccosum[c]
Glucose	36.2	45.8
Mannose	11.7	6.7
Galactose	tr[d]	n.d.
Glucosamine and N-acetylglucosamine	30.4	30.0
Protein	7.8	7.4
Lipid	6.6	3.3
Phosphate	0.1	n.d.
Galactosamine	n.d.[e]	0.4
Recovery (%)	92.8	93.6

[a]Results recorded as percent dry weight of cell walls.
[b]*Source*: Ref. 123.
[c]*Source*: Ref. 159.
[d]tr, trace.
[e]n.d., not determined.

Table 8 Composition of *Sporothrix schenckii* Cell Walls

Component[a]	Yeast form	Mycelial form
Glucose	29.3	24.2
Mannose	21.9	12.7
Galactose	Trace	Trace
L-Rhamnose	9.6	7.1
Glucosamine	7.0	7.0
Protein	14.4	21.7
Lipid	18.0	26.0
Phosphate	0.7	1.2
Recovery (%)	100.9	99.9

[a]Results recorded as percent dry weight of cell walls; isolate 1099.18 was used in the original report. Data calculated from Ref. 138.

Both of the *C. albicans* cell wall studies referred to in Table 6 utilized acidic conditions during defatting, a procedure which is now known to lead to a loss of phosphodiester-linked mannose residues. Lowered recovery of wall components is also due to the use of alkali to fractionate cell walls, with consequent loss of base-labile oligomannosides. For these reasons, the values calculated for the mannan content of the cell walls (ranging from 16.6% to 24.9% of the mural dry weight) are most likely underestimates.

The analyses of the dermatophytes (Table 7) are among the more rigorously accomplished cell wall studies. Objective criteria for purity were observed and levels for lipid and protein are reasonably low. Both dimorphic forms of *Sporothrix schenckii* are reported to contain high lipid levels accounting for about one-fourth of the total weight of mycelial form walls (Table 8). As no detergents or lipid solvents were used

Table 9 Composition of *Coccidioides immitis* M11 Cell Walls

Component[a]	Spherules	Mycelia
Glucose[b]	66	55
Mannose	27	42
3-O-methylmannose	8	2
Galactose	Trace	3
N-acetylglucosamine[c]	28	33
Protein (amino acids)	9	18

[a]Spherules grown in Converse medium; mycelial cells grown in mannitol-Converse medium. *Source:* Ref. 178.

[b]Sugars recorded as percent of neutral sugar content.

[c]N-acetylglucosamine and amino acids determined on sodium dodecyl sulfate-treated, pronase-digested, defatted cell wall preparations. Figures for N-acetylglucosamine and protein are percent dry weight of cells.

Table 10 Comparison of Selected Components of the *Histoplasma capsulatum* Yeast-Form Cell Wall Chemotypes 1 and 2

Component	Chemotype-1 strain[a]			Chemotype-2 strain[b]		
	SwA	SwB	A811	G184A	G184B	105
Glucose	19.8-32.6	17.2-19.8	39.7	17.8-45.3	49.1-74.0	72.5
Mannose	n.d.[c]	1.0-2.2	3.3	5.8	5.4	2.9
Galactose	n.d.	0.6	1.1	2.3	2.3	1.3
N-acetyl-glucosamine	37.6-46.1	37.6-53.7	29.8	12.3-18.5	11.5-12.3	16.8
Protein	11.0	25.0	14.5	22.8	7.1	9.4

[a]Figures represent % dry weight of cell walls. Source of data on these strains: Refs. 50, 51, 142, 155.
[b]Figures represent % dry weight of cell walls. Source of data on these strains: Refs. 50, 51, 89, 142, 155.
[c]n.d., not determined.

during the preparation of these walls, it is not possible to judge what proportion of these lipids is readily extractable. Long periods of shaking cells with glass beads, i.e., 20 min, in the Braun cell homogenizer, may be excessive. Cell walls of *Coccidioides immitis* were extracted with organic solvents, SDS, and pronase before analysis (Table 9). Spherules have a chitin content that is almost two times higher than mycelial walls. This finding is consistent with results reported with other systemic dimorphic pathogens where the chitin content of the tissue form is higher than that of the saprophytic form (Table 2). The use of pronase to remove protein that is not covalently linked to the cell wall matrix does not seem advisable because the specificity of that enzyme is too broad to exclude attack on covalent structural glycoprotein.

 Histoplasma capsulatum presents a most formidable challenge to cell wall investigation because of the multiple variables that may account for small but significant changes in the mural composition. Chiefly, there is the influence of dimorphism, but other factors

Table 11 Fluctuations in Major Glycans of the Cell Wall in the Yeast and Mycelial Forms of *Histoplasma capsulatum*[a]

Chemotype[b]	Form[c]	GM[d]	α-1,3-Glucan	β-1,3-Glucan[e]	Chitin
1	Y	2.2	0	19.8	37.6
	M	6.6	0	10.6	24.6
2	Y	7.7	41.5	36.0	11.5
	M	24.7	0	18.8	25.5

[a]Results presented as percent of dry weight of cell walls.
[b]Data on Chemotype 1 were obtained with *H. capsulatum* SwB: *Source*: Ref. 50: Data on Chemotype 2 were obtained with *H. capsulatum* G184B: *Source*: Ref. 89.
[c]Y, yeast form; M, mycelial form.
[d]GM, galactomannan. Mannose content of intact walls (galactose not quantitated).
[e]Glucose content of intact walls assuming all glucose in the M form is β-1,3-glucan.

are also important, such as (1) the occurrence of four surface factors and five yeast-form serotypes which are recognized by immunofluorescence cross-staining and adsorption [92]; (2) two yeast-form chemotypes with markedly different cell walls (Table 10); and (3) mating types that influence the conversion of isolates to the yeast form [103]. The adsorption of antiserum to *H. capsulatum* yeast forms with *Blastomyces dermatitidis* has two possible results. The 1,4-serotype of *H. capsulatum* contains determinants that cross-react with *B. dermatitidis* so that after adsorption the antiserum is no longer capable of immunofluorescent staining of *H. capsulatum*. Antiserum to the other major *H. capsulatum* yeast-form serotype 1,2,3,4 retains the ability to strain the homologous isolate after adsorption with *B. dermatitidis* because factors 2,3 are specific for *H. capsulatum*. There has not been a systematic attempt to identify the nature of the cell-wall factors that account for serotypes. It is known that galactomannan (GM) is a mural antigen that is shared by the two species, so one may infer that factors 1,4 reside in the GM. The identity of factors 2,3 is not known. Chemotypes of *H. capsulatum* yeast forms are a major discovery resulting from studies by Domer [50,51] and Pine and Boone [134]. Certain isolates (chemotype-2) of *H. capsulatum* contain high amounts of α-1,3-glucan which is completely absent in other isolates. The estimates of α-1,3-glucan content of chemotype-2 walls are 46.5% in isolate G184B [89] and 27.3% in strain 105 [141]. A second neutral polysaccharide, β-1,3-glucan, occurs in both chemotypes. Chemotype-1 walls of the A811 isolate contain 18.1% glucose liberated by β-1,3-glucanase; 21.3% of the mural glucan of the SW B isolate is alkali- and water-soluble and is probably β-1,3-glucan [51]. The value for the β-1,3-glucan in chemotype 2 varies from 20% in the 105 isolate [141] to 31% in the isolate G184B [89].

There is a variation ranging from 29.8% to 53.7% in the chitin content of chemotype-1 walls of two isolates (Table 11). The chitin content of chemotype-2 walls is reduced. The overall impression is that yeast-form chemotype-1 walls have no α-1,3-glucan and an elevated chitin content, but that chemotype-2 walls have a large α-1,3-glucan component and a reduction in chitin. So far as is known, serotype 1,4 correlates with chemotype 2 and serotype 1,2,3 with a chemotype-1 profile [141,142]. The major shortcoming of these studies is that, thus far, few isolates have been examined so that only tentative conclusions can be drawn.

The cell wall components should be regarded in their macromolecular form to address properly the question of fluctuations during morphogenesis. That is, it is useful to extract and quantitate the GM and soluble glucans of both the α- and β-configurations. This was accomplished for the G184B isolate of chemotype 2 [89], and partial data for chemotype 1 are also available (Table 11). The results suggest that GM and β-1,3-glucan are elevated in mycelial form walls of both chemotypes and that the α-1,3-glucan content is elevated in yeast forms of chemotype 2, possibly at the expense of chitin. The mycelial form of chemotype 2 contains no α-1,3-glucan. The chitin content of yeast forms of chemotype 1 is higher than that found in the corresponding mycelial forms. Important groundowrk has been laid for definitive studies of the cell wall of *H. capsulatum*. The relationships of chemotype, serotype, and mating type will benefit from further investigations. Confirmatory and new information about cell wall correlates of dimorphism can be anticipated.

The yeast form of *Paracoccidioides brasiliensis* contains α-1,3-glucan which is absent from the mycelial forms. A culture passaged on laboratory medium became attenuated in virulence and contained only 3% of α-1,3-glucan which is negligible when compared with 40% which occurs in the wild type [156]. But the neutral sugar component remained at a constant level because of an increase in GM in the mutant. The mutant

Table 12 Cell Wall Composition of Yeast and Mycelial Forms of *Paracoccidioides brasiliensis* 7193 and *Blastomyces dermatitidis* BD64

Component[a]	*P. brasiliensis*[b]		*B. dermatitidis*[c]	
	Yeast form	Mycelial form	Yeast form	Mycelial form
Total neutral sugar	37.2-44.4	37.5-38.0	36.2-47.1	43.5-51.0[d]
N-acetylglucosamine	32.2-40.2	11.7-18.0	37-48	13.9-22.8
Protein (amino acid)	8.6-11.2	20.6-37.0	7.1-7.8	10.9-26.8
Lipid	10.0	8.1	5.5	9.3
Phosphate	0.15-0.16	0.47-0.5	0.12-0.14	0.08-0.36

[a]Percent dry weight of cell walls.
[b]Values calculated from Ref. 88,90.
[c]Values calculated from Ref. 87,90.
[d]Glucose, 39.2%; galactose, 3.9%; mannose, 7.8%.

retained the ability to produce large amounts of α-1,3-glucan in vitro whem stimulated with fetal calf serum, so that the biochemical lesion was regulatory rather than a deletion in the glucan synthetic pathway [156]. GM, the only mural glycan known to be antigenic, comprises 5% of the dry weight of the wild-type yeast-form walls and 16.6% of the weight of walls of the mycelial form. In other respects, *P. brasiliensis* conforms to the general pattern of the primary systemic fungal pathogens (Table 12) in that the yeast-form cell wall is higher in chitin than that of mycelial form. The high values for protein in the mycelial walls justify further attempts to determine if it is readily extractable with detergents or covalently linked.

The culture referred to originally as *P. brasiliensis* 7193 [88,90] and more recently known as IVIC Pb 9 or ATCC 36324 was used for early work in the cell wall composition of *P. brasiliensis* [156,157]. More recent cell wall analysis of a second wild-type,

Table 13 Composition of *Paracoccidioides brasiliensis* IVIC Pb 73 Cell Walls

Component[a]	Total wall		Alkali-insoluble fraction		Alkali-soluble water-soluble		Alkali-soluble acid-precipitable	
	M[b]	Y	M	Y	M	Y	M	Y
Neutral sugar	50.1	33.5	33.1	6.8	13.0	0.4	3.9	26.3
Glucose	18.6	33.1	11.6	6.8	3.0	0	3.9	26.3
Galactose	23.8	0	16.1	0	7.7	0	0	0
Mannose	7.6	0.4	5.4	0	2.2	0.4	0	0
Amino sugar	5.9	29.8	5.8	29.8	0	0	0	0
Amino acid	20.7	23.3	3.4	22.6	17.3	0.3	<1	<1
Recovery (%)	76.7	86.6						

[a]Calculated as percent dry weight of cell walls: *Source*: Ref. 157.
[b]M, mycelial; Y, yeast.

IVIC 73 [157], indicates that revisions will be necessary in our concept of the cell wall composition of this and, by extension, of other systemic dimorphic fungal pathogens. Milder conditions of acid hydrolysis of the wall fractions appear to preserve a substantial galactose component that was not detected in the earlier analyses (Tables 12 and 13). Galactose is the most prevalent hexose in the mycelial form wall of *P. brasiliensis* IVIC 73, and it occurs in both alkali-soluble and insoluble fractions. Under conditions that preserve galactofuranoside linkages, the amino sugar content of the mycelial-form walls is revised to only 5.8% of the dry weight. Morphogenesis to the yeast form causes an increase in the chitin component which becomes *five times* higher, or 29.8% of the cell wall.

Both alkali-soluble and -insoluble glucans from yeast and mycelial forms of *Blastomyces dermatitidis* were exposed to the mixed glycosidases of snail digestive juice or the exo-β-1,3-glucanase of the Basidiomycete QM806 [87]. Snail digestive juice contains glucanases, mannanase, and chitinase, but has low proteolytic activity. It entirely lacks α-1,3-glucanase [133]. The alkali-soluble, acid-precipitable glucan of yeast forms was attacked to only a minor extent (5%) by snail digestive juice, increasing the dextrorotation of the product. About half of the alkali-resistant cell wall of the yeast form was susceptible to snail digestive juice but the analogous wall fraction from the mycelial forms was more susceptible (89%). The Basidiomycete's exo-β-1,3-glucanase completely removed the glucan from the alkali-resistant cell wall of mycelial forms but only a minor portion was recovered as glucose. This is probably because this enzyme is able to bypass β-1,6-branch points yielding gentiobiose [133]. About 27% of the mycelial form wall is an alkali-soluble, acid-precipitable, highly dextrorotatory glucan. The β-1,3-glucan present in the alkali-insoluble fraction was accessible by first digesting chitin with commercial chitinase. After this treatment, the insoluble glucan became soluble in dilute alkali. This provides indirect evidence that chitin and β-1,3-glucan are linked covalently, an idea that has been confirmed more recently [160] in another fungus. The results of chemical and enzymatic analysis are in accord with the proposal that the glycans of the yeast form wall of *B. dermatitidis* are a major α-1,3-glucan comprising nearly 95% of the polymeric glucose, and the remaining portion is a β-1,3-glucan. Chitin comprises about 37% of the yeast-form wall. In the mycelial forms, the α-1,3-glucan and chitin contents are reduced with corresponding increase in β-1,3-glucan. Galactomannan is also increased in mycelial-form walls. Two wall compositional analyses of the same isolate of *B. dermatitidis* have been reported [87,90] (Table 12). It appears that the more recent analysis gives a more accurate picture, because the protein and chitin contents are in closer alignment with what is expected in the walls of the systemic dimorphic fungi. In contrast to *P. brasiliensis*, α-1,3-glucan is more easily demonstrated in the cell walls of *B. dermatitidis* mycelial forms. The alkali-soluble protein fraction of *B. dermatitidis* walls has been discussed above.

X. CONCLUSIONS

The cell walls of fungi pathogenic for humans and animals is a legitimate subject for further investigations because the functions of the wall are important for host-fungus interactions. The mural outer layers consisting of readily soluble mannans are the principal surface antigens. Superficial protein microfibrils of *Candida albicans* that are lost during work-up in conventionally prepared walls supply an important function in mediating adherence to the mucosae. The wall provides a microenvironment for periplasmic enzymes that also have an antigenic role, one that is probably more de-pendent than peptidomannans on T-lymphocyte modulation. The fibrillar and more chemically inert mural matrix composed of glucans and chitin are a physical barrier to host phagocytes, but one whose significance has not been clarified. There is much cir-cumstantial evidence in histoplasmosis that the residual cell walls cannot be cleared and that the ensuing granulomatous reaction contributes to immunopathology.

Some stages of wall synthesis can be blocked by antibiotics, for example, the inhibition of chitin synthesis by polyoxin. Fungi are vulnerable at the sites of budding or at the hyphal apex, but the selective interruption of wall synthesis as a rational means of chemo-therapy has not been realized.

Walls of mechanically disrupted cells are purified by differential centrifugation in detergent solutions. Standard criteria for purity, such as removal of extraneous lipid and protein, have been supplemented by the novel use of IR spectra, two-dimensional PAGE, and ^{13}C-NMR as devices for monitoring purification. The selection of a method of purification is influenced by the sometimes incompatible goals of cell wall analysis. Thus, the preparation of superficial layers of the wall and isolation of periplasmic en-zymes should avoid cell disruption. Antigenic analysis of the mural glycans requires dis-ruption and exposure to detergents but should minimize exposure to extremes of pH and heat. Analysis of the chemical composition is carried out with walls purified with stronger detergents and proteinases.

Mannans of fungi can be classified as mural, capsular, or secreted. The first category is the most diverse, whereas true capsular mannan is restricted in the pathogenic fungi to the glucuronoxylomannan of *Cryptococcus neoformans*. Actively secreted mannans are not well recognized in the pathogenic genera, but the galactoxylomannan of *C. neo-formans* may belong to this type. The general plan of mannans is a comb-like structure composed of linear α-linked backbones with short oligosaccharides bearing antigenic determinants. Antigenic specificity resides in terminal nonreducing residues of mannose, galactose, fucose, xylose, rhamnose, glucuronic acid, or hexosamine. Noncarbohydrate determinants such as *O*-acetyl and *O*-phosphonomannan also contribute to antigenicity. Glycopeptide linkages in fungal cell walls occur as base-labile hydroxyamino acid esters and relatively more stable asparaginyl-glycosylamine bonds to GlcNAc. Bridges between β-1,3-glucan chains containing lysine and citrulline are connected to the chitin moiety, although proof of this linkage in the pathogenic genera is lacking.

Galactomannans are common antigens, widely distributed in the pathogenic fungal genera, in which acid-labile galactofuranosyl residues predominate. GMs vary in the extent of galactosyl substitution and in their ability to precipitate with Fehling solution. The occurrence of GMs in the primary systemic dimorphic genera hinders the attainment of diagnostic specificity, because of their cross-reactivity and persistence in culture supernates and cytoplasmic extracts.

Comparative analysis of the walls of the pathogenic fungi is still at an early stage despite much solid pioneering work. The gaps in knowledge can be addressed by adopt-ing more objective criteria for cell wall purity, more complete analysis of the constitu-ents under optimal conditions for hydrolysis of labile monosaccharides, and a compari-son of several isolates grown under readily reproducible conditions. The library of existing cell wall analyses should be increased with further definitive studies. An example of this is the need to determine the chemotypes of a larger number of *H. capsulatum* isolates so that studies to measure the effect of wall composition on pathogenicity can be initiated.

The present state of knowledge is consistent with a general model of the organization of the fungal cell wall. Superficial layers of protein microfibrils extend from the periphery of the wall and are loosely attached to readily soluble peptidomannans. The mannans are embedded in a fibrillar glucan-chitin matrix. α-1,3-glucans are present in the primary systemic pathogens and are enriched in the yeast forms. These short, thick fibrils are exterior to an interwoven network of fine fibrils of β-1,3-glucan and chitin. *Candida albicans* is a special case because it contains no α-1,3-glucan and the chitin content is low. Chitin is localized in the bud scars of this yeast-like fungus and only a minor amount is distributed along the lateral walls. The major structural component of *C. albicans* walls is β-1,3-glucan. Data obtained from fungi with a higher chitin content shows evidence for covalent glycopeptide linkages between β-1,3-glucan and chitin. In the mycelial forms of fungi, chitin is concentrated in the hyphal septa and is also abundant as a microcrystalline sleeve for the growing hypha. The wall is an important locus for enzymes and glucoenzymes that are present in the periplasmic space. Some, like acid phosphatase, are assayable in the intact cell, whereas others, like the acidic carboxyl proteinase of *C. albicans*, are secreted into the growth medium.

REFERENCES

1. Abrams, A., C. Baron, and H. P. Schnebli. 1974. The isolation of bacterial membrane ATPase and nectin. Methods Enzymol. *32*:428-439.
2. Anderson, K. S. 1978. Immunochemical and electron microscopy studies of mannoprotein from the yeast-form of *Histoplasma capsulatum*. First International Conference on Histoplasmosis, Atlanta, Ga., Am. College Chest Physicians (unpublished).
3. Arnold, W. N. 1972. The structure of the yeast cell wall-solubilization of a marker enzyme, β-fructofuranosidase, by the autolytic enzyme system. J. Biol. Chem. *247*:1161-1169.
4. Azuma, I., H. Kimura, F. Hirao, E. Tsubura, Y. Yamamura, and A. Misaki. 1971. Biochemical and immunological studies on *Aspergillus*. III. Chemical and immunological properties of glycopeptide obtained from *Aspergillus fumigatus*. Jpn. J. Microbiol. *15*:237-246.
5. Azuma, I., F. Kanetsuna, Y. Tanaka, Y. Yamamura, and L. M. Carbonell. 1974. Chemical and immunological properties of galactomannans obtained from *Histoplasma duboisii, Histoplasma capsulatum, Paracoccidioides brasiliensis,* and *Blastomyces dermatitidis*. Mycopathol. Mycol. Appl. *54*:111-125.
6. Bacon, J. S. D. 1981. Nature and disposition of polysaccharides within the cell envelope. In W. N. Arnold (Ed.), *Yeast Cell Envelopes, Biochemistry, Biophysics and Ultrastructure*, CRC Press, Boca Raton, Fla., pp. 85-96.
7. Baldo, B. A., T. C. Fletcher, and J. Pepys. 1977. Isolation of a peptidopolysaccharide from the dermatophyte *Epidermophyton floccosum* and a study of its reaction with human C-reactive protein and a mouse anti-phosphorylcholine myeloma serum. Immunology *32*:831-842.
8. Ballou, C. 1976. Structure and biosynthesis of the mannan component of the yeast cell envelope. Adv. Microb. Physiol. *14*:93-158.
9. Ballou, C. E. 1980. Genetics of yeast mannoprotein biosynthesis. In P. A. Sandford and K. Matsuda (Eds.), *Fungal Polysaccharides*, American Chemical Society, Washington, D.C., pp. 1-14.
10. Bardalaye, P. C., and J. H. Nordin. 1977. Chemical structure of galactomannan from the cell wall of *Aspergillus niger*. J. Biol. Chem. *252*:2584-2591.

11. Barker, S. A., C. N. D. Cruickshank, and J. H. Morris. 1963. Structure of a galactomannan-peptide allergen from *Trichophyton mentagrophytes*. Biochim. Biophys. Acta *74*:239-246.

12. Barker, S. A., O. Basarab, and C. N. D. Cruickshank. 1967. Galactomannan peptides of *Trichophyton mentagrophytes*. Carbohydr. Res. *3*:325-332.

13. Bartnicki-Garcia, S. 1968. Cell wall chemistry, morphogenesis and taxonomy of fungi. Annu. Rev. Microbiol. *22*:87-108.

14. Bartnicki-Garcia, S., and E. Lippman. 1982. Fungal cell wall composition. In A. I. Laskin and H. A. Lechevalier (Eds.), *CRC Handbook of Microbiology,* 2nd ed., Vol. IV, CRC Press, Boca Raton, Fla., pp. 229-252.

15. Bartnicki-Garcia, S., and W. J. Nickerson. 1962. Isolation, composition and structure of cell walls of filamentous and yeastlike forms of *Mucor rouxii*. Biochim. Biophys. Acta *58*:102-119.

16. Berger, L. R., and D. M. Reynolds. 1958. The chitinase system of a strain of *Streptomyces griseus*. Biochim. Biophys. Acta *29*:522-534.

17. Berkeley, R. C. W. 1980. Chitin, chitosan and their degradative enzymes. In A. C. N. Berkeley, G. W. Gooday, and D. C. Ellwood (Eds.), *Microbial Polysaccharides and Polysaccharases,* Academic Press, London, pp. 205-236.

18. Bhattacharjee, A. K., K. J. Kwon-Chung, and C. P. J. Glaudemans. 1979a. The structure of the capsular polysaccharide from *Cryptococcus neoformans* serotype D. Carbohydr. Res. *73*:183-192.

19. Bhattacharjee, A. K., K. J. Kwon-Chung, and C. P. J. Glaudemans. 1979b. On the structure of the capsular polysaccharide from *Cryptococcus neoformans* serotype C-II. Mol. Immun. *16*:531-532.

20. Bhattacharjee, A. K., K. J. Kwon-Chung, and C. P. J. Glaudemans. 1980. Structural studies on the major capsular polysaccharide from *Cryptococcus bacillisporus* serotype B. Carbohydr. Res. *82*:103-111.

21. Bhattacharjee, A. K., K. J. Kwon-Chung, and C. P. J. Glaudemans. 1981. Capsular polysaccharides from a parent strain and from a possible mutant strain of *Cryptococcus neoformans* serotype A. Carbohydr. Res. *95*:237-247.

21a. Biguet, J., P. Tran Van Ky, S. Andrieu, and T. Vaucelle. 1967. Premières caractérisation d'activités enzymatiques sur les immunoélectrophorégrammes des extraits antigéniques de *Histoplasma capsulatum*. Conséquences diagnostiques pratiques. Ann. Soc. Belge Méd. Trop. *47*:425-434.

22. Bishop, C. T., F. Blank, and P. E. Gardner. 1960. The cell wall polysaccharides of *Candida albicans*: Glucan, mannan, and chitin. Can. J. Chem. *38*:869-881.

23. Bishop, C. T., M. B. Perry, F. Blank, and F. P. Cooper. 1965. The water-soluble polysaccharides of dermatophytes. IV. Galactomannans I from *Trichophyton granulosum, Trichophyton interdigitale, Microsporum quinckeanum, Trichophyton rubrum,* and *Trichophyton schoenleinii.* Can. J. Chem. *43*:30-39.

24. Bishop, C. T., M. B. Perry, and F. Blank. 1966. The water-soluble polysaccharides of dermatophytes. V. Galactomannans II from *Trichophyton granulosum, Trichophyton interdigitale, Microsporum quinckeanum, Trichophyton rubrum,* and *Trichophyton schönleinii.* Can. J. Chem. *44*:2291-2297.

25. Bobbitt, T. F., and J. H. Nordin. 1970. Hyphal nigeran as a potential phylogenetic marker for *Aspergillus* and *Penicillium* species. Mycologia *70*:1201-1211.

26. Bowers, B., G. Levin, and E. Cabib. 1974. Effect of polyoxin D on chitin synthesis and septum formation in *Saccharomyces cerevisiae*. J. Bacteriol. *119*: 564-575.

27. Bull, A. T. 1970. Chemical composition of wild-type and mutant *Aspergillus nidulans* cell walls. The nature of polysaccharide and melanin constituents. J. Gen. Microbiol. *63*:75-94.

28. Bunting, L. A., J. B. Neilson, and G. S. Bulmer. 1979. *Cryptococcus neoformans*: gastrononic delight of a soil ameba. Sabouraudia *17*:225-232.

29. Cabib, E., and B. Bowers. 1971. Chitin and yeast budding. Localization of chitin in yeast bud scars. J. Biol. Chem. *246*:152-159.

30. Cabib, E., and E. M. Shematek. 1981. Structural polysaccharides of plants and fungi: comparative and morphogenetic aspects. In V. Ginsburg and P. Robbins (Eds.), *Biology of Carbohydrates*, Vol. 1, Wiley, New York, pp. 52-90.

31. Carbonell, L. M., F. Kanetsuna, and F. Gil. 1970. Chemical morphology of glucan and chitin in the cell wall of the yeast phase of *Paracoccidioides brasiliensis*. J. Bacteriol. *101*:636-642.

32. Chattaway, F. W., M. R. Holmes, and A. J. E. Barlow. 1968. Cell wall composition of the mycelial and blastospore forms of *Candida albicans*. J. Gen. Microbiol. *51*:367-376.

33. Chattaway, F. W., S. Shenolikar, and A. J. E. Barlow. 1974. The release of acid phosphatase and polysaccharide- and protein containing components from the surface of dimorphic forms of *Candida albicans* by treatment with dithiothreitol. J. Gen. Microbiol. *83*:423-425.

34. Chattaway, F. W., S. Shenolikar, and J. O'Reilly. 1976. Changes in the cell surface of the dimorphic forms of *Candida albicans* by treatment with hydrolytic enzymes. J. Gen. Microbiol. *95*:335-347.

35. Cherniak, R., E. Reiss, M. E. Slodki, R. D. Plattner, and S. O. Blumer. 1980. Structure and antigenic activity of the capsular polysaccharide from *Cryptococcus neoformans* serotype A. Mol. Immunol. *17*:1025-1032.

36. Cherniak, R., E. Reiss, and S. H. Turner. 1982. A galactoxylomannan antigen of *Cryptococcus neoformans* serotype A. Carbohydr. Res. *103*:239-250.

37. Cole, G. T. 1982. Cell wall structure and chemistry. 13th International Congress of Microbiology, Boston, Session 77 (unpublished).

38. Collins, M. S., D. Pappagianis, and J. Yee. 1977. Enzymatic solubilization of precipitin and complement fixing antigen from endospores, spherules and spherule fraction of *Coccidioides immitis*. In L. Ajello (Ed.), *Coccidioidomycosis, Current Clinical and Diagnostic Status*, Symposia Specialists, Miami, Fla., pp. 429-444.

39. Colonna, W. J., and J. O. Lampen. 1974. Structure of the mannan from *Saccharomyces* strain FH4C, a mutant constituitive for invertase biosynthesis. I. Significance of phosphate to the structure and refractoriness of the molecule. Biochemistry *13*:2741-2748.

40. Cope, J. E. 1980. The porosity of the cell wall of *Candida albicans*. J. Gen. Microbiol. *119*:253-255.

41. Cox, R. A., and G. K. Best. 1972. Cell wall composition of two strains of *Blastomyces dermatitidis* exhibiting differences in virulence for mice. Infect. Immun. *5*:449-453.

42. Cox, R. A., and H. W. Larsh. 1974. Isolation of skin-test-active preparations from yeast phase cells of *Blastomyces dermatitidis*. Infect. Immun. *10*:42-47.

43. Cox, R. A., and H. W. Larsh. 1974. Yeast and mycelial phase antigens of *Blastomyces dermatitidis*: comparison using disc gel electrophoresis. Infect. Immun. *10*:48-53.

44. Cox, R. A., L. R. Mills, G. K. Best, and J. F. Denton. 1974. Histological reactions to cell walls of an avirulent and a virulent strain of *Blastomyces dermatitidis*. J. Infect. Dis. *129*:179-186.

45. Davis, T. E., J. E. Domer, and L. Yuteh. 1977. Cell wall studies on *Histoplasma capsulatum* and *Blastomyces dermatitidis* using autologous and heterologous enzymes. Infect. Immun. *15*:978-987.

46. Deighton, F., R. A. Cox, N. K. Hall, and H. W. Larsh. 1977. In vivo and in vitro cell mediated immune responses to a cell wall antigen of *Blastomyces dermatitidis*. Infect. Immun. *15*:429-435.

47. Diamond, R. D., and R. Krzesicki. 1978. Mechanisms of attachment of neutrophils to *Candida albicans* pseudohyphae in the absence of serum and of subsequent damage to pseudohyphae by microbicidal processes of neutrophils in vitro. J. Clin. Invest. *61*:360-369.

48. Diamond, R. D., R. Krzesicki, and W. Jao. 1978. Damage to pseudohyphal forms of *Candida albicans* by neutrophils in the absence of serum in vitro. J. Clin. Invest. *61*:349-359.

49. Diamond, R. D. and C. C. Haudenschild. 1981. Monocyte mediated damage to hyphal and pseudohyphal forms of *Candida albicans* in vitro. J. Clin. Invest. *67*: 173-182.

50. Domer, J. E. 1971. Monosaccharide and chitin content of cell walls of *Histoplasma capsulatum* and *Blastomyces dermatitidis*. J. Bacteriol. *107*:870-877.

51. Domer, J. E., J. G. Hamilton, and J. C. Harkin. 1967. Comparative study of the cell walls of the yeastlike and mycelial phases of *Histoplasma capsulatum*. J. Bacteriol. *94*:466-474.

52. Domer, J. E., and S. A. Moser. 1980. Histoplasmosis—a review. Rev. Med. Vet. Mycol. *15*:159-182.

53. Evans, E. E., and J. F. Kessel. 1950. The antigenic composition of *Cryptococcus neoformans*. II. Studies with the capsular polysaccharide. J. Immunol. *67*:109-114.

54. Farkas, V. 1979. Biosynthesis of cell walls of fungi. Microbiol. Rev. *43*:117-144.

55. Fleet, G. H., and H. J. Phaff. 1974. Glucanases in *Schizosaccharomyces*. Isolation and properties of the cell wall-associated $\beta(1\rightarrow3)$ glucanases. J. Biol. Chem. *249*: 1717-1728.

56. Fleet, G. H., and D. J. Manners. 1976. Isolation and composition of an alkali-soluble glucan from the cell walls of *Saccharomyces cerevisiae*. J. Gen. Microbiol. *94*:180-192.

57. Fukazawa, Y., A. Nishikawa, M. Suzuki, and T. Shinoda. 1980. Immunochemical basis of the serological specificity of the yeast: Immunochemical determinants of several antigenic factors of yeasts. Zentralbl. Bakteriol. Parasitenkd. Infektionskr. Hyg., Abt. 1, Suppl. *8*:127-136.

58. Gander, J. E. 1974. Fungal cell wall glycoproteins and polysaccharides. Annu. Rev. Microbiol. *28*:103-119.

59. Gander, J. E., J. Beachy, C. J. Unkefer, and S. J. Tonn. 1980. Toward understanding the structure, biosynthesis, and function of a membrane-bound fungal glycopeptide—structural studies. In P. A. Sandford and K. Matsuda (Eds.), *Fungal Polysaccharides*, American Chemical Society, Washington, D.C., pp. 49-79.

60. Gander, J. E., and F. Fang. 1980. Toward understanding the structure, biosynthesis and function of a membrane-bound fungal glycopeptide—biosynthetic studies. In P. A. Sandford and K. Matsuda (Eds.), *Fungal Polysaccharides*, American Chemical Society, Washington, D.C., pp. 35-48.

61. Goihman-Yarh, M., E. Essenfeld-Yarh, M. C. de Albornoz, L. Yarzabal, M. H. de Gomez, B. San Martin, A. Ocanto, F. Gil, and J. Convit. 1980. Defect in digestive ability of polymorphonuclear leukocytes in paracoccidioidomycosis. Infect. Immun. *28*:557-566.

62. Gooday, G. W. 1977. Biosynthesis of the fungal cell wall—mechanisms and implications. J. Gen. Microbiol. *99*:1-11.

63. Goren, M. B., and G. M. Middlebrook. 1967. Protein conjugates of polysaccharide from *Cryptococcus neoformans*. J. Immunol. *98*:901-913.

64. Gorin, P. A. J., and J. F. T. Spencer. 1968. Galactomannans of *Trichosporon*

fermentans and other yeasts; proton magnetic resonance and chemical studies. Can. J. Chem. *46*:2299-2304.

65. Grappel, S. F., C. A. Buscavage, F. Blank, and C. T. Bishop. 1970. Comparative serological reactivities of twenty-seven polysaccharides from nine species of dermatophytes. Sabouraudia *8*:116-125.

66. Hall, N. K., F. Deighton, and H. W. Larsh. 1978. Use of an alkali-soluble water-soluble extract of *Blastomyces dermatitidis* yeast-phase cell walls and isoelectrically focused components in peripheral lymphocyte transformations. Infect. Immun. *19*:411-415.

67. Hasenclever, H. F. 1965. The antigens of *Candida albicans*. Am. Rev. Respir. Dis. *92*:150-158.

68. Hasenclever, H. F., and F. J. McAtee. 1977. Antigenic relationships of *Candida albicans, Saccharomyces telluris* and *Saccharomyces cerevisiae*. In A. M. Beemer, A. Ben-David, M. A. Klingberg, and E. S. Kuttin (Eds.), *Host Parasite Relationships in Systemic Mycoses,* S. Karger, Basel, pp. 126-137.

69. Hearn, V. M., and D. W. R. Mackenzie. 1979. The preparation and chemical composition of fractions from *Aspergillus fumigatus* wall and protoplasts possessing antigenic activity. J. Gen. Microbiol. *112*:35-44.

70. Hearn, V. M., and D. W. R. Mackenzie. 1981. Analysis of wall antigens of *Aspergillus fumigatus* by two dimensional immunoelectrophoresis. J. Med. Microbiol. *14*:119-129.

71. Hector, R. F., and D. Pappagianis. 1982. Enzymatic degradation of the walls of spherules of *Coccidioides immitis*. Exp. Mycol. *6*:136-152.

72. Holan, Z., K. Beran, and I. Miler. 1980. Preparation of zymosan from yeast cell walls. Folia Microbiol. *25*:501-504.

73. Horisberger, M., and J. Rosset. 1976. Localization of wheat germ agglutinin receptor sites on yeast cells by scanning electron microscopy. Experientia (Basel) *32*:998-1000.

74. How, M. J., M. T. Withnall, and C. N. D. Cruickshank. 1972. Allergenic glucans from dermatophytes. Part I. Isolation, purification and biological properties. Carbohydr. Res. *25*:341-353.

75. How, M. J., M. T. Withnall, and P. J. Somers. 1973. Allergenic glucans from dermatophytes. Part II. Enzymic degradation. Carbohydr. Res. *26*:21-31.

76. Howard, D. H. 1975. The role of phagocytic mechanisms in defense against *Histoplasma capsulatum*. In *Mycoses*. Proceedings of the Third International Conference on the Mycoses, Pan Am. Health Organ. Sci. Publ. No. 304, Washington, D.C., pp. 50-59.

77. Hunsley, D., and J. H. Burnett. 1970. The ultrastructural architecture of the walls of some hyphal fungi. J. Gen. Microbiol. *62*:203-218.

78. Hunsley, D., and G. W. Gooday. 1974. The structure and development of septa in *Neurospora crassa*. Protoplasma *82*:125-146.

79. Hunsley, D., and D. Kay. 1976. Wall structure of *Neurospora* hyphal apex— immunofluorescent localization of wall surface antigens. J. Gen. Microbiol. *95*: 233-248.

80. Jacobson, E. S., D. J. Ayers, A. C. Harrell, and C. C. Nicholas. 1982. Genetic and phenotypic characterization of capsule mutants of *Cryptococcus neoformans*. J. Bacteriol. *150*:1292-1296.

81. Jelsma, J., and D. R. Kreger. 1975. Ultrastructural observation of the (1 → 3)-β-D-glucan of fungal cell walls. Carbohydr. Res. *43*:200-203.

82. Johnston, I. R. 1965. The composition of the cell wall of *Aspergillus niger*. Biochem. J. *96*:651-658.

83. Johnston, I. R. 1965. The partial acid hydrolysis of a highly dextrorotatory fragment of the cell wall of *Aspergillus niger*. Biochem. J. *96*:659-664.

84. Jollès, P., I. Bernier, J. Berthou, D. Charlemagne, A. Faure, J. Hermann, J. Jollès, J-P. Périn, and J. Saint-Blancard. 1974. From lysozymes to chitinases: structural, kinetic and crystallographic studies. In E. F. Osserman, R. E. Canfield, and S. Beychok (Eds.), *Lysozyme,* Academic, New York, pp. 31-54.

85. Kamaya, T. 1970. Lytic action of lysozyme on *Candida albicans.* Mycopathol. Mycol. Appl. *42*:197-207.

86. Kanetsuna, F., and L. M. Carbonell. 1970. Cell wall glucans of the yeast and mycelial forms of *Paracoccidioides brasiliensis.* J. Bacteriol. *101*:675-680.

87. Kanetsuna, F., and L. M. Carbonell. 1971. Cell wall composition of the yeast-like and mycelial forms of *Blastomyces dermatitidis.* J. Bacteriol. *106*:946-948.

88. Kanetsuna, F., L. M. Carbonell, I. Azuma and Y. Yamamura. 1972. Biochemical studies on the thermal dimorphism of *Paracoccidioides brasiliensis.* J. Bacteriol. *110*:208-218.

89. Kanetsuna, F., L. M. Carbonell, F. Gil, and I. Azuma. 1974. Chemical and ultrastructural studies on the cell walls of the yeastlike and mycelial forms of *Histoplasma capsulatum.* Mycopathol. Mycol. Appl. *54*:1-13.

90. Kanetsuna, F., L. M. Carbonell, R. E. Moreno, and J. Rodrigues. 1969. Cell wall composition of the yeast and mycelial forms of *Paracoccidioides brasiliensis.* J. Bacteriol. *97*:1036-1041.

91. Kaplan, W., S. L. Bragg, S. Crane, and D. G. Ahearn. 1981. Serotyping *Crypto-coccus neoformans* by immunofluorescence. J. Clin. Microbiol. *14*:313-317.

92. Kaufman, L., and W. Kaplan. 1961. Preparation of a fluorescent antibody specific for the yeast phase of *Histoplasma capsulatum.* J. Bacteriol. *82*:729-735.

93. Kaufman, L., and W. Kaplan. 1963. Serological characterization of pathogenic fungi by means of fluorescent antibodies. I. Antigenic relationships between yeast and mycelial forms of *Histoplasma capsulatum* and *Blastomyces dermatitidis.* J. Bacteriol. *85*:986-991.

94. Kessler, G., and W. J. Nickerson. 1959. Glucomannan-protein complexes from the cell walls of yeasts. J. Biol. Chem. *234*:2281-2285.

95. Kidby, D. K., and R. Davies. 1970. Invertase and disulphide bridges in the yeast wall. J. Gen. Microbiol. *61*:327-333.

96. Kind, L. S., P. K. Kaushal, and P. Drury. 1972. Fatal anaphylaxis-like reaction induced by yeast mannans in nonsensitized mice. Infect. Immun. *5*:180-182.

97. King, R. D., J. C. Lee, and A. L. Morris. 1980. Adherence of *Candida albicans* and other *Candida* species to mucosal epithelial cells. Infect. Immun. *27*:667-674.

98. King, R. 1982. Adherence of *Candida* cells. 13th International Congress of Microbiology, Boston, Session 63 (unpublished).

99. Kocourek, J., and C. E. Ballou. 1969. Method for fingerprinting yeast cell wall mannans. J. Bacteriol. *100*:1175-1181.

100. Kozel, T. R. 1977. Nonencapsulated variant of *Cryptococcus neoformans.* II. Surface receptors for cryptococcal polysaccharide and their role in inhibition of phagocytosis by polysaccharide. Infect. Immun. *16*:99-106.

101. Kozel, T. R., and J. Cazin, Jr. 1971. Nonencapsulated variant of *Cryptococcus neoformans.* I. Virulence studies and characterization of soluble polysaccharides. Infect. Immun. *3*:287-294.

102. Kwon-Chung, K. J., I. Polacheck, and J. E. Bennett. 1982. Improved diagnostic medium for separation of *Cryptococcus neoformans* var. *neoformans* (Serotypes A & D) and *Cryptococcus neoformans* var. *gattii* (Serotypes B & C). J. Clin. Microbiol. *15*:535-537.

103. Kwon-Chung, K. J., R. J. Weeks, and H. W. Larsh. 1974. Studies on *Em-monsiella capsulata* (*Histoplasma capsulatum*). II. Distribution of the two mating types in 13 endemic states of the United States. J. Epidemiol. *99*:44-49.

104. Laxalt, K. A., and T. R. Kozel. 1979. Chemotaxigenesis and activation of the alternative complement pathway by encapsulated and nonencapsulated *Cryptococcus neoformans*. Infect. Immun. *26*:435-440.

105. Lee, W. L., and K. O. Lloyd. 1975. Immunological studies on a yeast peptidogalactomannan. Nature of antigenic determinants reacting with rabbit antisera and those involved in delayed hypersensitivity in guinea pigs. Arch. Biochem. Biophys. *171*:624-630.

106. Lehmann, P. F., and E. Reiss. 1980. Detection of *Candida albicans* mannan by immunodiffusion, counterimmunoelectrophoresis and enzyme-linked immunoassay. Mycopathologia *70*:83-88.

107. Lloyd, K. O. 1972. Molecular organization of covalent peptido-phospho-polysaccharide complex from the yeast form of *Cladosporium werneckii*. Biochemistry *11*:3884-3890.

108. Longbottom, J. L., and J. Pepys. 1964. Pulmonary aspergillosis: diagnostic and immunological significance of antigens and c-substance in *Aspergillus fumigatus*. J. Pathol. Bacteriol. *88*:141-151.

109. Macdonald, F., and F. C. Odds. 1980. Purified *Candida albicans* proteinase in the serological diagnosis of systemic candidiasis. JAMA *243*:2409-2411.

110. Mahadevan, P. R., and E. L. Tatum. 1965. Relationship of the major constituents of the *Neurospora crassa* cell wall to wild-type and colonial morphology. J. Bacteriol. *90*:1073-1081.

111. Mahedevan, P. R., and E. L. Tatum. 1967. Localization of structural polymers in the cell wall of *Neurospora crassa*. J. Cell Biol. *35*:295-302.

112. Marchessault, R. H., and J. Deslandes. 1980. Texture and crystal structure of fungal polysaccharides. In P. A. Sandford and K. Matsuda (Eds.), *Fungal Polysaccharides,* American Chemical Society, Washington, D.C., pp. 221-250.

113. Matsunaga, T., A. Okubo, M. Fukami, S. Yamazaki, and S. Toda. 1981. Identification of beta-galactofuranosyl residues and their rapid internal motion in the *Penicillium ochro-chloron* cell wall probed by ^{13}C-NMR. Biochem. Biophys. Res. Commun. *102*:524-530.

114. Merrifield, E. H., and A. M. Stephen. 1980. Structural investigations of two capsular polysaccharides from *Cryptococcus neoformans*. Carbohydr. Res. *86*: 69-76.

115. Miyazaki, T., T. Yadomae, H. Yamada, O. Hayashi, I. Suzuki, and Y. Ohshima. 1980. Immunochemical examination of the polysaccharides of mucorales. In P. A. Sandford and K. Matsuda (Eds.), *Fungal Polysaccharides,* American Chemical Society, Washington, D.C., pp. 81-94.

116. Michell, A. J., and G. Scurfield. 1967. Composition of extracted fungal cell walls as indicated by infrared spectroscopy. Arch. Biochem. Biophys. *120*:628-637.

117. Molano, J., B. Bowers, and E. Cabib. 1980. Distribution of chitin in the yeast cell wall. An ultrastructural and chemical study. J. Cell Biol. *85*:199-212.

118. Monreal, J., and E. T. Reese. 1969. The chitinase of *Serratia marcescens*. Can. J. Microbiol. *15*:689-696.

119. Moser, S. A., and J. D. Pollack. 1978. Isolation of glycopeptides with skin test activity from dermatophytes. Infect. Immun. *19*:1031-1046.

120. Murphy, J. W., and G. C. Cozad. 1972. Immunological unresponsiveness induced by cryptococcal capsular polysaccharide assayed by the hemolytic plaque technique. Infect. Immun. *5*:896-901.

121. Nakajima, T., and C. E. Ballou. 1974. Characterization of the carbohydrate fragments obtained from *Saccharomyces cerevisiae* mannan by alkaline degradation. J. Biol. Chem. *249*:7679-7684.

122. Nickerson, W. J. 1963. Symposium on biochemical basis of morphogenesis in fungi. IV. Molecular basis of form in yeasts. Bacteriol. Rev. *27*:305-324.

123. Noguchi, T., Y. Kitazima, Y. Nozawa, and Y. Ito. 1971. Isolation, composition and structure of cell walls of *Trichophyton mentagrophytes*. Arch. Biochem. Biophys. *146*:506-512.

124. Noguchi, T., Y. Banno, T. Watanabe, Y. Nozawa, and Y. Ito. 1975. Carbohydrate composition of the isolated cell walls of dermatophytes. Mycopathologia *55*:71-76.

125. Notario, V., T. G. Villa, and J. R. Villanueva. 1979. Cell wall associated 1,4-β-D-xylanase in *Cryptococcus albidus* var. *aerius*: In situ characterization of the activity. J. Gen. Microbiol. *114*:415-422.

126. Nurminen, T., E. Oura, and H. Suomalainen. 1970. The enzymic composition of the isolated cell wall and plasma membrane of baker's yeast. Biochem. J. *116*:61-69.

127. Odds, F. C., and J. C. Hierholzer. 1973. Purification and properties of a glycoprotein acid phosphatase from *Candida albicans*. J. Bacteriol. *114*:257-266.

128. Okubo, Y., T. Ichikawa, and S. Suzuki. 1980. Immunochemistry of *Candida albicans* mannan. In P. A. Sandford and K. Matsuda (Eds.), *Fungal Polysaccharides*, American Chemical Society, Washington, D.C., pp. 95-112.

129. Okubo, Y., N. Shibata, T. Ichikawa, S. Chaki, and S. Suzuki. 1981. Immunochemical study on bakers' yeast mannan prepared by fractional precipitation with cetyltrimethylammonium bromide. Arch. Biochem. Biophys. *212*:204-215.

130. Orenstein, N. S. 1971. Cell wall molecular architecture in baker's yeast. Ph.D. Dissertation, Rutgers University, New Brunswick, New Jersey.

131. Ottaviano, P. J., H. E. Jones, J. Jaeger, R. D. King, and D. Bibel. 1974. Trichophytin extraction: Biological comparison of trichophytin extracted from *Trichophyton mentagrophytes* grown in a complex medium and a defined medium. Appl. Microbiol. *28*:271-275.

132. Peat, S., W. J. Whelan, and T. E. Edwards. 1961. Polysaccharides of bakers' yeast. IV. Mannan. J. Chem. Soc. (London), Part 1, pp. 29-34.

133. Phaff, H. T. 1977. Enzymatic yeast cell wall degradation. In R. E. Feeney (Ed.), *Food Proteins: Improvement Through Chemical and Enzymatic Analysis*, American Chemical Society, Washington, D.C., pp. 244-282.

134. Pine, L., and C. J. Boone. 1968. Cell wall composition and serological activity of *Histoplasma capsulatum* serotypes and related species. J. Bacteriol. *96*:789-798.

135. Pine, L. 1977. Histoplasma antigens: Their production, purification and uses. In A. M. Beemer, A. Ben-David, M. A. Klingberg, and E. S. Kuttin (Eds.), *Proceedings of the 21st OHOLO Biological Conference*, Ma'alot Israel, Contributions Microbiology Immunology, Vol. 3, S. Karger, Basel, pp. 138-168.

136. Pine, L., H. Gross, G. Bradley-Malcolm, J. R. George, S. B. Gray, and C. W. Moss. 1977. Procedures for the production and separation of *H* and *M* antigens in histoplasmin: Chemical and serological properties of the isolated products. Mycopathologia *61*:131-141.

137. Potgieter, H. J., and M. Alexander. 1965. Polysaccharide components of *Neurospora crassa* hyphal walls. Can. J. Microbiol. *11*:122-125.

138. Previato, J. O., P. A. J. Gorin, and L. R. Travassos. 1979. Cell wall composition in different cell types of the dimorphic species *Sporothrix schenckii*. Exp. Mycol. *3*:83-91.

139. Pugh, D., and R. A. Cawson. 1978. The surface layer of *Candida albicans*. Microbios *23*:19-23.

140. Řeháček, J., J. Beran, and V. Bičik. 1969. Disintegration of microorganisms and preparation of yeast cell walls in a new type disintegrator. Appl. Microbiol. *17*:462-466.

141. Reiss, E. 1977. Serial enzymatic hydrolysis of cell walls of two serotypes of yeast-form *Histoplasma capsulatum* with α(1→3)-glucanase, β(1→3) glucanase, pronase, and chitinase. Infect. Immun. *16*:181-188.

142. Reiss, E., S. E. Miller, W. Kaplan, and L. Kaufman. 1977. Antigenic, chemical, and structural properties of cell walls of *Histoplasma capsulatum* yeast-form chemotypes 1 and 2 after serial enzymatic hydrolysis. Infect. Immun. *16*:690-700.

143. Reiss, E., W. O. Mitchell, S. H. Stone, and H. F. Hasenclever. 1974. Cellular immune activity of a galactomannan-protein complex from mycelia of *Histoplasma capsulatum*. Infect. Immun. *10*:802-809.

144. Reiss, E., and P. F. Lehmann. 1979. Galactomannan antigenemia in invasive aspergillosis. Infect. Immun. *25*:357-365.

145. Reiss, E., and W. J. Nickerson. 1974. Characterization of two melanins produced by *Phialophora verrucosa*. Sabouraudia *12*:193-201.

146. Reiss, E., D. G. Patterson, L. W. Yert, J. S. Holler, and B. K. Ibrahim. 1981. Structural analysis of mannans from *Candida albicans* serotypes A and B and from *Torulopsis glabrata* by methylation gas chromatography mass spectrometry and exo-α-mannanase. Biomed. Mass Spectrom. *8*:252-255.

147. Reiss, E., S. H. Stone, and H. F. Hasenclever. 1974. Serological and cellular immune activity of peptidoglucomannan fractions of *Candida albicans* cell walls. Infect. Immun. *9*:881-890.

148. Remold, H., H. Fasold, and F. Staib. 1968. Purification and characterization of a proteolytic enzyme from *Candida albicans*. Biochim. Biophys. Acta *167*:399-406.

149. Robertson, A. J., J. H. Gerlach, G. H. Rank, and L. C. Fowke. 1980. Yeast cell wall, membrane, and soluble marker polypeptides identified by comparative two-dimensional electrophoresis. Can. J. Biochem. *58*:565-572.

150. Rosenberger, R. F. 1976. The cell wall. In J. E. Smith and D. R. Berry (Eds.), The Filamentous Fungi, Vol. 2, Wiley, New York, pp. 328-344.

151. Roy, I., and J. W. Landau. 1972. Protein constituents of cell walls of the dimorphic phases of *Blastomyces dermatitidis*. Can. J. Microbiol. *18*:473-478.

152. Rüchel, R. 1981. Properties of a purified proteinase from the yeast *Candida albicans*. Biochim. Biophys. Acta *659*:99-113.

153. Ruiz-Herrera, J., and S. Bartnicki-Garcia. 1974. Synthesis of cell wall microfibrils in vitro by a "soluble" chitin synthetase from *Mucor rouxii*. Science *186*:357-359.

154. San-Blas, G. 1982. The cell wall of fungal human pathogens: its possible role in host-parasite relationships—a review. Mycopathologia *79*:159-184.

155. San-Blas, G., D. Ordaz, and F. J. Yegres. 1978. *Histoplasma capsulatum*: chemical variability of the yeast cell wall. Sabouraudia *16*:276-284.

156. San-Blas, G., and F. San-Blas. 1977. *Paracoccidioides brasiliensis*: Cell wall structure and virulence. Mycopathologia *62*:77-86.

157. San-Blas, G., and F. San-Blas. 1982. Variability of cell wall composition in *Paracoccidioides brasiliensis*: A study of two strains. Sabouraudia *20*:31-40.

158. Schwarz, J. 1981. *Histoplasmosis*, Praeger, New York. 472 pp.

159. Shah, V. K., and S. G. Knight. 1968. Chemical composition of hyphal walls of dermatophytes. Arch. Biochem. Biophys. *127*:229-234.

160. Sietsma, J. H., and J. G. H. Wessels. 1979. Evidence for covalent linkages between chitin and β-glucan in a fungal wall. J. Gen. Microbiol. *114*:99-108.

161. Skujins, J. J., H. J. Potgieter, and M. Alexander. 1965. Dissolution of fungal cell walls by a streptomycete chitinase and β(1-3) glucanase. Arch. Biochem. Biophys. *111*:358-364.

162. Stagg, C. M., and M. S. Feather. 1973. The characterization of a chitin-associated D-glucan from the cell walls of *Aspergillus niger*. Biochim. Biophys. Acta *320*:64-72.

163. Stewart, P. R., and P. J. Rogers. 1978. Fungal dimorphism: A particular ex-

pression of cell wall morphogenesis. In J. E. Smith and D. R. Berry (Eds.), *The Filamentous Fungi*, Vol. 3, Wiley, New York, pp. 164-196.

164. Summers, D. F., A. P. Grollman, and H. F. Hasenclever. 1964. Polysaccharide antigens of the *Candida* cell wall. J. Immunol. *92*:491-499.

165. Sunayama, H. 1970. Studies on the antigenic activities of yeasts. IV. Analysis of the antigenic determinant groups of the mannan of *Candida albicans* serotype A. Jpn. J. Microbiol. *14*:27-39.

166. Suzuki, S. 1981. Antigenic determinants. In W. N. Arnold (Ed.), *Yeast Cell Envelopes: Biochemistry, Biophysics, and Ultrastructure*, Vol. I, CRC Press, Boca Raton, Fla., pp. 85-96.

167. Suzuki, S., and H. Sunayama. 1968. Studies on the antigenic activities of yeasts. II. Isolation and inhibition assay of the oligosaccharides from acetolysate of mannan of *Candida albicans*. Jpn. J. Microbiol. *12*:413-422.

168. Szaniszlo, P. J., B. H. Cooper, and H. S. Voges. 1972. Chemical compositions of the hyphal walls of three chromomycosis agents. Sabouraudia *10*:94-102.

169. Taylor, I. F. P., and D. S. Cameron. 1973. Preparation and quantitative analysis of fungal cell walls. Strategy and tactics. Annu. Rev. Microbiol. *27*:243-260.

170. Torres-Bauza, L. J., and W. S. Riggsby. 1980. Protoplasts from yeast and mycelial forms of *Candida albicans*. J. Gen. Microbiol. *119*:341-349.

171. Tran Van Ky, P., C. Torck, T. Vaucelle, and F. Floch. 1969. Etude comparée sur immunoelectrophoregramme des enzymes de l'extrait antigenique d'*Aspergillus fumigatus* révélés par des sérums experimentaux et des sérums de malades atteints d'aspergillose. Sabouraudia 7:73-84.

172. Travassos, L. R., and K. O. Lloyd. 1980. *Sporothrix schenckii* and related species of *Ceratocystis*. Microbiol. Rev. *44*:683-721.

173. Tronchin, G., D. Poulain, J. Herbaut, and J. Biguet. 1981. Localization of chitin in the cell wall of *Candida albicans* by means of wheat germ agglutinin. Fluorescence and ultrastructural studies. Eur. J. Cell Biol. *26*:121-128.

174. Troy, F. A., and H. Koffler. 1969. The chemistry and molecular architecture of the cell walls of *Penicillium chrysogenum*. J. Biol. Chem. *244*:5563-5576.

175. Walborg, Jr., E. F. 1978. Current concepts of glycoprotein structure. In E. F. Walborg, Jr. (Ed.), *Glycoproteins and Glycolipids in Disease Processes*, American Chemical Society, Washington, D.C., pp. 1-20.

176. Wheat, R., and E. Scheer. 1977. Cell walls of *Coccidioides immitis*: Neutral sugars of aqueous alkaline extract polymers. Infect. Immun. *15*:340-341.

177. Wheat, R., T. Terai, A. Kiyomoto, N. F. Conant, E. P. Lowe, and J. Converse. 1967. Studies on the composition and structure of *Coccidioides immitis* cell walls. In L. Ajello (Ed.), *Coccidioidomycosis*, Papers from the Second Symposium on Coccidioidomycosis, University of Arizona Press, Tucson, pp. 237-242.

178. Wheat, R. W., C. Tritschler, N. F. Conant, and E. P. Lowe. 1977. Comparison of *Coccidioides immitis* arthrospore, mycelium and spherule cell walls and influence of growth medium on mycelial cell wall composition. Infect. Immun. *17*:91-97.

179. Whistler, R. L., and J. N. BeMiller. 1958. Alkaline degradation of polysaccharides. Adv. Carbohydr. Chem. *13*:289-329.

180. Wilson, D. E., J. E. Bennett, and J. W. Bailey. 1968. Serologic grouping of *Cryptococcus neoformans*. Proc. Soc. Exp. Biol. Med. *127*:820-832.

181. Winterburn, P. J. 1974. Polysaccharide structure and function. In A. T. Bull, J. R. Lagnado, J. O. Thomas, and K. F. Tipton (Eds.), *Companion to Biochemistry*, Longman, London, pp. 307-342.

182. Young, E., and F. J. Roth. 1979. Immunological cross-reactivity between a glycoprotein isolated from *Trichophyton mentagrophytes* and human isoantigen A. J. Invest. Dermatol. *72*:46-51.

183. Yu, R. J., C. T. Bishop, F. P. Cooper, Fl Blank, and H. F. Hasenclever. 1967.

Glucans from *Candida albicans* (serotype B) and from *Candida parapsilosis*. Can. J. Chem. *45*:2264-2267.

184. Yu, R. J., S. R. Harmon, S. F. Grappel, and F. Blank. 1971. Two cell-bound keratinases of *Trichophyton mentagrophytes*. J. Invest. Dermatol. *56*:27-32.

185. Zonneveld, B. J. M. 1971. Biochemical analysis of the cell wall of *Aspergillus nidulans*. Biochim. Biophys. Acta *249*:506-514.

3

Subcellular Particles in Pathogenic Fungi

Jill Adler-Moore / California State Polytechnic University, Pomona, California

I. INTRODUCTION

Many genera and species of fungi contain extrachromosomal, nonhost, encapsidated, double-stranded ribonucleic acid (dsRNA). These subcellular particles are usually similar morphologically to spherical, dsRNA, isometric viruses found in other types of eucaryotic cells, e.g., the reoviruses [21], but some of the particles demonstrate atypical viral morphology. For example, in the plant pathogen, *Endothia parasitica*, pleomorphic particles have been detected in hypovirulent fungal strains that contain dsRNA (Fig. 1) [40]. In some cases, virus particles cannot be demonstrated in fungi from which dsRNA has been extracted consistently. Examples of such fungi include strains of *Rhizoctonia solani* [33] and *Ustilago maydis* [57]. Terms such as "virus-like particle" (VLP) and "plasmid" have, therefore, been used for some of these subcellular particles.

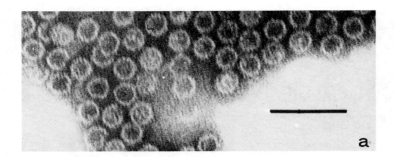

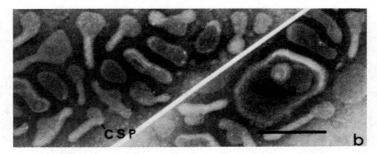

Figure 1 Electron micrographs of partially purified particulate suspensions, negatively stained in 2% phosphotungstic acid. (a) Sample prepared following density-gradient centrifugation from *Penicillium stoloniferum,* strain ATCC 14586. Bar = 100 nm. (b) Sample prepared before density gradient centrifugation from *Endothia parasitica* strain H_1; CSP = club-shaped particle; LMB = large membrane-like body. Bar = 200 nm. (From Ref. 40.)

The relationship between the particles and their fungous hosts can either be deleterious or harmless to the fungus. In *Agaricus bisporus,* virus infection is associated with a dieback disease of the mushroom. Virus-infected strains of *Saccharomyces cerevisiae* and *U. maydis,* called killer strains, produce a toxin that kills sensitive strains of the same or different species. In the majority of fungi, however, virus infection produces no obvious morphological or physiological changes [22].

Another subject of interest is the effect of a virus infection on the pathogenicity of a fungus for its plant or animal host. In the plant pathogen, *E. parasitica,* virus infection is associated with hypovirulence of infected fungal strains for chestnut trees [40]. In those fungi that infect mammals, the presence of dsRNA viruses could have some effect on the interferon production by the mammalian host since dsRNA is a potent interferon inducer [42].

In the following discussion, attention will be focused on fungous subcellular particles and their associated nucleic acid, and special consideration will be given to virus infection of fungi that cause human disease.

II. CHARACTERISTICS OF FUNGAL VIRUSES

A. Morphology

The virus particles in fungi vary in size from approximately 20 nm to 200 nm in diameter, but the majority of them are 25-50 nm in diameter [22]. Most of the

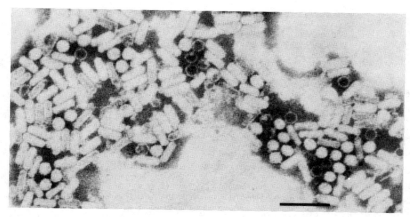

Figure 2   Bacilliform particles, 19 nm wide and 50 nm long, with a few spherical particles (25 nm), extracted from diseased, cultivated mushrooms, *Agaricus bisporus,* and negatively stained with phosphotungstic acid. Bar = 100 nm. (From Ref. 80.)

particles are spherical, although there are some that are rod-shaped (*A. bisporus*) (Fig. 2), Herpes-like (*Thraustochytrium* sp.), pleomorphic (*E. parasitica*) [18], and, in one case (*Penicillium* sp.) even phage-shaped [79].

B. Biochemistry

The capsid polypeptides of different particles range in molecular weight from 25,000 to 130,000 and most of the particles contain dsRNA [22]. Investigators have also reported detecting single-stranded RNA (ssRNA) in particles isolated from *Penicillium stoloniferum* [26]. The individual dsRNA species characterized thus far range in molecular weight from 0.27×10^6 to 6.3×10^6. Many of the particles are considered to be cytoplasmic, multicomponent viruses because several subpopulations of particles, each encapsidating a different-sized nucleic acid, can be isolated from a given fungous strain, and a given subpopulation may contain from one to eight dsRNA components [22].

C. Serology

Viruses isolated from different fungal species are usually serologically distinct, although exceptions to this generalization have been reported, such as the serological relatedness between *Aspergillus foetidus* and *A. niger*. Viruses from different strains within the same species of fungus are usually serologically identical, but in some instances, there may be more than one serological type of viral protein capsid produced within the same fungal strain [63]. In both *P. stoloniferum* and *A. foetidus,* the multicomponent viral subpopulations are enclosed in two serologically distinct capsids [18].

D. Infectivity

The viruses can be transmitted to uninfected strains by protoplast fusion, by heterocaryon formation, or by sexual mating. Protoplasts are made by treating the fungus with a variety of snail gut enzymes, and the protoplasts from infected and uninfected strains are mixed together. There is mixing of cytoplasmic material in the cells that fuse, and

when the cell walls of the protoplasts are regenerated, viruses can be extracted from
the newly infected strain. Heterocaryon formation, the fusion of the mycelium from
two fungal strains, has also been used as a means of viral transmission [21,59]. This
technique can only be used if the strains to be fused have the necessary compatibility
factors and these factors have not yet been definitely characterized [34].

When opposite mating-type strains undergo sexual union, the cytoplasms of the
strains are mixed and viruses can thereby be transmitted from an infected to an uninfected strain. This technique has been used in the study of virus infections such as
that in *S. cerevisiae* [84]. However, in other fungi such as *E. parasitica* [36],
Gaeumannomyces graminis [71], and *Helminthosporium maydis* [16], the viruses are
not transmitted to the ascopore progeny and thus, the technique may be used to cure
the fungi of their infection. Other methods used to cure a fungus of its virus infection
include heating to 40°C [13,82] and treatment of the fungus with cycloheximide [78],
but these latter procedures do not eliminate virus infection entirely.

III. CHARACTERISTICS OF SPECIFIC VIRUSES FROM FUNGI

A. *Aspergillus*

Among the *Aspergillus* species, *A. foetidus* viruses have been studied the most extensively. There are two electrophoretically distinct viruses: slow (Afv-S) virus and
fast (AfV-F) virus. The two viruses contain different-sized dsRNA segments, serologically
unrelated protein capsids with different molecular weights and amino acid compositions,
as well as viral subpopulations with different densities [27]. The *A. foetidus* viruses are
also electrophoretically and serologically identical to the viruses from *A. niger* [24]. In
A. flavus (ATCC 14586), VLPs, 27 nm in diameter, can be extracted in large quantities
from the mycelium (Fig. 3) but none of these particles contains any nucleic acid [88].
Double-stranded RNA has been extracted from several laboratory strains of *A. fumigatus,*
but no definite evidence for the presence of VLPs has yet been obtained (J. Adler,
unpublished data).

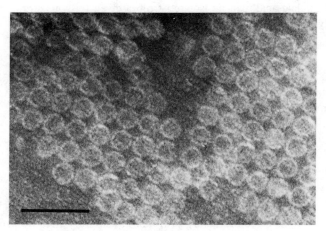

Figure 3 Virus-like particles containing no nucleic acid extracted from *Aspergillus
flavus* (NRRL A12268) and negatively stained with phosphotungstic acid. Bar =
100 nm.

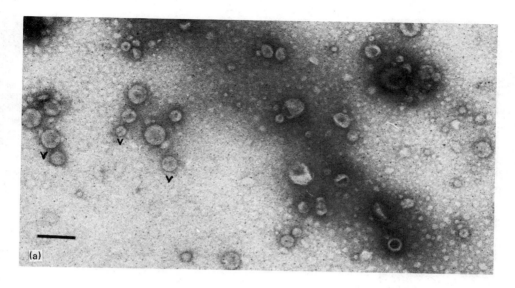

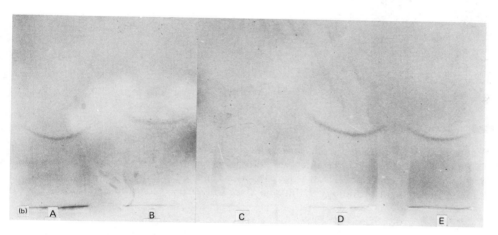

Figure 4 (a) Spherical virus-like particles, extracted from *Histoplasma capsulatum*, partially purified by sucrose density-gradient centrifugation, and negatively stained with phosphotungstic acid; V = virus-like particle. Bar = 210 nm. (b) dsRNA from *Penicillium chrysogenum* (ATCC 9480), mol wt 2.0×10^6 (A), and from *Penicillium stoloniferum* (ATCC 14586), mol wt 1.0×10^6 (B); dsRNA from the yeast phase of *Histoplasma capsulatum* incubated with RNase in (C) dilute sodium chloride, sodium citrate buffer (0.1 SSC), and (D) SSC buffer; dsRNA from the yeast phase of *H. capsulatum* with no RNase treatment (E).

B. *Penicillium*

Viruses have been detected in many species of *Penicillium*. The viruses extracted from strains of *P. stoloniferum* can be separated into two immunological types [25,26]. No viral capsids have been detected which contain polypeptide components of both immunological types of viruses, even though these two types of viruses can replicate within the same fungal cell [3,19].

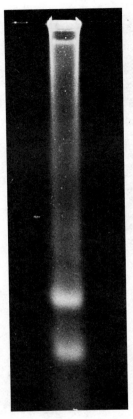

Figure 5 dsRNA extracted from *Torulopsis glabrata,* electrophoresed through a 5% SDS-polyacrylamide gel, and stained with ethidium bromide. (Photograph courtesy of Y. Koltin, Department of Microbiology, Tel Aviv University, Ramat Aviv, Israel, and J. Kandel, Department of Biology, California State University, Fullerton, California).

Viruses have been extracted from strains of *P. chrysogenum.* Three distinct molecular weight (mol wt) segments of dsRNA (2.18×10^6, 1.99×10^6, and 1.89×10^6) can be isolated from these viruses. Each of the segments is encapsidated individually [86]. The peptide molecular weight of the particles has been estimated to be 130,000 ± 5% [23]. The capsids of the particles are serologically related to those of *P. brevicompactum* and of *P. cyaneofulvum* [47].

C. *Histoplasma capsulatum*

Spherical VLPs, 60 nm, 80 nm, and 115 ± 10 nm in diameter, have been isolated from the yeast phase of strains of *Histoplasma capsulatum* (Fig. 4a) and dsRNA with a mol wt of approximately 1.5×10^6 has been extracted from these particles [2,4] (Fig. 4b). Purification of significant quantities of these particles has been difficult since these VLPs seem to be unstable when isolated by procedures routinely used for extraction of other fungal viruses such as those from *S. cerevisiae* and from *Penicillium* spp.

However, varying concentrations of the dsRNA can be readily extracted from several isolates of *H. capsulatum* [86].

D. The Yeasts

Since strains of *S. cerevisiae* can produce killer toxin if they are infected with certain dsRNA viruses, some investigators have looked for viruses in pathogenic yeast by screening them for their ability to produce a toxin that would kill sensitive *S. cerevisiae* cells. This ability to produce a killer toxin has been reported in strains of *Candida* [69], in strains of *Torulopsis (Candida) glabrata* that kill sensitive *S. cerevisiae* and *T. glabrata* cells [30,52,77], and in strains of *Pichia, Kluyveromyces,* and *Hansenula* [69]. Kandel and Koltin (unpublished data) have detected the presence of dsRNA species in killer strains of *T. glabrata* (Fig. 5). Nesterova et al. [65] extracted VLPs (100 ± 20 nm in diameter) from strains of *Candida tropicalis*, but did not report finding any dsRNA in those strains.

IV. RELATIONSHIP OF VIRUS TO FUNGAL HOST

A. Altered Fungal Growth

Although the presence of viruses and/or dsRNA in fungi is not usually associated with alterations in fungal metabolism, those systems in which these changes do occur have been studied extensively.

Alteration of fungal growth associated with the presence of viruses and/or dsRNA has been reported in a few fungi. Mushroom dieback disease or mushroom virus disease, characterized by reduction in yield of mushrooms, as well as abnormal and depressed fruiting of mushrooms, is caused by infection of the fungus with three types of virus particles: two sizes of spherical particles, 25 nm and 34 nm in diameter, and rod-shaped particles, 19 nm in width and 50 nm in length (Fig. 6). The role of each of these three types of viruses in the etiology of the disease has not yet been clarified since it has been very difficult to obtain adequate amounts of purified virus of each type. The instability of the 34-nm particles during purification has been a problem, and virus-infected mushroom tissue is not readily cultivated under sterile laboratory conditions since the infected mycelium often grows very slowly [80].

When nucleic acids are extracted from the diseased mushrooms infected with all three types of viruses, six species of dsRNA are observed following polyacrylamide gel electrophoresis of the preparations. Detection of these dsRNA species can be a useful method for diagnosing viral infections in cultivated mushrooms [64].

The formation of localized, lytic plaques in *Penicillium chrysogenum* cultures, after 4 weeks incubation, is associated with the presence of dsRNA viruses in these fungi (Fig. 7) [61]. When heterocaryons of genetically marked strains [60] were used to study this phenomenon, it was shown that plaque formation depended upon: (1) the presence of a high virus titer; (2) a nuclear host mutation of the wild-type strains that resulted in the loss of lysis resistance; and (3) fungal growth on an unbuffered medium that has a high lactose concentration. Plaque formation has also been observed in virus-infected strains of *P. citrinum* [11] and *P. variabile* [14].

Certain strains of *Rhizoctonia solani*, a plant pathogen that causes various diseases [9], are characterized by degenerative changes such as irregular culture appearance, minimal or no sclerotia production, and a very slow rate of growth [31]. Double-

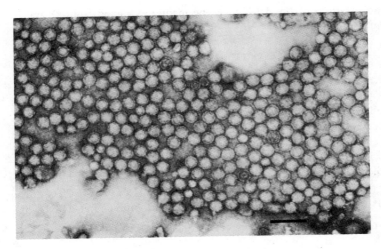

Figure 6 Typical virus preparation extracted and pelleted from fruit bodies of diseased mushrooms, *Agaricus bisporus*, showing mainly spherical particles, 34 nm in diameter, with some spherical particles, 25 nm in diameter, and a few bacilliform particles, 19 X 50 nm. Bar = 100 nm. (From Ref. 80.)

stranded RNA, detected in these strains, is not present in healthy fungus isolates, although no virus particles have been extracted from either healthy or diseased isolates [33]. A healthy hyphal tip isolate (No. 180HT5) of one of these diseased strains (189a) could be converted to the diseased condition by anastomosis with the original strain (189a). Since the diseased isolates have reduced virulence, their potential for use in biological control has been examined. Strain 189a mixed in soil with strain 189HT5 in laboratory tests prevented sugar beet seedling damping off [32].

B. Killer Toxin Production

In some fungi, the presence of viruses and/or dsRNA is not associated with altered growth, but with the synthesis and secretion of an unusual metabolite, the killer toxin. Strains of *S. cerevisiae* that contain both 1.4×10^6 mol wt dsRNA (M dsRNA) and 3.4×10^6 mol wt dsRNA (L dsRNA) [48], encapsidated within virus particles, produce a killer toxin that is lethal to other strains of the same or different species of yeasts. These killer strains are resistant to the toxin activity that kills sensitive strains (Fig. 8). There is significantly more L dsRNA than M dsRNA in a given cell; Wickner [84] estimated that the ratio is about 10:1. In vitro translation studies have shown that the M dsRNA codes for the killer toxin [15]. Since M dsRNA is only found in those strains that also contain L dsRNA, the former may require the L dsRNA for replication. Hopper et al. [48] have demonstrated that the L dsRNA in vitro codes for a product identical to the capside polypeptide of the virus particle that encapsidates both these dsRNA species. Herring and Bevan [45] demonstrated the presence of a capside-associated polymerase which may also be coded for by this L dsRNA since the dsRNA species is large enough to code for both the polymerase and the capside polypeptide.

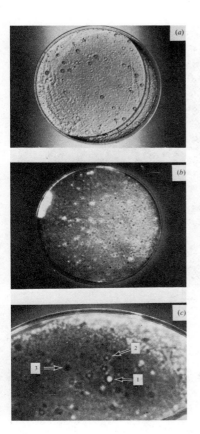

Figure 7 Late plaque formation in *Penicillium chrysogenum*: (a) C6 strain, surface of culture after 2 weeks of incubation; (b) C6 strain, after 4 weeks of incubation, bottom of Petri plate observed by transmitted light; (c) closeup of (b), arrows indicate differences in plaque morphology, i.e., clear (1), turbid with clear center (2), and turbid (3). (From Ref. 61.)

The loss of the killer phenotype and of M dsRNA is associated with recessive mutations in at least 29 different nuclear genes [12,35,83], but no yeast mutants lacking the L dsRNA have been isolated. Buck [22] suggested that L dsRNA may have a greater affinity than M dsRNA for components needed by both species for replication, and that possibly products produced by mutant genes might lower the concentration of certain factors to the extent that M dsRNA can no longer replicate.

Two other nuclear mutants, *kex 1* and *kex 2,* render the strains carrying M dsRNA incapable of secreting killer toxin [85]. There are also nuclear mutations that give rise to "suicide" or nontoxin-resistant strains carrying the M dsRNA. These *rex* mutants produce toxin to which they are not resistant [83]. Alternatively, a nuclear mutant of sensitive cells which lack M dsRNA, called *sek,* produces cells that are resistant to killer toxin when they have intact cell walls, but are sensitive to the toxin as sphaeroplasts [29]. Other nuclear mutant strains of sensitive cells have been isolated and are called *kre* mutants; they are resistant to the killer toxin activity [5].

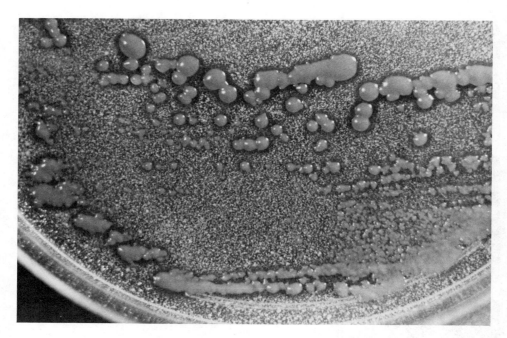

Figure 8 Killer strain of *Saccharomyces cerevisiae* streaked on a lawn of sensitive cells of *S. cerevisiae*. Note the zones of inhibition (plaques) surrounding the killer colonies. (Photograph courtesy of C. Bellinger, Department of Biological Sciences, California State Polytechnic University, Pomona, California.)

When the M dsRNA of killer strains is altered, mutants with unusual phenotypes can be detected. One such type, designated a neutral strain, cannot produce active toxin, but is resistant to the toxin's killing activity [12,81]. This strain contains a dsRNA species with the same mol wt as the M dsRNA (1.4×10^6) which suggests that there is either a very minor alteration in this dsRNA or in another gene necessary for the production of active toxin [15]. Other mutations produce superkiller strains which have increased killing ability and about 2.5 times more M dsRNA than normal killer strains [78,81].

Suppressive nonkiller mutants have also been isolated. Although they lack M dsRNA, they do have the L dsRNA as well as another smaller dsRNA(S) which is less than 1×10^6 [78,81]. It is possible that the S dsRNA suppresses replication of M dsRNA by preferentially using replication factors such as RNA polymerase [22].

The killer toxin from one strain has been purified by Palfree and Bussey [67]. It is a protein with a mol wt of 11,500. The mode of action of the toxin seems to involve changes in the permeability of the plasma membrane which after a lag period results in leakage of K^+ and ATP from whole cells [28,74]. Sphaeroplasts are also sensitive to the purified killer toxin, and it would be interesting to determine if killer toxin had any effect(s) on other eucaryotic organisms that lack cell walls, e.g., mammalian cells.

The ability to produce killer toxins is not limited to *S. cerevisiae,* as noted previously, but the only other well-characterized killer system is that occurring in the

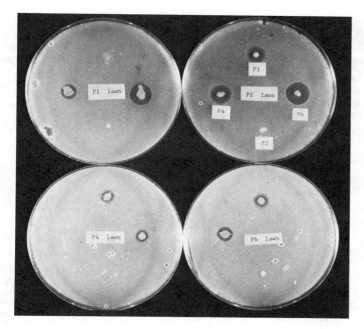

Figure 9 The *Ustilago maydis* killer system. (Upper right plate) Inhibitory effects of P1, P4, and P6 killers of *Ustilago maydis* on a lawn of sensitive P2 *U. maydis*. (Upper left and lower plates) Sensitivity of each killer to the two other killers. (From Ref. 56.)

corn smut pathogen, *U. maydis*. As in the *Saccharomyces* system, killer strains inhibit replication of sensitive strains in the same or different species [55]. Production of the toxin is associated with the presence of dsRNA virus particles in the fungus [56,87]. In the *U. maydis* system, there are three different *Ustilago* killer strains, designated P1, P4, and P6. A given strain is resistant to its own toxin, but sensitive to the toxin of the other two strains, and each killer phenotype is associated with specific dsRNA species (Fig. 9) [56]. When *U. maydis* strains having different killer phenotypes are mated, the progeny's ability to produce one or both killer toxins is lost [56]. Unlike the *S. cerevisiae* killer system, production of an active killer toxin is not dependent on host nuclear genes. All three *Ustilago* toxins are proteins with the same molecular weight, about 10,000 [51], but antisera to P6 killer toxin does not react serologically with P1 and P4 killer proteins.

C. Fungal Pathogenicity

Another potential consequence of the presence of dsRNA viruses in either plant or animal pathogenic fungi is an effect that this infection would have on the pathogenicity of the fungus for its host. Such an effect has been studied in strains of *E. parasitica*, the cause of chestnut blight. Hypovirulent strains of this fungus contain two to five major dsRNA components (mol wts of 4.4×10^6 to 6.2×10^6), which are not detectable in virulent strains of this fungus [49]. When the dsRNA is transmitted by fungal anastomosis to a virulent strain, the recipient converts to hypovirulence [8]. Extracts of the converted strain contain the dsRNA components present in the original

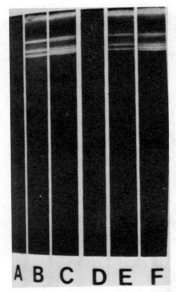

Figure 10 Major dsRNA components extracted from 0.5 g of a virulent (V) strain of *Endothia parasitica* (A,D); a hypovirulent (H_1) strain of this fungus (B,E); and a hypovirulent (H_2) strain produced following conversion of the virulent strain with strain H_1 (C,F), electrophoresed on 5% polyacrylamide gels, and stained with ethidium bromide. (From Ref. 40.)

hypovirulent strain (Fig. 10) [40]. Double-stranded RNA in this fungus is associated with the presence of pleomorphic, club-shaped particles with spherical heads (50-90 nm in diameter) and protrusions (25-300 nm in length). Since most fungal viruses are icosahedral, these pleomorphic particles may represent either an unusual type of fungal virus or the cellular site of accumulation of dsRNA.

Several studies that demonstrate a marked immunomodulating effect of unencapsidated fungal viral dsRNA on the mammalian immune system have been done. The dsRNA from *P. chrysogenum* viruses has been used as an effective adjuvant of antibody titer when it is given 24 h following immunogen inoculation, but it is most effective when administered simultaneously with the immunogen at the same inoculation site [39]. If dsRNA is inoculated into animals 24 h before an immunogen, however, it can have a marked immunosuppressive effect [39]. The immunosuppressive and immunopotentiating effects of dsRNA are also related to the concentration of dsRNA given. When 15 μg or less of dsRNA is inoculated into mice intraperitoneally followed immediately by an intraperitoneal immunogen inoculation, the antibody levels are suppressed, but 100 μg of dsRNA similarly administered is associated with enhanced antibody levels [46,90].

Inhibition of in vitro growth of lymphoma and sarcoma cells by mouse and rat peritoneal macrophages has been associated with treatment of these cells with dsRNA from *P. chrysogenum* viruses [6,7,68]. Alterations in the macrophages rather than release of any cytotoxic factor from the macrophages seems to be responsible for these effects [7].

Although relatively large doses of dsRNA (e.g., 500 μg) can produce marked toxicity in certain animals such as mice [1] and rats and dogs [41], primates seem to exhibit

Table 1 Colony-Forming Units (CFU)/Spleen of C57/B16 Mice Infected Sublethally with *Histoplasma capsulatum* and Treated with Mycoviral dsRNA Extracted from *Penicillium chrysogenum*

Group[a]	Mycoviral dsRNA (μg/mouse)[b]	CFU/spleen[c]	P[d]
1	—	28,750	—
2	10	3,075	<0.05
3	25	33	<0.05
4	50	42	<0.05
5	100	47	<0.05

[a]C57/B16 female mice, 9-10 weeks old, were used in all treatment groups. A sublethal dose of *H. capsulatum* (1×10^6 yeast cells) was inoculated intraperitoneally into each mouse (6 mice/group).

[b]Mice were given an intravenous inoculation of mycoviral dsRNA, extracted from *Penicillium chrysogenum*, 24 h following inoculation with *H. capsulatum*.

[c]Colony-forming units (CFU)/spleen represent the mean CFU/spleen for all mice in a given treatment group (6 mice/group).

[d]P represents a comparison between the mean CFU/spleen of each group with the mean CFU/spleen of the control group (no dsRNA treatment) analyzed by the Student's t-test.

minimal toxicity to this substance. It should be noted that many of the biological effects of dsRNA in mammals are observed at nontoxic concentrations of dsRNA.

Worthington and Hasenclever [89] reported that mice treated with 100 μg of poly-inosinic:polycytidylic (poly I:C) 1 day before infection with the fungi, or treated with 100 μg of poly I:C 1 day before the fungal injection, 1 day after the injection, and then every 2 days until a total of seven doses was given, demonstrated very severe *Candida albicans* and *Coccidioides immitis* infections. Since the dosage and inoculation schedule of dsRNA treatment markedly affects the immunomodulating activities of this molecule, later studies have shown that different dosages and inoculation schedules for the dsRNA treatment could decrease fungal virulence. When 50 μg or 100 μg of dsRNA extracted from the fungus *P. chrysogenum* were inoculated into C57B1/6 mice 24 h after challenge with a sublethal dose of *H. capsulatum,* the number of colony-forming units/spleen from dsRNA-treated mice was significantly less than the number of colony-forming units from the spleens of mice that were only challenged with the *Histoplasma capsulatum* (Table 1) (J. Olson and J. P. Adler, unpublished data).

The mechanism of action of dsRNA that might help to explain some of its biological effects could be related to its ability to induce interferon. Interferon induction in mice can be obtained by intraperitoneal injection of only 5 μg per mouse of dsRNA from *P. stoloniferum* viruses [10]; as little as 0.01 μg of dsRNA per mouse injected intravenously can induce measurable amounts of interferon [54].

For many years, only the antiviral effect of interferon was known [43]. Interferon makes host cells resistant to virus infection [62] by inducing the formation of other antiviral substances [70,91], such as endogenous, dsRNA-dependent, protein kinase which inhibits initiation of protein synthesis in the cells and which activates an endogenous nuclease that degrades viral mRNA [20,58,92]. Interferon-treated cells in the presence of ATP and dsRNA also produce another substance, iso-oligoadenylate,

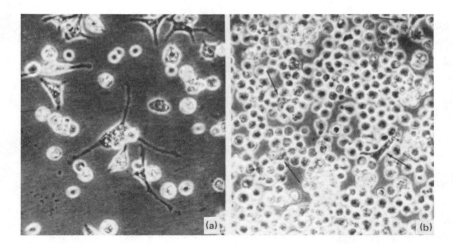

Figure 11 (a) Interferon (IF)-treated macrophages 72 h after challenge with MBL-2 leukemia cells. Macrophages appear well spread out, with granulation of cytoplasm. Very few viable leukemia cells were present (phase contrast, 250X). (b) Normal control macrophages 72 h after challenge with MBL-2 leukemia cells. Granulation was less marked in macrophages (arrows) with no evidence of dead cells or phagocytized debris. Leukemia (rounded) cells grow unhindered (phase contrast, 250X). (From Ref. 72. Vol. 197, pp. 674-676 © 1977 by the American Association for the Advancement of Science.)

which after a lag of 10 to 15 min inhibits protein synthesis in both L-cell extracts and reticulocyte lysates [53].

But interferon has other biological activities besides that of viral inhibition. It can inhibit normal and tumor cell growth [44]. Interferon can inhibit the humoral response if it is given prior to or approximately at the time of immunogen inoculation [50], but it can enhance the antibody response if it is administered a day or two after sensitization of the animal with the immunogen [50]. Similarly, interferon can inhibit the development of cellular immunity if it is given to the animal at or prior to the time of antigen exposure [37,38], but others have reported that interferon administration has been associated with enhanced cellular immunity that might be related, in part, to its ability to activate NK cells [38,44,73].

Interferon can increase the cytotoxicity of peritoneal macrophages for leukemia cells by a mechanism that does not seem to involve phagocytosis, and macrophages treated with interferon show accelerated spreading and marked cytoplasmic granulation (Fig. 11). Human interferon has been shown to increase degranulation of mast cells coated with IgE following contact with antigen or anti-IgE [49]. Interferon can also increase the toxicity of dsRNA for mammalian cells if cells are first treated with small amounts of interferon, and then incubated with either natural or synthetic dsRNA. A marked cytotoxic effect is seen in these cells a few hours after exposure to the dsRNA [75,76].

It is apparent from this review that little work has been done to elucidate the possible role of exogenously administered dsRNA and interferon on the course of fungal infections. These studies also suggest that the presence of dsRNA within the fungal pathogen may have some important effects on fungal virulence within the host. If pathogenic fungi, parasitized by dsRNA viruses, are destroyed by the host, some of the dsRNA from this fungus might be released into the host tissue in quantities sufficient to affect the host's immune response. Recent work has demonstrated that hypovirulent strains of *H. capsulatum* had 33% to 50% more dsRNA/g of fungal tissue than did hypervirulent strains of this fungus [66]. Further research in this area should help us to understand some of the complex interactions between fungal pathogens and their mammalian hosts.

REFERENCES

1. Absher, M., and W. R. Stinebring. 1969. Toxic properties of a synthetic double-stranded RNA. Endotoxin-like properties of poly I, poly C, an interferon stimulator. Nature (Lond.) *223*:715-717.

2. Adler, J. P. 1979. Screening for viruses in human pathogenic fungi. In H. P. Molitoris, M. Hollings, and H. A. Wood (Eds.), *Fungal Viruses,* Springer-Verlag, Berlin, pp. 129-137.

3. Adler, J. P., and D. W. Mackenzie. 1972. Intrahyphal localization of *Penicillium stoloniferum* viruses by fluorescent antibody. Abstr. Annu. Meet. Am. Soc. Microbiol., 1972, 68.

4. Adler, J. P., and U. Dempwolff. 1980. Double-stranded RNA associated with VLPs in *Histoplasma capsulatum.* Abstr. Annu. Meet. Am. Soc. Microbiol., 1980, 273.

5. Al-Aidroos, K. 1975. Biochemical genetics of the killer system in *Saccharomyces cerevisiae.* Ph.D. thesis, McGill University.

6. Alexander P. 1974. Multiple mechanisms involved in the antitumor action of endotoxin and double-stranded RNA. Johns Hopkins Med. J. *3*:321-332.

7. Alexander, P., and R. Evans. 1971. Endotoxin and double-stranded RNA render macrophages cytotoxic. Nature (Lond.) *232*:76-78.

8. Anagnostakis, S. L., and P. R. Day. 1979. Hypovirulence conversion in *Endothia parasitica.* Phytopathology *69*:1226-1229.

9. Baker, K. F., and C. A. Martinson. 1970. Epidemiology of diseases caused by *Rhizoctonia solani.* In J. R. Parmenter (Ed.), *Rhizoctonia solani, Biology and Pathology,* University of California Press, Berkeley, pp. 125-148.

10. Banks, G. T., K. W. Buck, E. B. Chain, F. Himmelweit, J. E. Marks, J. M. Tyler, M. Hollings, F. T. Last, and O. M. Stone. 1968. Viruses in fungi and interferon stimulation. Nature (Lond.) *218*:542-545.

11. Benigni, R., G. Ignazzitto, and L. Volterra. 1977. Double-stranded ribonucleic acid viruses in *Penicillium citrinum.* Appl. Environ. Microbiol. *34*:811-814.

12. Bevan, E. A., A. J. Herring, and D. J. Mitchell. 1973. Preliminary characterization of two species of dsRNA in yeast and their relationship to the "killer" character. Nature (Lond.) *245*:81-86.

13. Bevan, E. A., and D. J. Mitchell. 1979. The killer system in yeast. In P. A. Lemke (Ed.), *Viruses and Plasmids in Fungi,* Marcel Dekker, New York, pp. 161-199.

14. Borre, E., L. E. Morgantini, V. Ortali, and A. Tonolo. 1971. Production of lytic plaques of viral origin in *Penicillium.* Nature (Lond.) *229*:568-569.

15. Bostian, K. A., J. E. Hopper, D. T. Rogers, and D. J. Tipper. 1980. Translational analysis of the killer-associated virus-like particle dsRNA genome of *Saccharomyces cerevisiae*: M dsRNA encodes toxin. Cell *19*:403-414.

16. Bozarth, R. F. 1977. Biophysical and biochemical characterization of virus-like particles containing a high molecular weight dsRNA from *Helminthosporium maydis.* Virology *80*:149-157.

17. Bozarth, R. F. 1979. Physicochemical properties of mycoviruses: an overview. In H. P. Molitoris, M. Hollings, and H. A. Wood (Eds.), *Fungal Viruses,* Springer-Verlag, Berlin, pp. 48-61.

18. Bozarth, R. F. 1979. The physico-chemical properties of mycoviruses. In P. A. Lemke (Ed.), *Viruses and Plasmids in Fungi,* Marcel Dekker, New York, pp. 43-91.

19. Bozarth, R. F., H. A. Wood, and A. Mandelbrot. 1971. The *Penicillium stoloniferum* virus complex: two similar double-stranded RNA virus-like particles in a single cell. Virology *45*:516-523.

20. Brown, G. E., B. Lebleu, M. Kawakita, S. Shaila, G. C. Sen, and P. Lengyel. 1976. Increased endonuclease activity in an extract from mouse Ehrlich ascites tumor cells which had been treated with a partially purified interferon preparation: dependence on double-stranded RNA. Biochem. Biophys. Res. Commun. *69*: 114-122.

21. Buck, K. W. 1979. Replication of double-stranded RNA mycoviruses. In P. A. Lemke (Ed.), *Viruses and Plasmids in Fungi,* Marcel Dekker, New York, pp. 93-160.

22. Buck, K. W. 1980. Viruses and killer factors of fungi. In G. W. Gooday, D. Lloyd, and A. P. J. Trinci (Eds.), *The Eukaryotic Microbial Cell,* Society for General Microbiology Symposium 30. Cambridge University Press, Cambridge, pp. 329-374.

23. Buck, K. W., and R. F. Girvan. 1977. Comparison of the biophysical and biochemical properties of *Penicillium cyaneo-fulvum* virus and *Penicillium chrysogenum* virus. J. Gen. Virol. *34*:145-154.

24. Buck, K. W., R. F. Girvan, and G. Ratti. 1973. Two serologically distinct double-stranded ribonucleic acid viruses isolated from *Aspergillus niger.* Biochem. Soc. Trans. *1*:1138-1140.

25. Buck, K. W., and G. F. Kempson-Jones. 1970. Three types of virus particles in *Penicillium stoloniferum.* Nature (Lond.) *225*:945-946.

26. Buck, K. W., and G. F. Kempson-Jones. 1973. Biophysical properties of *Penicillium stoloniferum* virus. J. Gen. Virol. *18*:223-235.

27. Buck, K. W., and G. Ratti. 1977. Molecular weight of double-stranded RNA: a re-examination of *Aspergillus foetidus* virus S RNA components. J. Gen. Virol. *37*:215-219.

28. Bussey, H., and D. Sherman. 1973. Yeast killer factor: ATP leakage and coordinate inhibition of macromolecular synthesis in sensitive cells. Biochim. Biophys. Acta *298*:868-875.

29. Bussey, H., D. Sherman, and J. M. Somers. 1973. Action of yeast killer factor: a resistant mutant with sensitive spheroplasts. J. Bacteriol. *113*:1193-1197.

30. Bussey, H., and N. Skipper. 1975. Membrane-mediated killing of *Saccharomyces cerevisiae* by glycoproteins from *Torulopsis glabrata.* J. Bacteriol. *124*:476-483.

31. Castanho, B., and E. E. Butler. 1978. *Rhizoctonia* decline: a degenerative disease of *Rhizoctonia solani.* Phytopathology *68*:1505-1510.

32. Castanho, B., and E. E. Butler. 1978. *Rhizoctonia* decline: studies on hypovirulence and potential use in biological control. Phytopathology *68*: 1511-1514.

33. Castanho, B., E. E. Butler, and R. J. Shepherd. 1978. The association of double-stranded RNA with *Rhizoctonia* decline. Phytopathology *68*:1515-1519.

34. Caten, C. E. 1972. Vegetative incompatibility and cytoplasmic inheritance in fungi. J. Gen. Microbiol. *72*:221-229.

35. Cohn, M. S., C. W. Tabor, H. Tabor, and R. B. Wickner. 1978. Spermidine or spermine requirement for killer double-stranded RNA plasmid replication in yeast. J. Biol. Chem. *253*:5225-5227.

36. Day, P. R., J. A. Dodds, J. E. Elliston, R. A. Jaynes, and S. L. Anagnostakis. 1977. Double-stranded RNA in *Endothia parasitica*. Phytopathology *67*:1393-1396.

37. DeMaeyer-Guignard, J., A. Cachard, and E. DeMaeyer. 1975. Delayed-type hypersensitivity to sheep red blood cells: inhibition of sensitization by interferon. Science *190*:574-576.

38. DeMaeyer, E., and J. DeMaeyer. 1977. Effect of interferon on cell-mediated immunity. Tex. Rep. Biol. Med. *35*:370-374.

39. Dewdney, J. M. 1976. Clinical and veterinary application of double-stranded ribonucleic acid from fungal viruses. In D. A. Hems (Ed.), *Biologically Active Substances—Exploration and Exploitation*, Wiley, Chichester, pp. 149-169.

40. Dodds, J. A. 1980. Association of type 1 viral-like dsRNA with club-shaped particles in hypovirulent strains of *Endothia parasitica*. Virology *107*:1-12.

41. Field, A. K. 1973. Interferon induction by polynucleotides. In W. A. Carter (Ed.), *Selective Inhibitions of Viral Functions*, CRC Press, Cleveland, pp. 149-176.

42. Friedman, R. M. 1981. Production of interferons. *Interferons: A Primer*, Academic, New York, pp. 25-45.

43. Friedman, R. M. 1981. Mechanisms of antiviral action. *Interferons: A Primer*, Academic, New York, pp. 47-71.

44. Friedman, R. M. 1981. Other actions of interferons. *Interferons: A Primer*, Academic, New York, pp. 73-88.

45. Herring, A. J., and E. A. Bevan. 1977. Yeast virus-like particles possess a capsid-associated single-stranded RNA polymerase. Nature (Lond.) *268*:464-466.

46. Hewitt, C. W., and J. P. Adler. 1982. Murine immunosuppression with mycoviral dsRNA. Immunopharmacology. *5*:103-109.

47. Hollings, M. 1978. Mycoviruses: viruses that infect fungi. Adv. Virus Res. *22*:1-53.

48. Hopper, J. E., K. A. Bostian, L. B. Rowe, and D. J. Tipper. 1977. Translation of the L species double stranded RNA genome of the killer-associated virus-like particles of *Saccharomyces cerevisiae*. J. Biol. Chem. *252*:9010-9017.

49. Ida, S., J. J. Hooks, R. P. Siraganian, and A. L. Notkins. 1977. Enhancement of immunoglobulin E mediated histamine release from human basophils by viruses: role of interferon. J. Exp. Med. *145*:892-906.

50. Johnson, H. M. 1977. Effect of interferon on antibody formation. Tex. Rep. Biol. Med. *35*:357-369.

51. Kandel, J., and Y. Koltin. 1978. Killer phenomenon in *Ustilago maydis*: comparison of the killer proteins. Exp. Mycol. *2*:270-278.

52. Kandel, J. S., and T. A. Stern. 1979. The killer phenomenon in pathogenic yeast. Antimicrob. Agents Chemother. *15*:568-572.

53. Kerr, I. M., R. E. Brown, and A. G. Hovanessian. 1977. Nature of inhibitor of cell-free protein synthesis formed in response to interferon and double-stranded RNA. Nature (Lond.) *268*:540-542.

54. Kleinschmidt, W. J., L. F. Ellis, R. M. Van Frank, and E. B. Murphy. 1968. Interferon stimulation by a double stranded RNA of a mycophage in statolon preparations. Nature (Lond.) *220*:167-168.

55. Koltin, Y., and P. R. Day. 1975. Specificity of *Ustilago maydis* killer proteins. Appl. Microbiol. *30*:694-696.

56. Koltin, Y., and P. R. Day. 1976. Inheritance of killer phenotypes and double-stranded RNA in *Ustilago maydis*. Proc. Natl. Acad. Sci. U.S.A. *73*:594-598.

57. Koltin, Y., and P. R. Day. 1976. Suppression of the killer phenotype in *Ustilago maydis*. Genetics *82*:629-637.

58. Lebleu, B., G. C. Sen, S. Shaila, B. Cabrer, and P. Lengyel. 1976. Interferon, double-stranded RNA, and protein phosphorylation. Proc. Natl. Acad. Sci. U.S.A. *73*:3107-3111.

59. Lecoq, H., M. Boissonnet-Memes, and P. Delhotal. 1979. Infectivity and trans-
     mission of fungal viruses. In H. P. Molitoris, M. Hollings, and H. A. Wood (Eds.),
     Fungal Viruses, Springer-Verlag, Berlin, pp. 34-47.

60. Lemke, P. A. 1975. Biochemical and biological aspects of fungal viruses. In T.
     Hasegawa (Ed.), *Proc. 1st International Congress of IAMS,* Vol. 3, Science
     Council of Japan, Tokyo, pp. 380-395.

61. Lemke, P. A., C. A. Nash, and S. W. Pieper. 1973. Lytic plaque formation and
     variation in virus titre among strains of *Penicillium chrysogenum.* J. Gen.
     Microbiol. *76*:265-275.

62. Lindenmann, J., D. C. Burke, and A. Isaacs. 1957. Studies on the production,
     mode of action and properties of interferon. Br. J. Exp. Pathol. *38*:551-562.

63. Lister, R. M. 1979. Serological screening for fungal viruses. In H. P. Molitoris,
     M. Hollings, and H. A. Wood (Eds.), *Fungal Viruses,* Springer-Verlag, Berlin, pp.
     150-164.

64. Marino, R., K. N. Saksena, M. Schuler, J. E. Mayfield, and P. A. Lemke. 1976.
     Double-stranded RNA from *Agaricus bisporus.* Appl. Environ. Microbiol. *31*:
     433-438.

65. Nesterova, G. F., Y. U. Kyarner, and Y. O. Soom. 1973. Virus-like particles in
     Candida tropicalis. Mikrobiologiya *42*:162-164.

66. Newton, K., J. P. Adler, and D. H. Howard. 1982. Relationship between dsRNA
     concentration and virulence in *Histoplasma capsulatum.* Abstr. Annu. Meet. Am.
     Soc. Microbiol. 1982, 336.

67. Palfree, R. G. E., and H. Bussey. 1979. Yeast killer toxin: purification and
     characterization. Biochemistry *93*:487-493.

68. Parr, I., E. Wheeler, and P. Alexander. 1973. Similarities of the anti-tumour
     actions of endotoxin, lipid A and double-stranded RNA. Br. J. Cancer *27*:370-
     389.

69. Philliskirk, G., and T. W. Young. 1975. The occurrence of killer character in
     yeasts of various genera. Antonie van Leeuwenhoek J. Microbiol. Serol. *41*:147-
     151.

70. Radke, K. L., C. Colby, J. R. Kates, H. M. Krider, and D. M. Prescott. 1974.
     Establishment and maintenance of the interferon-induced antiviral state: studies
     in enucleated cells. J. Virol. *13*:623-630.

71. Rawlinson, C. J., D. Hornby, V. Pearson, and J. M. Carpenter. 1973. Virus-like
     particles in the take-all fungus, *Gaeumannomyces graminis.* Ann. Appl. Biol.
     74:197-209.

72. Schultz, R. M., J. D. Papamatheakis, and M. A. Chirigos. 1977. Interferon:
     an inducer of macrophage activation by polyanions. Science *197*:674-676.

73. Senik, A., J. P. Kolb, A. Orn, and M. Gidlund. 1980. Study of the mechanism
     for *in vitro* activation of mouse NK cells by interferon. Scand. J. Immunol. *12*:
     51-60.

74. Skipper, N., and H. Bussey. 1977. Mode of action of yeast toxin: energy re-
     quirement for *Saccharomyces cerevisiae* killer toxin. J. Bacteriol. *129*:668-677.

75. Stewart, W. E., II, E. DeClercq, A. Billiau, J. Desmyter, and P. DeSomer. 1972.
     Increased susceptibility of cells treated with interferon to the toxicity of poly-
     riboinosinic-polyribocytidylic acid. Proc. Natl. Acad. Sci. U.S.A. *69*:1851-1854.

76. Stewart, W. E., II, E. DeClercq, and P. DeSomer. 1973. Specificity of interferon-
     induced enhancement of toxicity for double-stranded ribonucleic acids. J. Gen.
     Virol. *18*:237-246.

77. Stumm, C., J. M. H. Hermans, E. J. Middlebeck, A. F. Croes, and G. J. M. L.
     DeVries. 1977. Killer-sensitive relationships in yeast from natural habitats.
     Antonie van Leeuwenhoek J. Microbiol. Serol. *43*:125-128.

78. Sweeney, K. T., A. Tate, and G. R. Fink. 1976. A study of the transmission and structure of double-stranded RNAs associated with the killer phenomenon in *Saccharomyces cerevisiae*. Genetics *84*:27-42.

79. Tikchonenko, T. I., G. A. Velikodvorskaya, A. F. Bobkova, Y. E. Bartschevich, E. P. Lebed, N. M. Chaplygina, and T. S. Maksimova. 1974. New fungal viruses capable of reproducing in bacteria. Nature (Lond.) *249*:454-456.

80. van Zaayen, A. 1979. Mushroom viruses. In P. A. Lemke (Ed.), *Viruses and Plasmids in Fungi,* Marcel Dekker, New York, pp. 239-324.

81. Vodkin, M., F. Katterman, and G. R. Fink. 1974. Yeast killer mutants with altered double-stranded ribonucleic acid. J. Bacteriol. *117*:681-686.

82. Wickner, R. B. 1974. "Killer character" of *Saccharomyces cerevisiae*: curing by growth at elevated temperatures. J. Bacteriol. *117*:1356-1357.

83. Wickner, R. B. 1974. Chromosomal and nonchromosomal mutations affecting the "killer character" of *Saccharomyces cerevisiae*. Genetics *76*:423-432.

84. Wickner, R. B. 1976. Killer of *Saccharomyces cerevisiae*: a double-stranded ribonucleic acid plasmid. Bacteriol. Rev. *40*(3):757-773.

85. Wickner, R. B., and M. J. Leibowitz. 1976. Two chromosomal genes required for killing expression in killer strains of *Saccharomyces cerevisiae*. Genetics *82*:429-442.

86. Wood, H. A., and R. F. Bozarth. 1972. Properties of virus-like particles of *Penicillium chrysogenum*: one double-stranded RNA molecule per particle. Virology *47*:604-609.

87. Wood, H. A., and R. F. Bozarth. 1973. Heterokaryon transfer of virus-like particles and a cytoplasmically inherited determinant in *Ustilago maydis*. Phytopathology *63*:1019-1021.

88. Wood, H. A., R. F. Bozarth, J. Adler, and D. W. Mackenzie. 1974. Proteinaceous virus-like particles from an isolate of *Aspergillus flavus*. J. Virol. *13*:532-534.

89. Worthington, M., and H. F. Hasenclever. 1972. Effect of an interferon stimulator, polyinosinic:polycytidylic acid, on experimental fungus infections. Infect. Immun. *5*:199-202.

90. Wright, C., J. P. Adler, and G. Roberts. 1981. Immunomodulation of C57/ black 6 mice by polyinosinic:polycytidylic acid (poly I:C) and fungal viral double-stranded RNA (dsRNA). Abstr. Annu. Meet. Am. Soc. Microbiol. 1981, 58.

91. Young, C. S. H., C. R. Pringle, and E. A. C. Follett. 1975. Action of interferon in enucleated cells. J. Virol. *15*:428-430.

92. Zilberstein, A., P. Federman, L. Shulman, and M. Revel. 1976. Specific phosphorylation *in vitro* of a protein associated with ribosomes of interferon-treated mouse L cells. FEBS Lett. *68*:119-124.

4

Phagocytic Mechanisms in Host Response

Jacob Fleischmann / UCLA School of Medicine, Los Angeles, California

Robert I. Lehrer / UCLA School of Medicine, Los Angeles, and VA Medical Center, West Los Angeles, California

I. INTRODUCTION

Phagocytic cells interact with fungi in several ways. They ingest spores or vegetative cells and sequester them in vacuoles whose pH, nutrient content, or ionic composition may be inimical to germination or growth. They generate, concentrate, or mobilize molecules capable of damaging fungal cells. Finally, in some instances they provide nurturing environments for well-adapted facultative intracellular parasites such as *Histoplasma capsulatum*.

It is worth recalling that the pioneering, century-old observations of Eli Metchnikoff that established the biological importance of phagocytic defenses concerned a fungus, then called *Monospora bicuspidata*, and abdominal cavity phagocytes of the water flea *Daphnia*. More recently, many laboratories have charted the roles of phagocytic leukocytes in resistance to fungal infection.

Our chapter reviews fungicidal mechanisms of phagocytes and summarizes recent literature describing interactions between fungi and leukocytes. Readers seeking a more comprehensive treatment of leukocyte physiology, metabolism, and antimicrobial defenses will be aided by several excellent reviews [99,190,191].

It should be appreciated that information in this area, although increasing, is incomplete. A reasonable outline of the antifungal properties of granulocytes can be presented, but the functions of mononuclear phagocytes (blood monocytes, tissue macrophages) are imperfectly understood. In large part, this is due to the inherent complexity of the mononuclear phagocyte system. There are profound biochemical and physiological differences between blood monocytes and tissue macrophages, between macrophages in different tissue locales, and between mononuclear phagocytes of different host species. Even before the subtleties of "activation," subpopulations and alteration by artificial tissue culture systems are brought into play, adequate opportunities for confusion exist. Having raised the problem of fractional knowledge and imparted (or at least implied) the appropriate notes of caution, we begin by considering some specific aspects of phagocyte biology.

II. FUNGICIDAL MECHANISMS

Phagocytic cells express two general types of antimicrobial mechanisms: oxygen-dependent and oxygen-independent. The former class reflects the presence of an activatable, membrane-associated enzyme system, NAD(P)H oxidase [64,98]. Phagocytosis or appropriate membrane perturbation by soluble or particulate stimuli results in activation of this oxidase, which catalyzes the following primary reaction: $NADPH + 2 O_2 \rightarrow NADP^+ + 2 O_2^- + H^+$. In this reaction, a molecule of reduced pyridine nucleotide is oxidized and two molecules of oxygen are reduced univalently, by one electron each, to form two molecules of superoxide anion.

Superoxide anions are relatively unstable and undergo rapid dismutation to hydrogen peroxide and oxygen, as follows: $2 O_2^- + 2 H^+ \rightarrow H_2O_2$. Dismutation occurs spontaneously, favored by low pH, or is enzymatically catalyzed by superoxide dismutases found in all eucaryotic and aerobic procaryotic cells [63].

Hydrogen peroxide and superoxide anions undergo additional reactions, especially when trace amounts of transition metal ions are present. For example, more powerful oxidizing species such as hydroxyl radicals $(OH^{\cdot})$ can be generated by the Fenton Reaction: $H_2O_2 + Fe^{2+} \rightarrow OH^{\cdot} + OH^- + Fe^{3+}$. Iron bound to the protein lactoferrin, a major constituent of neutrophil specific granules, can support hydroxyl radical generation in this process [1].

The congenital disorder, chronic granulomatous disease (CGD), has afforded a remarkable opportunity to examine the role of NAD(P)H oxidase and oxidative metabolism in phagocyte biology. Granulocytes and monocytes of affected subjects are usually totally deficient in ability to generate O_2^- and H_2O_2 via NAD(P)H oxidase, and their normally phagocytic leukocytes demonstrate selectively impaired microbicidal activity [99]. Impaired phagocyte fungicidal activity is thought to underlie the frequent occurrence of severe *Aspergillus* and *Candida* infections in CGD. A recent review reported 50 cases of systemic infection by fungi among 245 patients with CGD [28].

Not only do normal mammalian phagocytes respond to particulate stimuli such as fungi by greatly augmenting their oxygen consumption to produce molecules such as O_2^-, H_2O_2, and $OH^{\cdot}$ that can be directed against the fungal target, in addition, they may contain an enzyme, myeloperoxidase (MPO), that greatly potentiates the antimicrobial effects of H_2O_2.

As demonstrated by Klebanoff [97] and others, MPO-mediated antimicrobial activity in cell-free systems requires not only MPO, but also H_2O_2, and an oxidizable cofactor such as iodide or chloride ions. When microorganisms are exposed to MPO + H_2O_2 + I^-, the microbial targets are iodinated as well as killed [96]. When Cl^- ions replace I^-, conversion of amino acids to chloramines and aldehydes has been shown [173,199]. In addition, much evidence points to the production of hypochlorous acid, HOCl, both in cell-free systems [74] and by phagocytic normal human granulocytes. Cell-free MPO-H_2O_2-halide systems have been shown to kill various fungal spores, yeast cells, and hyphae in vitro [41,106a,120].

Myeloperoxidase is present in the primary (azurophil) granules of normal human neutrophils and is released both into phagocytic vacuoles and to the exterior when neutrophils are exposed to fungi, such as *Candida albicans,* under appropriate conditions. Although bone marrow promonocytes and most blood monocytes contain MPO, this enzyme disappears during their in vitro or in vivo maturation to macrophages. Eosinophils of many mammalian species, including man, contain a peroxidase enzyme that is structurally and genetically distinct from the neutrophil and monocyte enzyme [47a,162].

Detection of individuals with hereditary myeloperoxidase deficiency, an autosomal recessive trait, wherein affected homozygous subjects have neutrophils and monocytes totally devoid of MPO activity, has allowed careful dissection of the role of MPO in the antimicrobial arsenal of phagocytes. Although MPO appears to be essential for effective killing of *C. albicans* by human neutrophils and monocytes [42,112,118], other *Candida* species such as *C. parapsilosis, C. pseudotropicalis,* and *C. krusei* are killed effectively by MPO-deficient neutrophils [110]. Certain of these (*C. parapsilosis* and *C. pseudotropicalis*) are also killed normally by neutrophils from subjects with chronic granulomatous disease [110]. Several overall conclusions can be drawn from these observations. *Candida albicans* is relatively resistant to human neutrophils and its eradication requires both MPO and H_2O_2. Other *Candida* species are evidently killed by oxygen-independent neutrophil mechanisms that require neither MPO nor H_2O_2. These oxygen-independent mechanisms of human neutrophils are ineffective against *C. albicans.*

Myeloperoxidase-deficient monocytes are impaired in their ability to kill *C. albicans,* but are highly effective against *C. parapsilosis* and *C. pseudotropicalis.* Chronic granulomatous disease monocytes, which are unable to generate O_2^- and H_2O_2, can kill none of the aforementioned organisms. Thus, candidacidal activity in human monocytes appears to be invariably oxygen-dependent and to occur by MPO-dependent and MPO-independent pathways. The oxygen-independent candidacidal mechanisms of human neutrophils appear to lack direct functional counterparts in human blood monocytes. Sasada and Johnston recently reported studies on mouse peritoneal macrophages, also suggesting the primacy of oxygen-dependent killing mechanisms for *C. albicans* and *C. parapsilosis* in this cell type [164].

The ability of leukocytes to kill some fungi in the absence of oxidative metabolism may reflect the presence, in certain leukocytes, of proteins and peptides with intrinsic antifungal activity. Rabbit granulocytes, for example, possess a family of at least five arginine-rich, low molecular weight peptides ("lysosomal cationic proteins") that include *C. albicans* among their broad antimicrobial spectrum. Analogous peptides are present in guinea pig leukocytes [122]. Two related peptides, macrophage cationic peptides, MCP-1 and MCP-2, have been recovered from rabbit lung macrophages, where they constitute 1.7% of the total protein/peptide content of cells activated by a mycobacterial antigen [125]. MCP-1 and MCP-2 contain 33 amino acids each, differing in but a single amino acid residue [172]. They are highly fungicidal at concentrations ≥ 1 μg/ml in vitro against *Candida* species and *Cryptococcus neoformans*.

Although human neutrophils lack lysosomal cationic proteins of the type found in rabbit granulocytes, their granules do contain constituents with antifungal activity. Most prominent are several isozymes of a 25-28,000-dalton, highly cationic protein with chymotrypsin-like protease activity (chymotrypsin-like cationic protein, CLCP or cathepsin G) [139,140]. The fungicidal activity of CLCP resists treatments (boiling, covalently-bound active site inhibitors) that abrogate its enzyme activity, indicating the independence of these properties [122,139].

Other granulocyte constituents may also contribute to host defenses against fungi. Iron-free (apo)lactoferrin can, by tightly complexing iron necessary for optimal fungal growth, inhibit the growth of *Candida albicans* in vitro [95]. Apolactoferrin, prepared from human colostrum, has been reported to kill *C. albicans* in vitro [3]. *Coccidioides immitis* [29] and *Cryptococcus neoformans* [66] are reportedly susceptible to killing by lysozyme, a hydrolase found in granulocytes and macrophages of most species, including man [151]. These reports require confirmation.

Leukocytes contain phospholipases that can cleave membrane triglycerides to form free fatty acids and lysolecithins, intermediates that might participate in antifungal activity. Phospholipase A2, known to be activated by phagocytosis, would be a likely candidate for such a role [57].

At present, it is not known whether human monocytes or macrophages possess antifungal (or antimicrobial) components, other than lysozyme, analogous to any of those described above. This is an important area for future investigations.

III. SPECIFIC FUNGI

A. *Candida*

Fungi of the genus *Candida* have been used most commonly to probe the antifungal properties of phagocytes [113,114]. *Candida albicans,* an opportunistic human pathogen, most often reaches tissues via the circulation from the gastro intestinal tract [104] or from intravenous catheters.

Leukopenia, due to bone marrow suppressive disease or therapy, greatly reduces resistance to *C. albicans* infection. Although normal dogs tolerate 10^7 *C. albicans* organisms administered intravenously, injection of 10^6 organisms results in widespread disseminated candidiasis in leukopenic animals. Such impaired hosts are afforded substantial protection against *Candida* by granulocyte transfusions [161]. Studies with intraperitoneally placed diffusion chambers in mice also point to the important contribution of phagocytes to clearing sites of *C. albicans* in vivo [34]. The increased incidence of fungal infection among patients with phagocytic disorders such as CGD and myeloperoxidase deficiency suggests that intact phagocyte function contributes substantially in man to systemic defenses against *Candida* species.

Clearance of intravenously injected organisms from rabbit blood shows biphasic kinetics. Approximately 99% of the organisms leave the blood within 10 min, followed by a longer period of low-grade fungemia. Depending on route of injection, different organs predominate in clearance. After peripheral venous injections, lungs take up 45% of the total inoculum; after mesenteric vein injection, liver takes up almost 60% [4]. Mice injected with live, but not formalin-killed, *C. albicans* evidenced accelerated reticuloendothelial clearance of carbon particles [14].

Whole human blood is fungicidal for *C. albicans*, killing both blastoconidia and organisms bearing pseudohyphae up to 200 μm in length [35]. The candidacidal activity of blood is primarily attributable to its leukocytes, as neither plasma nor serum alone kill *C. albicans* [53]. Polymorphonuclear leukocytes play a principal role in resistance to experimental systemic candidiasis [85]. Thymus-dependent cell-mediated immunity appears not to contribute substantially, judged from studies with congenitally athymic (nude) mice [34,159].

In a quantitative vital staining (methylene blue) assay, polymorphonuclear leukocytes (PMNs) from normal human donors killed 29% ± 7.4% of ingested *C. albicans* after 60 min [117]. Serum, although required for efficient phagocytosis, did not facilitate killing of ingested organisms in one study [117], but did apparently do so in another [169]. As already noted, PMNs from patients with myeloperoxidase deficiency or CGD, have virtually no ability to kill ingested *C. albicans* [117].

In a different assay system, employing Giemsa staining of methanol-fixed preparations, human PMNs killed and degraded 28.1 ± 7.6% of ingested *C. albicans* after 2.5 h of incubation [107]. Human monocytes, studied in the presence of neutrophils by the same technique, killed and degraded 63.4 ± 10.2% of ingested organisms by 2.5 h [112]. Purified monocytes killed 27.2 ± 2.0% of ingested *C. albicans* in the absence of granulocytes [112]. A study employing colony counts to measure intracellular killing found a 58% and 50% rate for granulocytes and monocytes, respectively, after 60 min of incubation [126], confirming earlier results by this method [108].

As hyphal and pseudohyphal forms figure prominently in invasive candidiasis, phagocytic behavior also has been examined with these forms [39]. A comparison of monocytes and granulocytes, using yeast cells and pseudohyphae of *C. albicans* and yeasts of *C. tropicalis* and *Saccharomyces cerevisiae* as targets, revealed that monocytes ingested all but *C. albicans* pseudohyphae more rapidly than neutrophils. Intracellular killing was assessed by a fluorochromatic assay that we believe to be of uncertain validity and suggested that monocytes killed two to three times more of the targets than did neutrophils. The discrepancy was most marked with regard to *C. albicans* pseudohyphae [171]. In another study, *C. albicans* yeast cells were induced to germinate by cultivation in a mixture of human serum, cysteine, and sodium thioglycollate. Sixty minutes after mixing yeast cells or germlings with human PMNs, 92% of the yeasts and 9.5% of the germlings had been ingested. Candidacidal rates were 29% for yeast cells and 5.5% for germlings [168]. Hyphal *C. albicans* cells were also more resistant to killing by murine phagocytes in studies using in vivo diffusion chambers [34].

Radioisotopic studies demonstrated 53% inhibition by human neutrophils of [^{14}C]-cytosine uptake by pseudohyphal *C. albicans* in the absence of serum. Microscopic and metabolic studies showed that neutrophils attached and spread over the surface of pseudohyphae, degranulated, developed augmented oxidative metabolism and appeared to damage the organisms [42]. Neutrophils from patients with hereditary myeloperoxidase (MPO) deficiency and chronic granulomatous disease failed to damage hyphae when studied with the same isotope system. In vitro-generated (per)oxidizing molecular species, representing substances formed during the phagocyte's metabolic processes, were damaging to hyphae and inhibition of this system prevented fungal damage. These data suggest a primary role for the neutrophil's oxidative fungicidal system(s) in controlling tissue invasion by *C. albicans* [41] similar to that earlier shown for yeast-phase organisms. *Candida albicans* hyphae may be more than passive targets for host phagocytes. Leukocytes attach preferentially to live rather than dead hyphae, and growing *Candida* hyphae release low molecular weight anionic constituents that inhibit neutrophil attachment to live hyphae, as well as chemotaxis and respiratory burst activity [47].

The role of heat-stable and heat-labile (56°C, 30 min) serum components in phago-cytosis and killing has been studied. In one study [163], the heat-stable opsonic factor of normal human serum was believed to be naturally occurring, low-level anti-*Candida* IgG. High antibody concentrations, typically present in serum from individuals with chronic mucocutaneous candidiasis or some patients with disseminated candidiasis, inhibited candidacidal activity by normal neutrophils without significantly impairing phagocytic uptake [84,105,192]. Most studies have shown that complement enhances phagocytosis, and suggested that both classical and alternative systems are involved [60, 91,136,137,176,179,198]. Chemotaxis of PMNs is induced by components of *C. albicans* that include cell wall mannans [33,36,194].

Some data concerning in vivo candidacidal activity of macrophages is available. By 15 min after tail vein injection, *C. albicans* appears within murine hepatic macrophages. The ingested yeasts lose their gram stain reactivity by 48 h and PAS staining thereafter. Granulomas, possibly glucan-induced, persist for weeks [130].

Normal rat livers clear *C. albicans* from perfusates, but their candidacidal activity is negligible. Livers from animals that received prior vaccination with *Corynebacterium parvum* killed approximately 40% of the cleared *Candida albicans*. This fungicidal activity was reversed by silica, phenylbutazone, and iodoacetate [166]. Phenylbutazone, but not iodoacetate, is reported to inhibit killing of *C. albicans* by human blood mono-cytes [112]. In contrast, iodoacetate, but not phenylbutazone, blocked killing of *C. albicans* by rabbit lung macrophages [124]. Such discrepancies emphasize the heter-ogeneity of mononuclear phagocyte fungicidal mechanisms according to host species and/or tissue location.

In a murine model wherein diffusion chambers with different pore sizes (0.45 μm and 3 μm) were implanted intraperitoneally, killing of *C. albicans* required phagocytic cells. Thioglycollate-induced peritoneal macrophages from BALB/c mice restricted growth of *C. albicans,* but did not kill them. Macrophages from nude mice reduced the number of *C. albicans* by 80-90% in 24 h when added at high ($\geqslant$ 40:1) macrophage: yeast cell ratios [34].

More information deals with the in vitro performance of various macrophage popula-tions. Resident (unstimulated) mouse peritoneal macrophages, grown in tissue culture medium for 24 h, rapidly ingested six species of *Candida* in the presence of 10-20% homologous serum. Within 2 h, intracellular replication by germ tubes (*C. albicans*) or budding (other *Candida* spp.) was noted. By 24 h, macrophages cultured with *C. albicans* or *C. tropicalis* had been destroyed. In contrast, macrophages incubated with *C. parapsilosis, C. pseudotropicalis, C. krusei,* and *C. guilliermondii* remained viable for an additional 24-48 h. The authors speculated that macrophages were un-likely to contribute effectually toward host defenses against dissemination of candidal infections [180].

Ozato and Uesake used [^{3}H]leucine or [^{3}H]uridine uptake with radioautography to study the ability of caseinate-elicited mouse peritoneal macrophages to inhibit *C. albicans* [145]. By 2 h, ingested organisms displayed no isotope uptake, despite significant incorporation by extracellular fungi. Intracellular growth of *C. albicans* commenced by 3 h and resulted in rapid destruction of the macrophages.

Colony counting was used to compare resident peritoneal macrophages with cells obtained from lipopolysaccharide (LPS)- or *Bacille Calmette-Guérin* (BCG)-treated mice. Resident macrophages killed 10% of *C. albicans* in 3 h, compared with 27% for LPS-elicited cells and 23% for BCG-elicited cells. In contrast, *C. parapsilosis* was killed much more efficiently, as follows: resident macrophages, 72%; lipopolysaccharide-elicited cells, 84%; and BCG-elicited cells, 81% [164]. Muramyl dipeptide, a synthetic adjuvant, increased fungicidal activity of overnight-cultured mouse peritoneal macrophages against *C. albicans* in vivo [31] and *C. parapsilosis* in vitro [138].

Mouse alveolar macrophages were reported to ingest and kill 54.5% of *C. krusei* in the presence of nonimmune serum and complement factors. Macrophages from mice with parainfluenza-1 virus infections showed significantly diminished candidacidal ability, despite intact powers of ingestion [193].

Other investigators examined rabbit peritoneal and alveolar macrophages. In a study comparing normal alveolar macrophages with those obtained from *C. albicans*-immunized rabbits, immune macrophages in immune serum displayed the most effective ingestive powers, but immune and control macrophages were believed to have equivalent candidacidal activity [2]. Another study compared resident macrophages with macrophages elicited by prior in vivo injection of complete Freund's adjuvant (CFA). Resident (unelicited) alveolar macrophages destroyed approximately 28% of ingested *C. albicans* after 4 h, whereas resident peritoneal macrophages killed 15%. Peritoneal macrophages from animals pretreated with CFA manifested enhanced candidacidal activity (28% in 4 h), and CFA-elicited alveolar macrophages killed 32% of ingested *C. albicans* after 4 h [124]. In a limited study of antecedent BCG stimulation, BCG-elicited rabbit peritoneal and alveolar macrophages showed candidacidal activity for *C. albicans* that was similar to that of their unstimulated counterparts [69]. The study, which employed intracellular vital staining with methylene blue, reported higher estimates of macrophage candidacidal activity with 42-45% of ingested organisms killed in 1 h. An assay based on [^{3}H]leucine incorporation reported a 71-93% inhibition of macromolecular synthesis by *C. albicans* ingested by alveolar macrophages consistent with fungistatic and/or fungicidal activity [149].

Data on interactions of human macrophages with *Candida* spp. are limited. The ability of human alveolar macrophages to ingest *C. albicans* depends on energy provided by both oxidative and glycolytic metabolism. Although able to kill ingested *Listeria monocytogenes*, they failed to kill yeast cells of *C. albicans* [27]. In a study comparing smokers and nonsmokers, 18% of *C. pseudotropicalis* were killed in 90 min by alveolar macrophages from both groups [187]. Macrophages from human milk could ingest *C. albicans* in the presence of milk, but their candidacidal activity was not determined [158]. Immunofluorescence studies of tissues from patients with systemic candidiasis have shown damaged-appearing *Candida* within fixed macrophages [186]. Such observations could reflect either the intrinsic fungicidal competence of macrophages or merely uptake by macrophages of *Candida* rendered nonviable by other host factors. Macrophages, derived by cultivating human blood monocytes in vitro, retain their ability to take up and digest heat-killed *C. albicans* [142], but lose their ability to kill viable *C. albicans* yeast cells [106].

1. Clinical Studies

Myeloperoxidase deficiency may occur either as a congenital or acquired disorder. In hereditary myeloperoxidase deficiency, the enzyme is lacking in all neutrophils and monocytes. Eosinophils, which contain large amounts of a structurally distinct peroxidase, are unaffected and stain normally with peroxidase stains.

Hereditary myeloperoxidase deficiency, especially in association with diabetes mellitus, can predispose to serious systemic *Candida* infection. Although these patients have lifelong MPO deficiency, their *Candida* infections typically occur after the onset of diabetes, which may be clinically mild. Neutrophils from patients with hereditary MPO deficiency phagocytize *Candida* normally, but are greatly impaired in their ability to kill *C. albicans* and certain other *Candida* species, including *C. tropicalis, C. stellatoidea,* and *C. krusei* [23,110,118]. Myeloperoxidase-deficient neutrophils also kill selected bacteria at a reduced rate [22,121].

Recently, with the advent of automated equipment for analyzing blood counts by flow cytometry, it has become apparent that the incidence of MPO deficiency is higher than previously suspected. In a population of 60,000 patients tested at Stamford Hospital over 40 months, 28 MPO-deficient persons were identified. Fourteen of these had completely MPO-deficient leukocytes and the others had partially deficient cells. Only four of the affected persons had infectious problems. The most serious of these occurred in a 30-year-old woman with insulin-dependent diabetes mellitus, who developed fatal pneumonia caused by *C. albicans* and *C. parapsilosis.* Another patient, a 32-year-old man with partial MPO deficiency (50% of his neutrophils lacked MPO) developed an appendiceal abscess complicated by two episodes of bacteremia caused by *Bacteroides fragilis.* In vitro, the MPO-deficient neutrophils exhibited a markedly impaired ability to kill *C. albicans,* but only minor defects in killing *Staphylococcus aureus* [148].

Including the recent report of Parry et al. [148], a total of 29 individuals with complete hereditary myeloperoxidase deficiency have been reported. Five of these had evidently increased susceptibility to infection, manifested in four instances by systemic *Candida* infection [22,23,118,135,148]. Three of the four patients with systemic *Candida* infection also had diabetes mellitus. Given the unexpectedly high incidence, approximately one affected patient per 2100 population, of myeloperoxidase deficiency suggested by the Stamford, Connecticut, study and estimating the prevalence of diabetes to be approximately 2% [100], then approximately one individual per 100,000 would have both conditions coexisting. Such considerations lead us to agree with the views of Parry et al. [148] that diabetics in whom severe fungal infection develops should be screened for the presence of MPO deficiency. In addition, patients with known MPO deficiency who are diabetic or receive broad spectrum antibiotics should be observed closely for complicating systemic candidiasis.

A striking example of acquired myeloperoxidase deficiency was provided by a patient with refractory megaloblastic anemia. His PMNs, 99.2% of which were completely MPO-deficient, showed greatly impaired killing of ingested *C. albicans* and *C. tropicalis.* A bactericidal defect was present for *S. aureus,* but *Streptococcus faecalis* was killed normally by his PMNs. Unlike CGD neutrophils, his PMNs showed intact postphagocytic stimulation of oxygen consumption. The patient succumbed to fungal pneumonia, caused by *Aspergillus fumigatus, C. albicans,* and disseminated aspergillosis [123].

Acquired myeloperoxidase deficiency, sometimes noted in conjunction with a number of hematologic disorders [123] is seldom complete and may coexist with other abnormalities of leukocyte composition or metabolism.

Neutrophils from healthy pregnant women ingested C. guilliermondii normally, but killed and degraded these organisms only 65% as well as normal controls, with recovery of neutrophil function by 6 weeks postpartum. Neutrophil myeloperoxidase activity was noted to be decreased to 55% of control levels during pregnancy [56]. Although MPO and H_2O_2 form a potent candidacidal system, the fact that subjects genetically heterozygous for MPO deficiency have PMNs with intact ability to kill C. albicans makes it unlikely that any transient candidacidal defect of pregnancy is solely attributable to decreased MPO levels.

An unusual case report describes an otherwise healthy 15-year-old female who developed severe disseminated candidiasis including fungemia, gastric perforations, and peritonitis. Her normally phagocytic neutrophils consistently killed C. albicans approximately half as well as controls. The cause of this defect, which persisted for a year after her clinical recovery, was not established despite extensive testing [181]. Her neutrophils were neither MPO-deficient, nor did they appear to lack the chymotrypsin-like cationic proteins also reported to be active against C. albicans. Their microbicidal defect was selective; Staphylococcus aureus, Escherichia coli, Group-D Streptococcus, and C. parapsilosis were all killed with normal efficacy.

Patients with neoplasms are predisposed to systemic candidal infections especially while receiving immunosuppressive therapy. Polymorphonuclear leukocytes from patients with acute leukemias are generally able to ingest C. albicans normally, but frequently manifest decreased candidacidal activity [68,119,160]. Polymorphonuclear leukocytes from patients with chronic granulocytic leukemia have been reported to kill C. albicans [68] but not C. guilliermondii [55] normally. Subjects with myeloid metaplasia, polycythemia vera, untreated metastatic solid tumors, Hodgkin's disease, and other lymphomas had PMNs with normal candidacidal activity for C. albicans. Patients receiving chemotherapy or radiation therapy for these conditions often had PMNs with diminished candidacidal activity [119]. Another study using C. guilliermondii to study PMNs from patients with various leukemias and lymphomas noted the frequent occurrence (12 of 24 patients) of candidacidal defects, frequently corrected in vitro by addition of levamisole [25].

Although neonates, generally considered to be relatively immunocompromised hosts, were reported to have neutrophils with decreased candidacidal activity [197], this finding has not been confirmed [143,150]. Malnourished children, known to harbor large concentrations of Candida spp. in their upper intestinal tracts, were found to have neutrophils with significantly decreased neutrophil candidacidal activity [189].

2. Other Studies

The effects of various antibiotics on the ability of phagocytes to ingest and kill C. albicans have been reported. Sulfonamides interfered with killing of ingested C. albicans by PMNs by inhibiting with myeloperoxidase-mediated reactions [24,90, 108]. Penicillin, tetracycline, chloramphenicol, and gentamicin did not interfere with PMN candidacidal activity in one study [90], although five aminoglycosides (including gentamicin) inhibited this function in another [61].

Prostaglandin E_1 (PGE_1) and theophylline, substances that modulate intracellular cAMP levels, inhibit the candidacidal activity (C. albicans) of human neutrophils [15] and monocytes [112]. Phenylbutazone is, in vitro, a potent inhibitor of human PMN

[111] and monocyte candidacidal [112] and digestive [141] activity. As hydrocortisone lacks such activity in granulocytes [93,111], the ability of such corticosteroids to inhibit chemotactic entry of leukocytes into *Candida*-infected tissues may underlie its in vivo impairment of anti-*Candida* defenses [39,127]. Corticosteroids have been reported to inhibit candidacidal activity by human monocytes in vitro in some experiments [157] but not in others [112].

Escherichia coli endotoxin reportedly reduced ingestion and degradation of ^{125}I-labeled *C. albicans* by human monocytes [73]. Hyperosmolar conditions decreased ingestion and killing of *C. albicans* by human neutrophils in vitro [92]. Normal phagocytosis but decreased cidal activity against *C. albicans* has been reported in PMNs from children with thalassaemia [54]. Amphotericin B-resistant *C. tropicalis* developed in a patient whose neutrophils displayed diminished candidacidal activity, most marked in autologous serum, against both *C. tropicalis* and *C. albicans* [48].

Human eosinophils ingest and kill *C. albicans* in vitro at a rate similar to neutrophils, and their phagocytic activity also depends on immunoglobulin and complement components [86,87,109]. Eosinophils from subjects with CGD have an impaired ability to kill *C. albicans* [109].

Relatively few studies have examined the candidacidal activity of monocytes in patients with various disorders, which is unfortunate given the ease whereby such studies can be performed [112,116]. A recent report that monocytes from patients with lepromatous leprosy have monocytes markedly deficient in ability to kill *C. pseudotropicalis* (MPO-independent, H_2O_2-dependent killing in monocytes) warrants verification and further exploration [58].

The chronic mucocutaneous candidiasis syndrome has attracted considerable attention. Affected patients often have severe *Candida* infections, localized to skin and mucous membranes, but show little or no tendency for systemic candidiasis [53]. Their predisposing defects, presumed to arise from abnormalities of lymphocyte function and lymphocyte/macrophage interaction, have been recently reviewed and will not be considered here [94,182].

B. *Cryptococcus neoformans*

Cryptococcus neoformans typically initiates infection after inhalation of its yeast cells [50] or basidiospores [51] into the upper or lower respiratory tract. In tissue, organisms manifest a prominent polysaccharide capsule that serves as a major factor contributing to their virulence. The negatively-charged, uronic acid-rich capsular material forms a barrier, masking opsonizing components such as immunoglobulin attached to the yeast cell wall, and interfering with uptake by phagocytes both sterically [129] and electrostatically [103]. Nonencapsulated mutants of *C. neoformans* have low virulence for mice [20], and induce marked inflammatory responses in vivo [59], in contrast to the minimal cellular response incited by normally encapsulated strains.

After experimental respiratory infection of mice or rats, cryptococci can be identified in the lung alveoli and alveolar septae. Although many organisms are rapidly destroyed by an influx of neutrophils, surviving fungi generate large capsules and—as the inflammatory response dwindles—lie within granulomas containing mononuclear and epithelioid cells [65].

Cryptococci can be killed both intracellularly and extracellularly by phagocytes. The former activity depends on serum opsonins, with both immunoglobulin and complement components participating, depending on the leukocyte type and host species under investigation.

Nonencapsulated *C. neoformans* yeasts are ingested by normal mouse peritoneal macrophages in the absence of serum opsonins, but addition of purified human IgG or serum substantially increases uptake [102]. Although heat-labile serum components did not enhance the opsonic effect of IgG in these experiments, they did facilitate phagocytosis of *C. neoformans* by thioglycollate [184] and glycogen-elicited [129] macrophages. Transmission and scanning electron micrographs demonstrating the interactions of *C. neoformans* with resident and "exudate" peritoneal macrophages of guinea pigs and rabbits have been published [147].

Human neutrophils and monocytes required ≥10% serum for maximal phagocytosis of poorly and well-encapsulated *C. neoformans* in vitro. Heat-labile serum components stimulated ingestion, high concentrations of free capsular polysaccharide impaired it [43]. The early classical complement components, C1, C2, and C4, are required for optimal rates of uptake, but the alternative complement system (properdin and factor B) and late-acting complement components C3-9 appear to be of greater significance for ingestion of this organism [45].

Mice genetically deficient in C5 [155] and guinea pigs depleted of late complement components by cobra venom factor [44] exhibit shortened survival, relative to controls, after experimental cryptococcal infection. In contrast, C4-deficient guinea pigs show normal survival in such experiments [44].

Normal human blood leukocytes can kill *C. neoformans* in vitro [43,185]. After 2 h, viability of an inoculum of *C. neoformans* was reduced 46% by neutrophils and 59% by monocytes. Studies with inhibitors and cell-free models suggested that myeloperoxidase and H_2O_2 contributed to the fungicidal events in this system [43]. Neutrophils from patients with CGD, deficient in oxidative metabolism, had markedly diminished activity against *C. neoformans*. Cells from patients with cryptococcal infection behaved normally in vitro. As capsule size increased, ingestion and killing diminished. Neutrophils were more sensitive to this effect than were monocytes. Normal or antibody-containing serum was not directly cryptococcocidal [43], in contrast to an earlier, unconfirmed report [185].

When human blood monocytes are placed in tissue culture, they differentiate into cells with morphologic and functional features of macrophages. Such tissue cultured macrophages can ingest *C. neoformans* yeast cells, but fail to kill them. Indeed, after a few hours, intracellular fungi grow more rapidly than extracellular yeast cells. Macrophages derived by culturing blood monocytes from normal subjects and patients with cryptococcal infections behaved similarly [40]. The authors noted that the macrophage monolayers remained more resistant to destruction by the intracellularly replicating cryptococci if nonadherent lymphocytes were retained during preparation of the cultures. Macrophage monolayers established from mice with nonspecifically enhanced resistance to intracellular infections better resisted destruction by cryptococci than did control macrophage monolayers [40].

Resident rat peritoneal macrophages have been reported to ingest *C. neoformans* in the presence of native, but not heat-inactivated serum. Efficiency of uptake was inversely related to capsule size. Although most ingested yeasts resisted intracellular killing, a substantial number failed to multiply upon subsequent agar culture [132]. Cryptococcal isolates were observed to vary in their susceptibility to macrophages. Phagocytosis of *C. neoformans* by alveolar macrophages has also been examined [19, 89].

The relationship of free capsular polysaccharide (CP) to phagocytic defenses has attracted considerable interest. Addition of CP to incubation mixtures of granulocytes and nonencapsulated *C. neoformans* decreased ingestion substantially [18,101]. This effect was specific for *C. neoformans*. Ingestion of *E. coli, S. aureus, Saccharomyces cerevisiae*, and *Candida* spp. was unaffected. Although these effects are of considerable scientific interest, the high levels of CP required for their display make their pathophysiologic significance uncertain [43].

If cryptococci are injected intraperitoneally into mice, an inflammatory response develops within a few hours. Neutrophils predominate, and a few of these can be seen phagocytizing fungi. By 24-48 h, the cell population shifts to a predominantly mononuclear pattern that persists for a week or more. A "phagocyte ring response" occurs, wherein rosettes of phagocytes encircle encapsulated cryptococci. The host cells consist, at first, of granulocytes. Later, combinations of granulocytes and mononuclear cells, and finally only macrophages surround the pathogenic yeasts [65,170]. Evidence of lysosomal enzyme release by the macrophages and extracellular destruction of some of the organisms has been presented [88]. Extracellular killing of *Cryptococcus neoformans* by human blood mononuclear leukocytes in vitro has also been reported [38]. In this system, killing was dependent on specific antibody and effected by a subpopulation of adherent cells.

The role of the reticuloendothelial system in Swiss albino mice was studied with intravenously inoculated *C. neoformans*. Stimulation with BCG markedly increased resistance to doses as high as $100 \times LD_{50}$. Intravenous silica decreased carbon clearance, increased mortality, and increased the number of viable cryptococci recovered from organs of animals 24 days or longer after infection [134]. Hairless and athymic nude (*nu/nu*) BALB/c and Swiss mice were much more susceptible to *C. neoformans* than were their heterozygous, immunologically intact *Nu*/x littermates [72], suggesting the great importance of thymus-dependent immune functions in resistance to cryptococcosis, in contrast to their evident dispensability with regard to systemic *Candida albicans* infection [34,159].

C. *Coccidioides immitis*

Coccidioides immitis, a fungus endemic to the southwestern United States, produces highly infectious arthroconidia, contributing to the relatively limited number of in vitro studies with this organism.

Human neutrophils are attracted to *C. immitis* mycelium in vitro, avidly ingesting arthroconidia and limiting subsequent mycelial growth [6]. Intraleukocytic mycelial fragments remain viable, subsequently rounding up to form spherules and endospores. Examination of tissues from human and experimental murine coccidioidomycosis suggests that neutrophils, by promoting spherule and endospore formation in vivo, may actually increase tissue damage by this organism, despite their attraction to and ingestion of endospores in vivo.

The cellular response to intranasal infection of mice with *C. immitis* arthroconidia includes an influx of mononuclear cells and granulocytes, and increased numbers of both phagocytic cell classes can be recovered by tracheobronchial lavage [165]. Mature, thick-walled spherules are typically surrounded by a granulomatous response rich in epithelioid cells [6]. Rupture of the spherules with endospore release initiates a brisk influx of neutrophils, with ensuing phagocytosis.

Human monocytes ingested killed endospores of *C. immitis* in the presence of serum at the same rate, whether they came from a coccidioidin-reactive or nonreactive person [37]. Ingestion of heat-killed arthroconidia by human and canine neutrophils was examined in a rather crude system that did not distinguish opsonic from cellular factors involved in fungal uptake [195]. The authors reported increased phagocytosis by neutrophils from vaccinated dogs and coccidioidin-reactive humans, relative to their controls.

Alveolar macrophages lavaged from rhesus macaques could phagocytize endospores and arthroconidia of *C. immitis,* but were unable to reduce their viability or impede their development into spherules. Addition of alveolar lining material, complement, or immune serum did not induce fungicidal ability. *Coccidioides immitis* appeared to inhibit phagosome/lysosome fusion, perhaps explaining this result [11]. It might be significant that, despite their swinging from a branch close to man's on the evolutionary tree, rhesus monkeys have leukocytes that are virtually devoid of lysozyme [151], an abundant constituent of human leukocytes and one reported to damage coccidioidal spherules [29,30].

Peritoneal macrophages from normal mice have been reported to ingest arthroconidia and endospores of *C. immitis* without significantly affecting their viability or manifesting phagosome-lysosome fusion. Addition of lymphocytes from immune mice to non-immune macrophages resulted in killing of approximately half the ingested arthroconidia or endospores by 4 h. Lymphocytes from normal mice showed little enhancing ability. A significant increase in phagosome-lysosome fusion, assessed by the somewhat controversial acridine orange technique [71], accompanied and may have been responsible for the salutary effects of immune lymphocytes on macrophage performance [12]. Studies with anti-Thy 1.2 serum plus guinea pig complement provided evidence that T cells were required for the macrophage enhancement. As Howard et al. had earlier reported in analogous studies with *Histoplasma capsulatum* [83], immune lymphocytes lacked direct effect on the fungal targets.

D. *Histoplasma capsulatum*

Histoplasma capsulatum, a facultative intracellular parasite [77], is usually acquired via the respiratory tract wherefrom it may disseminate. With few exceptions, e.g., endocarditis, histopathological studies consistently demonstrate the organisms within the cytoplasm of macrophages only. Degenerating fragments of organisms are often observed in healed primary lesions. In sharp contrast, disseminated histoplasmosis lesions show no degenerating fungi within the macrophages. This has led to a hypothesis that the primary failure in disseminated histoplasmosis may be failure of macrophages to kill *H. capsulatum* [70]. Conversely, effective macrophage fungicidal activity promotes containment and localization of the infection.

Studies with glycogen-elicited, in vitro-cultivated mouse peritoneal macrophages and yeast phase *H. capsulatum* have been done. In the presence of normal human serum, 61% of macrophages ingested yeast cells by 3 h. A tinctorial method revealed no evident cidal activity, and showed that the fungi multiplied intracellularly with a generation time of 10.3 h [77]. Similar results were obtained with guinea pig peritoneal macrophages and serum. Neither exposing the yeasts to specific antibodies and complement nor immunizing the animals with formalin-killed yeasts altered the above results [78]. Also, studies with ^{3}H-labeled leucine showed protein synthesis by intracellular fungi, clearly a sign of their continued viability [81].

As earlier studies with mouse macrophages immunized against *H. capsulatum* had shown inhibition of intracellular fungal growth [75,133], further studies were done to clarify this inconsistency. Peritoneal macrophages from immunized mice, parasitized 1 h after harvest, inhibited intracellular growth. However, if macrophages were fed fungi after 48 h of cell culture, no inhibition was noted. In addition, inhibitory capacity was significantly reduced if 1 h ex vivo macrophages were washed prior to fungal ingestion. Nonimmune or 48-h cell culture macrophages acquired inhibitory capacity after exposure to purified lymphocytes from immune mouse peritoneal exudates. This occurred even if lymphocytes were added after fungal ingestion, suggesting the lymphocyte effect was exerted on macrophages rather than fungi [83]. Supernatants from cultures of immune or mitogen-stimulated lymphocytes were ineffective in improving macrophage performance [82]. After their liberation from macrophages, the inhibited fungi were noted to be viable, both by eosin-Y dye exclusion and by germination on 1% casein hydrolysate agar.

Material solubilized by repetitively freezing and thawing a lysosome-rich fraction of normal rabbit alveolar macrophages inhibited protein synthesis by *H. capsulatum*. Organisms incubated in the extract for at least 20 h showed cytopathic changes and a significant decrease in their viability [21]. An electron microscopic study of unstimulated, nonimmune hamster peritoneal macrophages revealed that within 1 h or ingestion, unaltered *H. capsulatum* organisms were present within tight phagolysosomes. Subsequently, two classes of larger vacuoles were apparent. One type lacked acid phosphatase, suggesting its failure to interact with host cell lysosomes. The other was multilocular and contained acid phosphatase. The authors hypothesized its source to be lysosomes from other degenerated phagocytes ingested with the fungus, suggesting successive phagocytosis of the same fungus by different macrophages [49].

Guinea pig peritoneal PMNs phagocytize *H. capsulatum* only in the presence of fresh serum. After 3 h incubation, 87% of ingested yeasts appeared killed, as judged by the tinctorial method [79]. As *H. capsulatum* is an intracellular parasite, the susceptibility of ingested organisms to amphotericin B has been studied. When incubated with murine peritoneal PMNs, 33 of 34 strains showed diminished susceptibility to amphotericin B [10]. In contrast, *Histoplasma* within murine [76] and guinea pig peritoneal macrophages [183] were susceptible to amphotericin B added to the medium.

E. Other Yeastlike Fungi

Other yeastlike fungi have been used occasionally to study phagocytes. *Torulopsis glabrata*, found among the normal gastrointestinal and urogenital flora, is an increasingly recognized opportunistic human pathogen. In the presence of human serum, stimulated mouse peritoneal macrophages phagocytized 70-80% of an inoculum of *T. glabrata* in 3 h. Although serum alone retarded fungal growth, viable cells increased significantly in 8 h of incubation. In contrast, ingested fungi increased only slightly after 24 h, indicating inhibition by the macrophages [80]. Adding iron to the medium diminished the fungistatic effect of serum but not that of macrophages. No definite killing of intracellular organisms was demonstrated [144].

Human neutrophils, in presence of serum, phagocytized *T. glabrata*, and by 4 h, 81.4% of ingested organisms were killed. Unconjugated bilirubin (4×10^{-5} M) decreased the percentage killed to 40.9% without affecting phagocytosis [188].

Blastomyces dermatitidis is typically acquired via and may disseminate from the respiratory tract. It causes suppurative and granulomatous lesions that usually contain significant numbers of granulocytes. Broth culture filtrates of *B. dermatitidis* stimulated granulocyte chemotactic activity significantly better than did filtrates from

H. capsulatum and *Cryptococcus neoformans*, two fungi that usually do not elicit granulocytes in infected tissue [177]. Serum from patients with *B. dermatitidis* infection has been reported to inhibit zymosan-stimulated PMN locomotion [153]. Human neutrophils in presence of serum phagocytized *B. dermatitidis* very efficiently and killed 29% after 3 h of incubation [177]. Studies with mice suggest an inhibitory role for macrophages, and virulence of fungus seems to be correlated with an ability to escape from this inhibition [16].

Leukocytes from patients infected by *Paracoccidioides brasiliensis* showed phagocytosis and killing of these organisms. Significantly increased killing occurred when serum from these patients was used, and this increase was specific for *P. brasiliensis* [154]. A more recent study found a decreased ability of neutrophils from patients with paracoccidioidomycosis to digest *P. brasiliensis*. There was a correlation with strain pathogenicity and decreased neutrophil killing [67].

Sporothrix schenckii, a biphasic fungus found on decaying vegetation, typically causes skin and subcutaneous infections. Human PMNs ingested and killed approximately 80% of an inoculum of yeast-phase *S. schenckii* in the presence of 10% native serum. The fungus was killed in vitro by a mixture of myeloperoxidase, H_2O_2, and iodide. Chloride ions could not replace iodide in this system [32]. These observations may related to the clinical efficacy of iodide in clinical sporotrichosis.

Although *Saccharomyces cerevisiae* is man's most pathogenic fungus, this arises almost exclusively from his proclivity for imbibing its metabolic by-products rather than from any intrinsic aggressiveness by the yeast. The organism is readily phagocytized and killed by murine peritoneal neutrophils, as well as by alveolar and splenic macrophages [175]. "Zymosan," an invaluable reagent for immunologists, is the delipidated, partially extracted residue of this organism.

F. *Aspergillus*

Spores of *Aspergillus* spp., widespread in nature, gain entry into the respiratory tract where, in immunocompromised hosts, they may germinate and cause severe infections often marked by vascular invasion that causes infarction and tissue necrosis.

In vivo models with inhaled spores are suggestive for a role by phagocytes in normal host defenses. Mice made to inhale spores of *A. flavus* developed only transient nonfatal pneumonitis without germination of spores. In cortisone-treated mice, spores rapidly germinated into hyphae, invading the entire lung and leading to death [174]. In a similar study with *A. fumigatus*, *A. flavus*, and *A. niger*, mice killed 1 day after exposure showed acute inflammatory reactions in their bronchial lumens. A macrophage response surrounded the bronchi after 4 days and complete clearance occurred after 6 days. No fungal hyphae could be demonstrated in lungs [13]. In another study, macrophages washed from the lungs of sacrificed animals revealed phagocytized spores. Up to 64% of macrophages contained an average of 7 spores per cell, with some having as high as 20 [62]. One study where low-grade germination of spores was observed found that even these were eventually cleared by normal mice, but not by ones treated with cortisone [196]. Electron microscopical studies of macrophages lavaged from lungs of mice that inhaled spores of *A. flavus* showed that spores within normal mouse cells remained dormant or became fragmented. Spores within macrophages of steroid-treated mice showed evidence of germination after 2-4 h [131].

Human neutrophils and monocytes required unheated serum for efficient phagocytosis in vitro. The intracellular organisms showed no change in size, morphological characteristics, or staining characteristics for up to 3 h of incubation. After lysis of leukocytes, all spores were found to be viable in a germination medium [120].

Interaction of neutrophils with hyphal forms of *A. fumigatus* has been studied with more optimistic results. Neutrophils attach to hyphae in the absence of serum and cause dramatic morphological changes, visible by light and electron microscopy, within 2 h. Uptake studies with radioisotopes demonstrated inhibition of fungal metabolism. Inhibitors of neutrophil motility and oxidative metabolism, prevented hyphal damage, further indicating a role for neutrophils [46]. A complement requirement for efficient phagocytosis has been reported [77].

A recent study involving both murine and human phagocytes suggested that macrophages form the first line of defense against the spores. Neutrophils protected against the hyphal form and inhibition of both systems was required to make the host susceptible to infection [167]. Rabbit alveolar macrophages are able to ingest *A. fumigatus,* and it appears that injection of animals with aflatoxin can reduce this phagocytic activity significantly [128,156].

A specific killing defect has been described involving the neutrophils of a 6-year-old boy who died from repeated *A. fumigatus* infections. Though his PMNs phagocytized spores of *A. fumigatus* well, they killed them at much lower rate as compared with controls. Metabolic responsiveness of his neutrophils was superior to CGD cells and they killed *Staphylococcus aureus* and *Candida albicans* normally [146]. A 26-year-old male with disseminated *Aspergillus* infection (*A. niger* and *A. fumigatus*) has been reported to have a granulocyte oxidative defect similar to CGD. He apparently acquired his infection from smoking marijuana contaminated with these organisms [26].

G. Zygomycetes

Mucormycosis, a fungal infection with devastating results in diabetics and immuno-compromised patients, is most commonly caused by species of *Rhizopus, Absidia,* and *Mucor.* In diabetics, usually with ketoacidosis, inhaled spores can give rise to rhino-cerebral infection. Necrotizing pneumonias, characterized by blood vessel invasion and infarctions, may also occur [115]. There is one report of a 13-year-old girl with CGD who died from disseminated mucormycosis in spite of prolonged amphotericin therapy [17].

As with *Aspergillus* spp., animal models suggest that inhaled spores do not germinate and are eliminated from lungs [5,152,178]. When large numbers of spores are instilled into nares of normal rabbits, mild local inflammatory reaction develops. When this is done to leukopenic [7] or alloxan-induced ketoacidotic diabetic rabbits, an infection resembling human rhinocerebral mucormycosis develops. Microscopic examination of inflamed tissues discloses neutrophil-rich exudates around hyphal elements in normal animals, and very few neutrophils in diabetic animals [8,9]. Endotoxin increases susceptibility of mice to intravenously injected *Absidia ramosa* [52].

Neutrophil studies showing damage to hyphal elements have also been done with *Rhizopus oryzae* with generally comparable results to those described for *Aspergillus fumigatus.* Polyanions, presumed to act by inhibiting neutrophil cationic proteins, inhibited fungal damage in this in vitro system [46]. Rabbit alveolar macrophages can ingest *R. oryzae* [128], but the fate of these ingested spores was not reported.

IV. CONCLUDING REMARKS

Given the ubiquity of fungi and the frequency of exposure to them, the rarity of systemic fungal disease is probably more remarkable than its occasional occurrence. Although numerous factors may contribute to the relatively low pathogenicity of fungi, their usual fate at the hands of phagocytic leukocytes figures importantly in host resistance. In recent years, many investigators have contributed toward defining relationships between various host cells and fungi. A general understanding of leukocyte fungicidal mechanisms has emerged, and a start in defining, on a molecular basis, specific pathogenic features of the organisms has been made. The extreme usefulness of fungi for probing immune and constitutive host effector mechanisms is becoming more widely recognized. Future progress in this area may contribute to advances in understanding and treating fungal diseases.

ACKNOWLEDGMENTS

This chapter is publication no. 46 of the Collaborative California Universities-Mycology Research Unit (CCU-MRU). The authors wish to thank the National Institutes of Health (NIAID and the National Cancer Institute) for research support (AI 16252 and CA 30526).

REFERENCES

1. Ambruso, D. R., and R. B. Johnston, Jr. 1981. Lactoferrin enhances hydroxyl radical production by human neutrophils, neutrophil particulate fractions and an enzymatic generating system. J. Clin. Invest. 67:352-360.
2. Arai, T., Y. Mikami, and K. Yokoyana. 1977. Phagocytosis of Candida albicans by rabbit alveolar macrophages and guinea pig neutrophils. Sabouraudia 15:171-177.
3. Arnold, R. R., M. Brewer, and J. J. Gauthier. 1980. Bactericidal activity of human lactoferrin: sensitivity of a variety of microorganisms. Infect. Immun. 28:893-898.
4. Baine, W. B., M. G. Koenig, and J. S. Goodman. 1974. Clearance of Candida albicans from the bloodstream of rabbits. Infect. Immun. 10:1420-1425.
5. Baisakh, K. M., D. S. Agarwal, B. Iyengar, and V. N. Bhatia. 1975. Experimental aspergillosis and phycomycosis in mice. Indian J. Med. Res. 63(12):1716-1731.
6. Baker, O., and A. I. Braude. 1956. A study of stimuli leading to the production of spherules in coccidioidomycosis. J. Lab. Clin. Med. 47:169-181.
7. Bauer, H., and W. H. Sheldon. 1957. Leukopenia with granulocytopenia in experimental mucormycosis (Rhizopus oryzae infection). J. Exp. Med. 106:501-508.
8. Bauer, H., J. F. Flanagan, and W. H. Sheldon. 1955. Experimental cerebral mucormycosis in rabbits with alloxan diabetes. Yale J. Biol. Med. 28:29-36.
9. Bauer, H., J. F. Flanagan, and W. H. Sheldon. 1956. The effects of metabolic alterations on experimental Rhizopus oryzae (mucormycosis) infection. Yale J. Biol. Med. 29:23-32.
10. Baum, G. L., and D. Artis. 1965. Susceptibility to amphotericin B of phagocytosed yeast cells of Histoplasma capsulatum. Am. J. Med. Sci. 249:211-215.
11. Beaman, L., and C. A. Holmberg. 1980. In vitro response of alveolar macrophages to infection with Coccidioides immitis. Infect. Immun. 28:594-600.

12. Beaman, L., E. Benjamini, and D. Pappagianis. 1981. Role of lymphocytes in macrophage-induced killing of *Coccidioides immitis* in vitro. Infect. Immun. *34*: 347-353.

13. Bhatia, V. N., and L. N. Mohapatra. 1969. Experimental aspergillosis in mice. Mykosen *12*(11):651-654.

14. Bird, D. C., and J. N. Sheagren. 1969. Evaluation of reticuloendothelial system phagocytic activity during systemic *Candida albicans* infection in mice (34401). Proc. Soc. Exp. Biol. Med. *133*:34-37.

15. Bourne, H. R., R. I. Lehrer, M. J. Cline, and K. L. Melmon. 1971. Cyclic 3′,5′-adenosine monophosphate in the human leukocyte: synthesis, degradation, and effects on neutrophil candidacidal activity. J. Clin. Invest. *50*:920-929.

16. Brummer, E., P. A. Morozumi, D. E. Philpott, and D. A. Stevens. 1981. Virulence of fungi: correlation of virulence of *Blastomyces dermatitidis* in vivo with escape from macrophage inhibition of replication in vitro. Infect. Immun. *32*: 864-871.

17. Bruun, J. N., C. O. Solberg, E. Hamre, C. J. Janssen, Jr., S. Thunold, and J. Eide. 1976. Acute disseminated phycomycosis in a patient with impaired neutrophil granulocyte function. Acta Pathol. Microbiol. Scand. Sect. C *84*:93-99.

18. Bulmer, G. S., and M. D. Sans. 1968. *Cryptococcus neoformans*. III. Inhibition of phagocytosis. J. Bacteriol. *95*:5-8.

19. Bulmer, G. S., and J. R. Tacker. 1975. Phagocytosis of *Cryptococcus neoformans* by alveolar macrophages. Infect. Immun. *11*:73-79.

20. Bulmer, G. S., M. D. Sans, and C. M. Gunn. 1967. *Cryptococcus neoformans*. I. Nonencapsulated mutants. J. Bacteriol. *94*:1475-1479.

21. Calderone, R. A., and E. Peterson. 1979. Inhibition of amino acid uptake and incorporation into *Histoplasma capsulatum* by a lysosomal extract from rabbit alveolar macrophages. J. Reticuloendothel. Soc. *26*:11-19.

22. Cech, P., A. Papathanassiou, G. Boreux, P. Roth, and P. A. Miescher. 1979. Hereditary myeloperoxidase deficiency. Blood *53*:403-411.

23. Cech, P., H. Stalder, J. J. Widmann, A. Rohner, and P. A. Miescher. 1979. Leukocyte myeloperoxidase deficiency and diabetes mellitus associated with *Candida albicans* liver abscess. Am. J. Med. *66*:149-153.

24. Chan, C. K., and E. Balish. 1978. Inhibition of granulocyte phagocytosis of *Candida albicans* by amphotericin B. Can. J. Microbiol. *24*:363-364.

25. Child, J. A., S. Martin, J. C. Cawley, and A. T. M. Ghoneim. 1978. Defective microbicidal function of neutrophils in haematological malignancies and lymphomas: correction by levamisole in vitro. Biomedicine *29*:159-161.

26. Chusid, M. J., P. G. Sohnle, J. N. Fink, and M. L. Shea. 1981. A genetic defect of granulocyte oxidative metabolism in a man with disseminated aspergillosis. J. Lab. Clin. Med. *97*:730-738.

27. Cohen, A. B., and M. J. Cline. 1971. The human alveolar macrophage: isolation, cultivation in vitro, and studies of morphologic and functional characteristics. J. Clin. Invest. *50*:1390-1398.

28. Cohen, M. S., R. E. Isturiz, H. L. Malech, R. K. Root, C. W. Wilfert, L. Gutman, and H. R. Buckley. 1981. Fungal infection in chronic granulomatous disease. The importance of the phagocyte in defense against fungi. Am. J. Med. *71*: 59-66.

29. Collins, M. S., and D. Pappagianis. 1973. Effects of lysozyme and chitinase on the spherules of *Coccidioides immitis* in vitro. Infect. Immun. *7*:817-822.

30. Collins, M. S., and D. Pappagianis. 1974. Lysozyme-enhanced killing of *Candida albicans* and *Coccidioides immitis* by amphotericin B. Sabouraudia *12*:329-340.

31. Cummings, N. P., M. J. Pabst, and R. B. Johnston, Jr. 1980. Activation of

macrophages for enhanced release of superoxide anion and greater killing of *Candida albicans* by injection of muramyl dipeptide. J. Exp. Med. *152*:1659-1669.

32. Cunningham, K. M., G. S. Bulmer, and E. R. Rhoades. 1979. Phagocytosis and intracellular fate of *Sporothrix schenckii.* J. Infect. Dis. *140*:815-817.

33. Cutler, J. E. 1977. Chemotactic factor produced by *Candida albicans.* Infect. Immun. *18*:568-573.

34. Cutler, J. E., and A. H. Poor. 1981. Effect of mouse phagocytes on *Candida albicans* in in vivo chambers. Infect. Immun. *31*:1110-1116.

35. Davies, R. R., and T. J. V. Denning. 1972. *Candida albicans* and the fungicidal activity of the blood. Sabouraudia *10*:301-312.

36. Denning, T. J. V., and R. R. Davies. 1973. *Candida albicans* and the chemotaxis of polymorphonuclear neutrophils. Sabouraudia *11*:210-221.

37. Deresinski, S. C., H. B. Levine, and D. A. Stevens. 1978. *Coccidioides immitis* endospores: phagocytosis by human cells. Mycopathologia *64*:179-181.

38. Diamond, R. D. 1974. Antibody-dependent killing of *Cryptococcus neoformans* by human peripheral blood mononuclear cells. Nature (Lond.) *247*:148-149.

39. Diamond, R. D. 1981. Mechanisms of host resistance to *Candida albicans.* In *Microbiology, 1981,* American Society for Microbiology, Washington, D.C., pp. 200-204.

40. Diamond, R. D., and J. E. Bennett. 1973. Growth of *Cryptococcus neoformans* within human macrophages in vitro. Infect. Immun. *7*:231-236.

41. Diamond, R. D., R. A. Clark, and C. C. Haudenschild. 1980. Damage to *Candida albicans* hyphae and pseudohyphae by the myeloperoxidase system and oxidative products of neutrophil metabolism in vitro. J. Clin. Invest. *66*:908-917.

42. Diamond, R. D., R. Krzesicki, and W. Jao. 1978. Damage to pseudohyphal forms of *Candida albicans* by neutrophils in the absence of serum in vitro. J. Clin. Invest. *61*:349-359.

43. Diamond, R. D., R. K. Root, and J. E. Bennett. 1972. Factors influencing killing of *Cryptococcus neoformans* by human leukocytes in vitro. J. Infect. Dis. *125*:367-375.

44. Diamond, R. D., J. E. May, M. Kane, M. M. Frank, and J. E. Bennett. 1973. The role of late complement components and the alternate complement pathway in experimental cryptococcosis (37580). Proc. Soc. Exp. Biol. Med. *144*:312-315.

45. Diamond, R. D., J. E. May, M. A. Kane, M. M. Frank, and J. E. Bennett. 1974. The role of the classical and alternate complement pathways in host defenses against *Cryptococcus neoformans* infection. J. Immunol. *112*:2260-2270.

46. Diamond, R. D., R. Krzesicki, B. Epstein, and W. Jao. 1978. Damage to hyphal forms of fungi by human leukocytes in vitro. Am. J. Pathol. *91*:313-323.

47. Diamond, R. D., F. Oppenheim, Y. Nakagawa, R. Krzesicki, and C. C. Haudenschild. 1980. Properties of a product of *Candida albicans* hyphae and pseudohyphae that inhibits contact between the fungi and human neutrophils in vitro. J. Immunol. *125*:2797-2804.

47a. Dri, P., R. Cramer, M. R. Soranzo, A. Comin, V. Miotti, and P. Patriarca. 1982. New approaches to the detection of myeloperoxidase deficiency. Blood *60*(2):323-327.

48. Drutz, D. J., and R. I. Lehrer. 1978. Development of amphotericin B-resistant *Candida tropicalis* in a patient with defective leukocyte function. Am. J. Med. Sci. *276*:77-92.

49. Dumont, A., and A. Robert. 1970. Electron microscopic study of phagocytosis of *Histoplasma capsulatum* by hamster peritoneal macrophages. Lab. Invest. *23*:278-286.

50. Duperval, R., P. E. Hermans, N. S. Brewer, and G. D. Roberts. 1977. Crypto-coccosis, with emphasis on the significance of isolation of *Cryptococcus neoformans* from the respiratory tract. Chest *72*:13-19.

51. Dykstra, M. A., and L. Friedman. 1978. Pathogenesis, lethality, and immunizing effect of experimental cutaneous cryptococcosis. Infect. Immun. *20*:446-455.

52. Eades, S. M., and M. J. Corbel. 1975. Enhancement of susceptibility to experimental phycomycosis by agents producing reticuloendothelial stimulation. Br. Vet. J. *131*:622-624.

53. Edwards, J. E. (Moderator), R. I. Lehrer, E. R. Stiehm, T. J. Fischer, and L. S. Young. 1978. Severe candidal infections. Clinical perspective, immune defense mechanisms, and current concepts of therapy. Ann. Intern. Med. *88*:91-106.

54. El Falaky, I. H., and H. M. Shoukry. 1977. Phagocytosis and intracellular killing of *Candida albicans* by polymorphonuclear leucocytes in thalassaemia. J. Egyptian Public Health Assoc. *LII* (5):317-329.

55. El-Maalem, H., and J. Fletcher. 1976. Defective neutrophil function in chronic granulocytic leukaemia. Br. J. Haematol. *34*:95-103.

56. El-Maallem, H., and J. Fletcher. 1980. Impaired neutrophil function and myeloperoxidase deficiency in pregnancy. Br. J. Haematol. *44*:375-381.

57. Elsbach, P., J. Goldman, and P. Patriarca. 1972. Phospholipid metabolism by phagocytic cells. VI. Observations on the fate of phospholipids of granulocytes and ingested *Escherichia coli* during phagocytosis. Biochim. Biophys. Acta *280*:33-44.

58. Estevez, M. E., L. Sen, R. Vadez, and L. M. Balina. 1980. Defective blood mononuclear phagocyte function in patients with leprosy. Int. J. Leprosy *47*:575-579.

59. Farmer, S. G., and R. A. Komorowski. 1973. Histologic response to capsule-deficient *Cryptococcus neoformans*. Arch. Pathol. *96*:383-387.

60. Ferrante, A., and Y. H. Thong. 1979. Requirement of heat-labile opsonins for maximal phagocytosis of *Candida albicans*. Sabouraudia *17*:293-297.

61. Ferrari, F. A., A. Pagani, M. Marconi, R. Stefanoni, and A. G. Siccardi. 1980. Inhibition of candidacidal activity of human neutrophil leukocytes by amino-glycoside antibiotics. Antimicrob. Agents Chemother. *17*:87-88.

62. Ford, S., and L. Friedman. 1967. Experimental study of the pathogenicity of aspergilli for mice. J. Bacteriol. *94*:928-933.

63. Fridovich, I. 1981. The biology of superoxide and superoxide dismutases-in brief. Prog. Clin. Biol. Res. *51*:153-172.

64. Gabig, T. G., and B. M. Babior. 1981. The killing of pathogens by phagocytes. Annu. Rev. Med. *32*:313-326.

65. Gadebusch, H. H. 1972. Mechanisms of native and acquired resistance to infection with *Cryptococcus neoformans*. Crit. Rev. Microbiol. (Feb.) *1*:311-320.

66. Gadebusch, H. H., and A. G. Johnson. 1966. Natural host resistance to infection with *Cryptococcus neoformans*. IV. The effect of some cationic proteins on the experimental disease. J. Infect. Dis. *116*:551-565.

67. Goihman-Yahr, M., E. Essenfeld-Yahr, M. C. deAlbornoz, L. Yarzabal, M. H. de Gomez, B. San Martin, A. Ocanto, F. Gil, and J. Convit. 1980. Defect of in vitro digestive ability of polymorphonuclear leukocytes in paracoccidioidomycosis. Infect. Immun. *28*:557-566.

68. Goldman, J. M., and K. H. Th'ng. 1973. Phagocytic function of leucocytes from patients with acute myeloid and chronic granulocytic leukaemia. Br. J. Haematol. *25*:299-308.

69. Gontijo, P. P., Jr., and L. G. Wayne. 1978. Phagocytic and antimicrobial activities of rabbit peritoneal and alveolar macrophages activated with *Mycobacterium bovis* BCG on *Candida albicans*. Rev. Latinoam. Microbiol. *20*:41-44.

70. Goodwin, R. A., Jr., J. L. Shapiro, G. H. Thurman, S. S. Thurman, and R. M. Des Prez. 1980. Disseminated histoplasmosis: clinical and pathologic correlations. Medicine 59 (1):1-33.

71. Goren, M. B., C. L. Swendsen, and J. Henson. 1980. Factors modifying the fusion of phagosomes and lysosomes: art, fact and artifact. In R. van Furth (Ed.), Mononuclear Phagocytes: Functional Aspects, Martinus Nijhoff, the Hague, pp. 999-1034.

72. Graybill, J. R., and D. J. Drutz. 1978. Host defense in cryptococcosis. II. Cryptococcosis in the nude mouse. Cell. Immunol. 40:263-274.

73. Hammerstrom, J., and G. Unsgaard. 1979. In vitro influence of endotoxin on human mononuclear phagocyte structure and function. Acta Pathol. Microbiol. Scand. Sect. C 87:381-389.

74. Harrison, J. E., and J. Schultz. 1976. Studies on the chlorinating activity of myeloperoxidase. J. Biol. Chem. 251:1371-1374.

75. Hill, G. A., and S. Marcus. 1960. Study of cellular mechanisms in resistance to systemic Histoplasma capsulatum infection. J. Immunol. 85:6-13.

76. Howard, D. H. 1960. Effect of mycostatin and fungizone on the growth of Histoplasma capsulatum in tissue culture. J. Bacteriol. 79:442-449.

77. Howard, D. H. 1964. Intracellular behavior of Histoplasma capsulatum. J. Bacteriol. 87:33-38.

78. Howard, D. H. 1965. Intracellular growth of Histoplasma capsulatum. J. Bacteriol. 89:518-523.

79. Howard, D. H. 1973. Fate of Histoplasma capsulatum in guinea pig polymorphonuclear leukocytes. Infect. Immun. 8:412-419.

80. Howard, D. H., and V. Otto. 1967. The intracellular behavior of Torulopsis glabrata. Sabouraudia 5:235-239.

81. Howard, D. H., and V. Otto. 1969. Protein synthesis by phagocytized yeast cells of Histoplasma capsulatum. Sabouraudia 7:186-194.

82. Howard, D. H., and V. Otto. 1977. Experiments on lymphocyte-mediated cellular immunity in murine histoplasmosis. Infect. Immun. 16:226-231.

83. Howard, D. H., V. Otto, and R. K. Gupta. 1971. Lymphocyte-mediated cellular immunity in histoplasmosis. Infect. Immun. 4:605-610.

84. Hurley, D. L., J. E. Balow, and A. S. Fauci. 1975. Experimental disseminated candidiasis. II. Administration of glucocorticoids, susceptibility to infection and immunity. J. Infect. Dis. 132:393-398.

85. Hurtrel, B., P. H. Lagrange, and J. C. Michel. 1980. Systemic candidiasis in mice. II. Main role of polymorphonuclear leukocytes in resistance to infection. Ann. Immunol. (Inst. Pasteur) 131:105-118.

86. Ishikawa, T., A. C. Dalton, and C. E. Arbesman. 1972. Phagocytosis of Candida albicans by eosinophilic leukocytes. J. Allergy Clin. Immunol. 49:311-315.

87. Ishikawa, T., M. C. Yu, and C. E. Arbesman. 1972. Electron microscopic demonstration of phagocytosis of Candida albicans by human eosinophilic leukocytes. J. Allergy Clin. Immunol. 50:183-187.

88. Kalina, M., Y. Kletter, A. Shahar, and M. Aronson. 1971. Acid phosphatase release from intact phagocytic cells surrounding a large-sized parasite. Proc. Soc. Exp. Biol. Med. 136:407-410.

89. Karaoui, R. M., N. K. Hall, and H. W. Larsh. 1977. Role of macrophages in immunity and pathogenesis of experimental cryptococcosis induced by the airbonre route. Part II. Phagocytosis and intracellular fate of Cryptococcus neoformans. Mykosen 20 (11):409-422.

90. Kernbaum, S. 1974. Pouvoir candidacide des polynucléaires neutrophiles humains et chimiothérapie antibactérienne. Pathol. Biol. (November) 22:789-794.

91. Kernbaum, S. 1975. Pouvoirs phagocytaire et fongicide envers Candida albicans

des polynucléaires neutrophiles humains en présence de sérum depourvu de C3 et C4. Ann. Microbiol. (Inst. Pasteur) *126A*:75-81.

92. Kernbaum, S. 1976. Effects of hyperosmolarity on candidacidal activity of human neutrophil polymorphonuclear leukocytes and on clumping of *Candida albicans* by human serum. Biomedicine *25*:109-114.

93. Kernbaum, S., and J.-L. Vilde. 1974. Etude du pouvoir candidacide des polynucleaires neutrophiles humains. Pathol. Biol. (Paris) January *22*:61-66.

94. Kirkpatrick, C. H., R. R. Rich, and J. E. Bennett. 1971. Chronic mucocutaneous candidiasis: model-building in cellular immunity. Ann. Intern. Med. *74*:955-978.

95. Kirpatrick, C. H., I. Green, R. R. Rich, and A. L. Schade. 1971. Inhibition of growth of *Candida albicans* by iron-unsaturated lactoferrin: relation to host defense mechanisms in chronic mucocutaneous candidiasis. J. Infect. Dis. *124*: 539-544.

96. Klebanoff, S. J. 1967. Iodination of bacteria: a bactericidal mechanism. J. Exp. Med. *126*:1063-1078.

97. Klebanoff, S. J. 1968. Myeloperoxidase-halide-hydrogen peroxide anti-bacterial system. J. Bacteriol. *95*:2131-2138.

98. Klebanoff, S. J. 1980. Oxygen metabolism and the toxic properties of phagocytes. Ann. Intern. Med. *93*:480-489.

99. Klebanoff, S. J., and R. A. Clark. 1978. *The Neutrophil: Function and Clinical Disorders,* North-Holland, Amsterdam.

100. Knowles, H. C., Jr., C. L. Meinert, and T. E. Prout. 1976. Diabetes mellitus: the overall problem and its impact on the public. In S. S. Fajans (Ed.), *Diabetes mellitus,* DHEW Publ. No. (NIH) 76-854, Washington, D.C., pp. 11-32.

101. Kozel, T. R. 1977. Non-encapsulated variant of *Cryptococcus neoformans*. II. Surface receptors for cryptococcal polysaccharide and their role in inhibition of phagocytosis by polysaccharide. Infect. Immun. *16*:99-106.

102. Kozel, T. R., and T. G. McGaw. 1979. Opsonization of *Cryptococcus neoformans* by human immunoglobulin G: role of immunoglobulin G in phagocytosis by macrophages. Infect. Immun. *25*:255-261.

103. Kozel, T. R., E. Reiss, and R. Cherniak. 1980. Concomitant but not causal association between surface charge and inhibition of phagocytosis by cryptococcal polysaccharide. Infect. Immun. *25*:295-300.

104. Krause, W., H. Matheis, and K. Wulf. 1969. Fungaemia and funguria after oral administration of *Candida albicans*. Lancet *1*:598-599.

105. Laforce, F. M., D. M. Mills, K. Iverson, R. Cousins, and E. D. Everett. 1975. Inhibition of leukocyte candidacidal activity by serum from patients with disseminated candidiasis. J. Lab. Clin. Med. *86*:657-666.

106. Lehrer, R. I. 1970. The fungicidal activity of human monocytes: a myeloperoxidase-linked mechanism. Clin. Res. *18*:408.

106a. Lehrer, R. I. 1969. Antifungal effects of peroxidase systems. J. Bacteriol. *99*: 361-365.

107. Lehrer, R. I. 1970. Measurement of candidacidal activity of specific leukocyte types in mixed cell populations. Infect. Immun. *2*:42-47.

108. Lehrer, R. I. 1971. Inhibition by sulfonamides of the candidacidal activity of human neutrophils. J. Clin. Invest. *50*:2498-2505.

109. Lehrer, R. I. 1971. Measurement of candidacidal activity of specific leukocyte types in mixed cell populations. Infect. Immun. *3*:800-802.

110. Lehrer, R. I. 1972. Functional aspects of a second mechanism of candidacidal activity by human neutrophils. J. Clin. Invest. *51*:2566-2572.

111. Lehrer, R. I. 1972. The fungicidal activity of human leukocytes. In R. G. Williams, Jr., and H. H. Fudenberg (Eds.), *Phagocytic Mechanisms in Health and Disease,* Intercontinental Medical Book Corp., New York, chapter 10, pp. 151-166.

112. Lehrer, R. I. 1975. The fungicidal mechanisms of human monocytes. I. Evidence for myeloperoxidase-linked and myeloperoxidase-independent candidacidal mechanisms. J. Clin. Invest. 55:338-346.

113. Lehrer, R. I. 1978. Host defense mechanisms against disseminated candidiasis, pp. 94-96. In J. E. Edwards, Jr. (Moderator), Severe candidal infections. Clinical perspective, immune defense mechanisms, and current concepts of therapy. Ann. Intern. Med. 89:91-106.

114. Lehrer, R. I. 1978 Metabolism and microbicidal function, pp. 79-82. In M. J. Cline (Moderator), Monocytes and macrophages: function and diseases. Ann. Intern. Med. 88:78-88.

115. Lehrer, R. I. (Moderator). 1980. Mucormycosis. Ann. Intern. Med. 93 (1):93-108.

116. Lehrer, R. I. 1981. Ingestion and destruction of Candida albicans. In D. A. Adams, H. Koren, and P. Edelson (Eds.), Methods for Studying Mononuclear Phagocytes, Academic, New York, pp. 693-708.

117. Lehrer, R. I., and M. J. Cline. 1969. Interaction of Candida albicans with human leukocytes and serum. J. Bacteriol. 98:996-1004.

118. Lehrer, R. I., and M. J. Cline. 1969. Leukocyte myeloperoxidase deficiency and disseminated candidiasis: the role of myeloperoxidase in resistance to Candida infection. J. Clin. Invest. 48:1478-1488.

119. Lehrer, R. I., and M. J. Cline. 1971. Leukocyte candidacidal activity and resistance to systemic candidiasis in patients with cancer. Cancer 27:1211-1217.

120. Lehrer, R. I., and R. G. Jan. 1970. Interaction of Aspergillus fumigatus spores with human leukocytes and serum. Infect. Immun. 1:345-350.

121. Lehrer, R. I., J. Hanifin, and M. J. Cline. 1969. Defective bactericidal activity in myeloperoxidase-deficient human neutrophils. Nature (Lond.) 223:78-79.

122. Lehrer, R. I., K. M. Ladra, and R. B. Hake. 1975. Nonoxidative fungicidal mechanisms of mammalian granulocytes: demonstration of components with candidacidal activity in human, rabbit, and guinea pig leukocytes. Infect. Immun. 11:1226-1234.

123. Lehrer, R. I., L. S. Goldberg, M. A. Apple, and N. P. Rosenthal. 1972. Refractory megaloblastic anemia with myeloperoxidase-deficient neutrophils. Ann. Intern. Med. 76:447-453.

124. Lehrer, R. I., L. G. Ferrari, J. Patterson-Delafield, and T. Sorrell. 1980. Fungicidal activity of rabbit alveolar and peritoneal macrophages against Candida albicans. Infect. Immun. 28:1001-1008.

125. Lehrer, R. I., D. Szklarek, M. E. Selsted, and J. Fleischmann. 1981. Increased content of microbicidal cationic peptides in rabbit alveolar macrophages elicited by complete Freund adjuvant. Infect. Immun. 33:775-778.

126. Leijh, P. C. J., M. T. van den Barselaar, and R. van Furth. 1977. Kinetics of phagocytosis and intracellular killing of Candida albicans by human granulocytes and monocytes. Infect. Immun. 17:313-318.

127. Louria, D. B., N. Fallon, and H. G. Browne. 1960. The influence of cortisone on experimental fungus infections in mice. J. Clin. Invest. 39:1435-1449.

128. Lundborg, M., and B. Holma. 1972. In vitro phagocytosis of fungal spores by rabbit lung macrophages. Sabouraudia 10:152-156.

129. McGaw, T. G., and T. R. Kozel. 1979. Opsonization of Cryptococcus neoformans by human immunoglobulin G: masking of immunoglobulin G by cryptococcal polysaccharide. Infect. Immun. 25:262-267.

130. Meister, H., B. Heymer, H. Schafer, and O. Haferkamp. 1977. Role of Candida albicans in granulomatous tissue reactions. II. In vivo degradation of C. albicans in hepatic macrophages of mice. J. Infect. Dis. 135:235-242.

131. Merkow, L. P., S. M. Epstein, H. Sidransky, E. Verney, and M. Pardo. 1971. The pathogenesis of experimental pulmonary aspergillosis. Am. J. Pathol. 62:57-66.

132. Mitchell, T. G., and L. Friedman. 1971. In vitro phagocytosis and intracellular fate of variously encapsulated strains of *Cryptococcus neoformans*. Infect. Immun. *5*:491-498.

133. Miya, F., and S. Marcus. 1961. Effect of humoral factors on in vitro phagocytic and cytopeptic activities of normal and "immune" phagocytes. J. Immunol. *86*: 652-668.

134. Monga, D. P. 1981. Role of macrophages in resistance of mice to experimental cryptococcosis. Infect. Immun. *32*:975-978.

135. Moosman, K., and A. Bojanowsky. 1975. Rezidivierende candidosis bei myelo-peroxydasemangel. Monatschr. Kinderheilkd. *123*:408-409.

136. Morelli, R., and L. T. Rosenberg. 1971. The role of complement in the phago-cytosis of *Candida albicans* by mouse peripheral blood leukocytes. J. Immunol. *107*:476-480.

137. Morrison, R. P., and J. E. Cutler. 1981. In vitro studies of the interaction of murine phagocytic cells with *Candida albicans*. J. Reticuloendothel. Soc. *29*:23-34.

138. Nozawa, R. T., R. Sekiguchi, and T. Yokota. 1980. Stimulation by conditioned medium of L-929 fibroblasts, *E. coli* lipopolysaccharide, muramyl dipeptide of candidacidal activity of mouse macrophages. Cell. Immunol. *53*:116-124.

139. Odeberg, H., and I. Olsson. 1975. Antibacterial activity of cationic proteins from human granulocytes. J. Clin. Invest. *56*:1118-1124.

140. Odeberg, H., and I. Olsson. 1976. Microbicidal mechanisms of human granulocytes: synergistic effects of granulocyte elastase and myeloperoxidase or chymotrypsin-like cationic protein. Infect. Immun. *14*:1276-1283.

141. Odegaard, A., and J. Lamvik. 1976. The effect of phenylbutazone and chloramphen-icol on phagocytosis of radiolabelled *Candida albicans* by human monocytes cultured in vitro. Acta Pathol. Microbiol. Scand. Sect. C *84*:37-44.

142. Odegaard, A., K. E. Viken, and J. Lamvik. 1974. Structural and functional proper-ties of blood monocytes cultured in vitro. Acta Pathol. Microbiol. Scand. Sect. G *82*:223-234.

143. Osease, R., and R. I. Lehrer. 1978. A micromethod for measuring neutrophil candidacidal activity in neonates. Pediatr. Res. *12*:828-829.

144. Otto, V., and D. H. Howard. 1976. Further studies on the intracellular behavior of *Torulopsis glabrata*. Infect. Immun. *14*:433-438.

145. Ozato, K., and I. Uesaka. 1974. The role of macrophages in *Candida albicans* in-fection in vitro. Jpn. J. Microbiol. *18* (1):29-35.

146. Pagani, A., R. Spalla, F. A. Ferrari, M. Duse, L. Lenzi, U. Bretz, M. Baggiolini, and A. G. Siccardi. 1981. Defective *Aspergillus* killing by neutrophil leucocytes in a case of systemic aspergillosis. Clin. Exp. Immunol. *43*:201-207.

147. Papadimitriou, J. M., T. A. Robertson, Y. Kletter, M. Aronson, and M. N-I. Walters. 1978. An ultrastructural examination of the interaction between macrophages and *Cryptococcus neoformans*. J. Pathol. *124*:103-109.

148. Parry, M. F., R. K. Root, J. A. Metcalf, K. K. Delaney, L. S. Kaplou, and W. J. Richar. 1981. Myeloperoxidase deficiency. Prevalence and clinical significance. Ann. Intern. Med. *95*:293-301.

149. Peterson, E. M., and R. A. Calderone. 1977. Growth inhibition of *Candida albicans* by rabbit alveolar macrophages. Infect. Immun. *15*:910-915.

150. Quie, P. G., and R. A. Chilgren. 1971. Acute disseminated and chronic mucocutan-eous candidiasis. Sem. Hematol. *8*:227-242.

151. Rausch, P. G., and T. G. Moore. 1975. Granule enzymes of polymorphonuclear neutrophils. A phylogenetic comparison. Blood *46*:913-919.

152. Reinhardt, D. J., W. Kaplan, and L. Ajello. 1970. Experimental cerebral zygomycosis in alloxan-diabetic rabbits. I. Relationship of temperature tolerance of selected zygomycetes to pathogenicity. Infect. Immun. *2* (4):404-413.

153. Repine, J. E., C. C. Clawson, F. L. Rasp, Jr., G. A. Sarosi, and J. R. Hoidal. 1978. Defective neutrophil locomotion in human blastomycosis: evidence for a serum inhibitor. Am. Rev. Respir. Dis. *118*:325-334.

154. Restrepo, M. A., and H. Vélez A. 1975. Efectos de la fagocitosis *in vitro* sobre el *Paracoccidioides brasiliensis*. Sabouraudia *13*:10-21.

155. Rhodes, J. C., L. S. Wicker, and W. J. Urba. 1980. Genetic control of susceptibility to *Cryptococcus neoformans* in mice. Infect. Immun. *29*:494-499.

156. Richard, J. L., and J. R. Thurston. 1975. Effect of aflatoxin on phagocytosis of *Aspergillus fumigatus* spores by rabbit alveolar macrophages. Appl. Microbiol. *30*: 44-47.

157. Rinehart, J. J., A. L. Sagone, S. P. Balcerzak, G. A. Ackerman, and A. F. LoBuglio. 1975. Effects of corticosteroid therapy on human monocyte function. N. Engl. J. Med. *292*:236-241.

158. Robinson, J. E., B. A. M. Harvey, and J. F. Soothill. 1978. Phagocytosis and killing of bacteria and yeast by human milk cells after opsonisation in aqueous phase of milk. Br. Med. J. *1*:1443-1445.

159. Rogers, T. J., E. Balish, and D. D. Manning. 1976. The role of thymus-dependent cell-mediated immunity in resistance to experimental disseminated candidiasis. J. Reticuloendothel. Soc. *20*:291-298.

160. Rosner, F., I. Valmont, P. J. Kozinn, and L. Caroline. 1970. Leukocyte function in patients with leukemia. Cancer *25*:835-842.

161. Ruthe, R. C., B. R. Anderson, B. L. Cunningham, and R. B. Epstein. 1978. Efficacy of granulocyte transfusions in control of systemic candidiasis in the leukopenic host. Blood *52*:493-498.

162. Salmon, S. E., M. J. Cline, J. Schultz, and R. I. Lehrer. 1970. Myeloperoxidase deficiency. Immunologic study of a genetic leukocyte defect. N. Engl. J. Med. *282*:250-253.

163. Sandhu, D. K., R. S. Sandhu, V. N. Damodaran, and H. S. Randhawa. 1970. Effect of cortisone on bronchopulmonary aspergillosis in mice exposed to spores of various *Aspergillus* species. Sabouraudia *8*:32-38.

164. Sasada, M., and R. B. Johnston, Jr. 1980. Macrophage microbicidal activity. Correlation between phagocytosis-associated oxidative metabolism and the killing of *Candida* by macrophages. J. Exp. Med. *152*:85-98.

165. Savage, D. C., and S. H. Madin. 1968. Cellular responses in lungs of immunized mice to intranasal infection with *Coccidioides immitis*. Sabouraudia *6*:94-102.

166. Sawyer, R. T., R. J. Moon, and E. S. Beneke. 1981. Trapping and killing of *Candida albicans* by *Corynebacterium parvum*-activated livers. Infect. Immun. *32*:945-950.

167. Schaffner, A., H. Douglas, and A. Braude. 1982. Selective protection against conidia by mononuclear and against mycelia by polymorphonuclear phagocytes in resistance to *Aspergillus*. J. Clin. Invest. *69*:617-631.

168. Scherwitz, C., and R. Martin. 1979. The phagocytosis of *Candida albicans* blastospores and germ tubes by polymorphonuclear leukocytes. Dermatologica *159*:12-23.

169. Schmid, L., and K. Brune. 1974. Assessment of phagocytic and antimicrobial activity of human granulocytes. Infect. Immun. *10*:1120-1126.

170. Schneerson-Porat, S., A. Shahar, and M. Aronson. 1965. Formation of histiocyte rings in response to *Cryptococcus neoformans* infection. J. Reticuloendothel. Soc. *2*:249-255.

171. Schuit, K. E. 1979. Phagocytosis and intracellular killing of pathogenic yeasts by human monocytes and neutrophils. Infect. Immun. *24*:932-938.

172. Selsted, M. E., D. M. Brown, R. J. DeLange, and R. I. Lehrer. 1983. Primary structures of MCP-1 and MCP-2, natural peptide antibiotics of rabbit lung macrophages. J. Biol. Chem. *258*:14485-14489.

173. Selvaraj, R. J., B. B. Paul, R. R. Strauss, A. A. Jacobs, and A. J. Sbarra. 1974. Oxidative peptide cleavage and decarboxylation by the MPO-H_2O_2-Cl⁻ antimicrobial system. Infect. Immun. 9:255-260.

174. Sidransky, H., and L. Friedman. 1959. The effect of cortisone and antibiotic agents on experimental pulmonary aspergillosis. Am. J. Pathol. 35:169-179.

175. Simpson, D. W., R. Roth, and L. D. Loose. 1979. A rapid, inexpensive and easily quantified assay for phagocytosis and microbicidal activity of macrophages and neutrophils. J. Immunol. Methods 29:221-226.

176. Sinski, J. T., G. L. Reed, L. M. Kelley, and R. LeFebvre. 1973. Macrophage migration technique using coccidioidin. Infect. Immun. 7:226-230.

177. Sixbey, J. W., B. T. Fields, C. N. Sun, R. A. Clark, and C. M. Nolan. 1979. Interactions between human granulocytes and *Blastomyces dermatitidis*. Infect. Immun. 23:41-44.

178. Smith, J. M. B. 1976. In vivo development of spores of *Absidia ramosa*. Sabouraudia 14:11-15.

179. Solomkin, J. S., E. L. Mills, G. S. Giebink, R. D. Nelson, R. L. Simmons, and P. G. Quie. 1978. Phagocytosis of *Candida albicans* by human leukocytes: opsonic requirements. J. Infect. Dis. 137:30-37.

180. Stanley, V. C., and R. Hurley. 1969. The growth of *Candida* species in cultures of mouse peritoneal macrophages. J. Pathol. 97:357-366.

181. Staples, P. J., J. Boujak, R. G. Douglas, Jr., and J. P. Leddy. 1977. Disseminated candidiasis in a previously healthy girl: implication of a leukocyte candidacidal defect. Clin. Immunol. Immunopathol. 7:157-167.

182. Stiehm, E. R. 1978. Chronic mucocutaneous candidiasis: clinical aspects, pp. 96-99. In J. E. Edwards, Jr. (Moderator), Severe candidal infections. Clinical perspective, immune defense mechanisms and current concepts of therapy. Ann. Intern. Med. 89:91-106.

183. Subbarathnam, S., and N. G. Miller. 1979. Comparative study of the effect of thiabendazole and fungizone on *Histoplasma capsulatum* in macrophages. Sabouraudia 17:331-338.

184. Swenson, F. J., and T. R. Kozel. 1978. Phagocytosis of *Cryptococcus neoformans* by normal and thioglycolate-activated macrophages. Infect. Immun. 21:714-721.

185. Tacker, J. R., F. Farhi, and G. S. Bulmer. 1972. Intracellular fate of *Cryptococcus neoformans*. Infect. Immun. 6:162-167.

186. Taschdjian, C. L., E. F. Toni, K. C. Hsu, M. S. Seelig, M. B. Cuesta, and P. J. Kozinn. 1971. Immunofluorescence studies of *Candida* in human reticuloendothelial phagocytes: implications for immunogenesis and pathogenesis of systemic candidiasis. Am. J. Clin. Pathol. 56:50-58.

187. Territo, M. C., and D. W. Golde. 1979. The function of human alveolar macrophages. J. Reticuloendothel. Soc. 25:111-120.

188. Thong, Y. H., D. Ness, and A. Ferrante. 1979. Effect of bilirubin on the fungicidal capacity of human neutrophils. Sabouraudia 17:125-129.

189. Tuck, R., V. Burke, M. Gracey, A. Malajczuk, and Sunoto. 1979. Defective *Candida* killing in childhood malnutrition. Arch. Dis. Child. 54:445-447.

190. van Furth, R. (Ed.). 1975. *Mononuclear Phagocytes in Immunity, Infection and Pathology*. Blackwell Scientific Publ., Oxford. (Collection of papers from the Second Conference on Mononuclear Phagocytes held in the Eysingahuis at Leiden, 2nd to 7th September 1973.)

191. van Furth, R. (Ed.). 1978. *Mononuclear Phagocytes: Functional Aspects of Mononuclear Phagocytes*, Klower, Boston.

192. Walker, S. M., and S. J. Urbaniak. 1980. A serum-dependent defect of neutrophil function in chronic mucocutaneous candidiasis. J. Clin. Pathol. 33:370-372.

193. Warr, G. A., and G. J. Jakab. 1979. Alterations in lung macrophage antimicrobial activity associated with viral pneumonia. Infect. Immun. 26:492-497.

194. Weeks, B. A., M. R. Escobar, P. B. Hamilton, and V. M. Fueston. 1976. Chemotaxis of polymorphonuclear neutrophilic leukocytes by mannan-enriched preparations of *Candida albicans*. Adv. Exp. Med. Biol. 73 (A):161-169.

195. Wegner, T. N., R. E. Reed, R. J. Trautman, and C. D. Beavers. 1972. Some evidence for the development of a phagocytic response by polymorphonuclear leukocytes recovered from the venous blood of dogs inoculated with *Coccidioides immitis* or vaccinated with an irradiated spherule vaccine. Am. Rev. Respir. Dis. 105:845-849.

196. White, L. O. 1977. Germination of *Aspergillus fumigatus* conidia in the lungs of normal and cortisone-treated mice. Sabouraudia 15:37-41.

197. Xanthou, M., E. Valassi-Adam, E. Kintzonidou, and N. Matsaniotis. 1975. Phagocytosis and killing ability of *Candida albicans* by blood leucocytes of healthy term and preterm babies. Arch. Dis. Child. 50:71-75.

198. Yamamura, M., and H. Valdimarsson. 1977. Participation of C3 in intracellular killing of *Candida albicans*. Scand. J. Immunol. 6:591-594.

199. Zgliczyński, J. M., T. Stelmaszyńska, J. Domański, and W. Ostrowski. 1971. Chloramines as intermediates of oxidative reaction of amino acids by myeloperoxidase. Biochim. Biophys. Acta 235:419-424.

Part Two

DETECTION, CONSERVATION, AND APPLICATION

5

Conservation, Collection, and Distribution of Cultures

Shung C. Jong and Winnifred B. Atkins / American Type Culture Collection, Rockville, Maryland

I. INTRODUCTION

Living fungous cultures are essential elements in the production of food, drugs, and chemicals; in assays of the quality, potency, and safety of many products used daily; in the diagnosis and treatment of mycoses that afflict man and animals; in comparative and taxonomic studies of new isolates; and in the education of students, physicians, and other paramedical and technical personnel. To provide suitable materials for these needs, it is essential to conserve authenticated and reliable strains of fungi, utilizing conservation techniques that will ensure their viability without contamination, variation, mutation, or deterioration.

Fungi are well known to have the capacity to develop rapid morphological and physiological changes in culture with frequent transfers on artificial media. Individual workers often lack facilities for permanently maintaining and preserving cultures in a satisfactory condition, and may have little need to maintain them after a piece of research has been completed. Thus, many important strains have been lost and become unavailable to other workers who wish to repeat or extend the work described in the literature. The benefits of deposition of fungous cultures in a central respository where facilities exist for long-term conservation and distribution have been recognized for more than a century. Such a centralized collection not only supplies reliable reference cultures but also provides full information on the background and properties of the strains. It can also provide an identification service for specific strains isolated by field workers, and act as an information clearing house, disseminating notes on morphology, physiology, biochemistry, pathogenicity, toxicology, and other special applications of the cultures.

II. MAINTENANCE AND PRESERVATION

According to Weiss [87], in keeping cultures of microorganisms, conservation implies both maintenance and preservation. Maintenance means keeping the culture alive and pure; and preservation means maintaining them at constant biological potentials for a prolonged period. Therefore, he emphasizes that the function of a culture collection should be to conserve cultures, not merely to maintain them. Methods available for maintenance and preservation of fungi have been reviewed and discussed by Fennell [35] and Onions [65], respectively. The traditional method of maintaining cultures is to grow them in an active state under optimum laboratory conditions on a suitable solid substrate using a system of periodic subculturing at reasonable intervals of time. To reduce frequent serial subculturing, the cultures may be maintained in a reduced metabolic state, which is achieved by storage at low temperatures, by covering with distilled water or mineral oil, and drying in soil or on silica gel. At present the most effective methods of conserving fungi in the culture collection are freeze-drying (lyophilization) and cryogenic freezing with liquid nitrogen.

A. Periodic Transfer

The majority of fungi can be maintained as living cultures if they are transferred from old cultures to fresh slants of a suitable substrate at fairly frequent intervals. This is a general practice for routinely growing cultures in the laboratory. Although it is a laborious and time-consuming operation, thousands of fungi have been maintained by this technique throughout the world. The major disadvantages of the technique are the high possibility of contamination by mites or microorganisms, the risks of deterioration, with subsequent loss of morphological characters and desired biochemical responses, and selection of either a mutant strain or a purely vegetative nonsporulating form.

Fungi are grown on test tube slants composed of an agar medium that favors a minimum of mycelial growth accompanied by the maximum development of their fructifications such as sexual and asexual spores and other propagative structures. A great many different culture media have been used for maintenance of a variety of fungi. Sabouraud's glucose agar [80], water agar [81], potato-carrot agar [54], and soil agar [85] are commonly used for pathogenic fungi. There is no doubt that in practically all cases the conditions of temperature, pH, and light also influence the growth and sporulation of fungi. The optimum cultivation conditions may vary between species of a given genus and even between strains of a single species. In general, the range of optimum conditions for sporulation is usually narrower than for mycelial development.

Transfer of propagative cells is then made from old cultures to fresh slants of a same medium at periodic intervals of time. Increased sporulation can be obtained with some strains if they are transferred from a medium rich in nutrients such as Sabouraud's agar to a weaker medium, corn meal (Difco 0386), or potato carrot agar. The interval between transfers depends largely on the peculiarities of the particular fungus, but also to some extent on external conditions, especially on the storage temperature. Transfer of room-temperature-maintained cultures once every month is sufficiently frequent for most of the pathogenic fungi, although certain species may remain viable for many years. To avoid rapid drying of the agar medium and to reduce the metabolic rate of the organism, the cultures may be kept in a refrigerator at about 5°C [36,45] or in a freezer at temperatures of about −10°C to −20°C [19,20]. Under these low-temperature conditions, the viability of most fungi is lengthened and the interval between transfers can be longer than at room temperature.

B. Oil Sealing

The value of maintaining fungous cultures under mineral oil or paraffin oil as means of insuring longevity for relatively small collections has been recognized since Sherf [78] first reported that cultures of *Fusarium* and *Alternaria* thus maintained were still viable after 6 months. The method consists simply of covering a young, vigorous colony on a slant of suitable agar medium with sterile mineral oil. High-quality oil of the medicinal grade is commonly used. The oil can be sterilized by autoclaving at 15 lb pressure for 2 h and then drying off any entrapped moisture by heating in a drying oven at 170°C for 1-2 h. The culture must be completely covered with a depth of about 1 cm of the sterile oil above the tip of the slant. The oil cultures are stored in the upright position at room temperature or in a refrigerator or cold room. We prefer to keep our oiled cultures of *Histoplasma*, *Paracoccidioides*, *Blastomyces*, and *Coccidioides* at room temperature.

The prime function of the mineral oil method is to prevent dehydration of the cultures and to decrease metabolic activity and growth of the fungi through reduced oxygen consumption [16,31]. It is widely applicable to strictly mycelial or non-sporulating forms to which the freezing and freeze-drying techniques cannot be applied.

Among the fungi pathogenic for humans, Buell and Weston [16] first reported a successful application of this method to cultures of *Microsporum*, *Epidermophyton*, *Trichophyton*, and *Phialophora* for 9 months. The cultures maintained under oil showed no signs of pleomorphism or other undesirable modification. At the Centers for Disease Control in Atlanta, Georgia, a wide variety of pathogenic fungi representing 15 genera and 34 species were conserved under oil by Ajello et al. [1] and observed to retain their viabilities for 2 years. Contrary to the report of Buell and Weston, pleomorphic changes occurred in cultures of *Epidermophyton floccosum*, *Trichophyton mentagrophytes*, and *T. tonsurans*. At the Division of Laboratories and Research, New York State Department of Health in Albany, Little and Gordon [55] maintained over 200 cultures of fungi, consisting primarily of human pathogens together with a few commonly encountered saprophytes, under oil for 12 years. Morphological transformation was observed in cultures of *Microsporum audouinii*, *M. gypseum*, *Trichophyton violaceum*, and *Epidermophyton floccosum*.

This technique is also effectively used in the control of mite contamination and in the elimination of mites contaminating the cultures. Norris [63] was the first to suggest this possibility, and others further confirmed the practical applicability [16, 36,42,88]. To get rid of mites, the infested cultures are covered with mineral oil in the usual manner for a period of 2-3 months and then transferred to appropriate agar media. The resulting cultures will be free of the mites.

C. Sterile Distilled Water as a Maintenance Medium

Castellani [21] first reported the maintenance of cultures of human pathogenic fungi in sterile distilled water for 12 months without apparent evidence of changing morphological and physiological characters. Test tubes of sterile distilled water were inoculated with thin layers of growing agar cultures. The tubes were sealed with Bunsen flame and kept at room temperature. In his later experiments, Castellani [22-25] simplified the original procedure by eliminating the sealing of the inoculated tubes and using cotton wool plugs. The reliability and usefulness of the method was emphasized by Benedek [9], who used commercially available physiologic salt solution in place of distilled water and small screw-capped bottles instead of cotton-plugged test tubes.

The effectiveness of Castellani's technique in conserving fungous cultures has been further demonstrated with human pathogens by McGinnis et al. [60], with plant pathogens by Boesewinkel [10], and for ectomycorrhizae by Marx and Daniel [56].

The advantages of the water cultures consist of the reduced necessity of continuous short-term subculturing and suppression of pleomorphic changes. The method is simple and needs little storage space. However, care must be taken not to allow the water to evaporate. McGinnis et al. [60] claim that the selection of actively sporulating cultures and adequate amount of suspension consisting of spores and hyphae are the most important factors influencing survival in water over a longer period of time.

D. Storage in Sterile Soil or Sand

Sterilized soil is an excellent desiccating substrate for conservation of living fungi in culture. This technique has been widely used in industrial laboratories for maintenance of commercially important cultures [35,39]. However, the most serious objection to this technique is that the considerable time lag before the onset of dormancy due to dryness induces nonsporulating variants to overgrow the wild type [11]. Furthermore, soil is a very complex mixture of varying composition and is difficult to standardize biologically.

Either moistened soil inoculated with a small volume of inoculum and followed by incubation [4] or dried soil inoculated with a large volume of spore suspension and followed by immediately drying [87] is in use for conserving fungous cultures. In the first case, soil is placed in cotton-plugged test tubes and moistened to a level of about 60% of its maximum water-holding capacity. The tubes are autoclaved four times at 15 lb pressure for 30 min on alternate days. The sterile soil is then inoculated with a fungous culture and incubated at the optimal temperature for growth. After the soil cultures have sufficiently grown, they are air-dried by allowing moisture to evaporate through the cotton plugs and then suitably sealed and stored in the refrigerator. This method permits the growth of the fungus and preserves propagative cells and mycelia.

If air-dried soil is to be used as an absorbent of spore suspension, it is transferred in convenient amounts to ordinary half-inch test tubes. The tubes are first given three 3-h sterilizations at 15 lb of pressure on alternate days, then heated in a drying oven until moisture-free, and finally tested for sterility by addition of yeast-malt extract broth (Difco 0711) to tubes selected at random. The sterilized soil must be stored in a desiccator until needed. To preserve a culture, a heavy aqueous suspension of spores is added to the sterilized soil, and the mixture is aseptically air-dried and stored in the refrigerator. This method obviously permits no growth and preserves only those spores introduced into the soil.

Using the soil culture technique, Ciferri and Redaelli [27] found that three species of dermatophytes were still viable after 3 years in soil and showed little pleomorphic change in transplants. Bakerspigel [5,6] also reported on the survival of a variety of pathogenic and saprophytic fungi, in loam, clay, sawdust, peat, sand, and other natural materials. All of the dermatophytes and systemic pathogens remained viable in loam for 13 months.

Although Miller [61], Cormack [28], Gordon [37], and Toussoun and Nelson [82] described the successful maintenance of certain *Fusarium* cultures in sterile soil, a few species do not appear to survive this treatment. In 1966, Booth [11] examined 800 strains of W. L. Gordon's *Fusarium* cultures which were maintained at the American Type Culture Collection by the soil culture method. The complete loss of the cultures of *F. nivale* and *F. decemcellulare* and a 90% loss of *F. avenaceum* cultures further indicated that this is not a satisfactory method for all *Fusarium* species.

Raper and Fennell [73] and Raper and Thom [74] respectively recommended the soil culture method as a means of preserving cultures of *Aspergillus* and *Penicillium*. *Aspergillus fischeri*, *A. sydowi*, and *Penicillium chrysogenum* were successfully maintained in soil by Greene and Fred [39] for over 2 years and *Aspergillus flavus*, *A. luteus*, and *A. niger* by Guida and doAmaral [41] for 5 years. Fennell et al. [36] found that all but 16 of 245 members of the Mucorales survived slightly over 2 years storage in soil culture and claimed that next to lyophilization the dried-soil culture technique was most efficient in maintaining viability.

E. Drying on Silica Gel

A method of drying and storing fungal spores over anhydrous silica gel was first described by Perkins [68], who considered it comparable to lyophilization for long-term preservation of *Neurospora crassa*. The Fungal Genetics Stock Center has, since 1962, employed this technique for preserving genetic stocks of *Aspergillus nidulans* and *Neurospora crassa* [7,64]. Bell and Hamalle [8] found that three insect pathogenic species, *Beauveria bassiana*, *Metarrhizium anisopliae*, and *Nomurea rileyi* (as *Spicaria rileyi*), retained viability and pathogenicity after their spores had been stored on silica-gel crystals in test tubes at −20°C for 3 years. Sleesman et al. [79] successfully maintained stock cultures of four isolates of *Helminthosporium maydis* (races T and O) on silica gel over a period of 12 months without loss of viability and pathogenicity. Elliott [32] reported that cultures of selected fungi, including representative isolates of 10 homothallic species of *Pythium*, had survived up to 4 years when agar discs of mycelium were dried over silica gel in sealed 0.5-ml ampoules. Viability of cultures was dependent on the strain of fungus and the medium on which it was grown before being dried.

Acrasis rosea [75], *Aspergillus parasiticus* [57], *Candida* spp. [66], *Claviceps paspali* [62], *Dictyostelium discoideum* [86], *Endothia parasitica* [71], *Rhodotorula* spp. [75], *Saccharomyces cerevisiae* [40], and *Ustilago maydis* [70] were also reported to survive dehydration on silica gel for 1-3 years.

Trollope [83] preserved 22 fungi on silica gel. Of those stored at room temperature, 77% survived 1 year or more. Storage at 4°C often increased the survival period about two- to threefold.

With incorporation of several changes to increase effectiveness, Perkins [69] has recently described his procedure in detail for preservation of *Neurospora* stock cultures. The 13 × 100-mm culture tubes plugged with cotton are filled to a 65-mm depth with silica gel. They are hot-air sterilized at 180°C for 2 h and then stored at room temperature in a moistureproof box to be ready for use. Davison Refrigeration Grade Silica gel (PA400, approximately 12-20 mesh size) without indicator dye is employed. Cultures are grown for a week on 4% agar slants containing appropriate nutrients. For conidiating strains, about 0.5 ml of sterile water is gently introduced in a sporulating culture and conidia are suspended by shaking, using a Vortex-type mixer. For nonconidiating strains, the aerial hyphae and mycelia are peeled off with a sterile blade and transferred to a 10 × 75-mm tube containing 0.5 ml of water, and then ground with a pipet or glass rod against the tube wall to obtain a creamy homogenate. About 0.5 ml of sterile nonfat milk is then added and stirred gently, and the entire suspension is pipetted dropwise over the silica gel in a prelabeled cotton-plugged tube. The tube is vibrated briefly with the mechanical mixer to distribute inoculum over as many particles as possible throughout the silica gel, and is then placed in an ice-water bath for 15 min. After 1 day at room temperature, the particles appear dry and the tube is sealed against moisture by covering the plug and mouth of tube with a 20-mm square of Parafilm. The sealed tubes are stored at 5°C or −20°C in a moistureproof box.

F. Freeze-Drying

Freeze-drying, commonly called lyophilization, has been highly recommended as an economical and effective means of conserving the viability and characteristics of living microorganisms. The ability of the cells to survive freeze-drying is critically dependent on the degree of freezing injury and the final water content. The cells to be dried are placed in ampoules and solidly frozen before being subjected to a very low pressure in a high vacuum. Thus, the available water in the form of an ice matrix is removed quickly via sublimation (i.e., ice transforms directly to vapor, by-passing the intermediary liquid phase), so that physical and chemical reactions cannot take place during the entire dehydration. The ampoules are then sealed under vacuum to prevent the re-entry of moisture into the desiccated preparations that are rendered chemically inert in the absence of most of the residual water. For the long-term conservation, refrigerated storage of freeze-dried preparations is preferable to storage at room temperature. Many types of freeze-drying apparatus are now commercially available.

The use of the freeze-drying technique to conserve fungi, including yeasts, is now well established. The cells capable of withstanding freeze-drying are the spores or dormant forms of fungi that regularly withstand dehydration in nature. Elser et al. [34] first successfully freeze-dried five strains of wine yeasts in blood serum without loss of physiological activity. At the Northern Regional Research Laboratory (NRRL) of the U.S. Department of Agriculture in Peoria, Illinois, Wickerham and Andreasen [90] successfully used the method to preserve 15 of 16 dermatophytes and other molds, and 95% of 384 yeasts and yeast-like fungi for a period of 1 year. Raper and Alexander [72] demonstrated that many strains of *Aspergillus*, *Penicillium*, and some members of the Mucorales remained viable for up to 40 months and a limited number of Fungi Imperfecti survived for 20 months. Since then, the freeze-drying technique developed at the NRRL has been successfully applied to the large and varied collection of fungous cultures [33,36,45,46,59].

The NRRL method may be summarized briefly. Fungi are grown on appropriate sporulating media in test tubes or petri dishes until abundant spores are produced. A heavy suspension of spores is prepared in sterile bovine serum or in dried skimmed milk reconstituted at double strength, and approximately 0.05-0.1 ml of the suspension is added to each of several sterile cotton-stopped, Pyrex glass tubes that have been properly labeled with glass-marking ink. The cotton plugs are replaced and the exposed cotton is burned off. The remaining plug is pushed down into the tube to a depth of about one-half inch to prevent possible contamination or loss of the dried pellet during processing. The tubes are inserted in rubber sleeves on a glass manifold and lowered into a bath of dry ice and methyl cellosolve at a temperature of about −40°C to −50°C where the spore suspensions are completely frozen within a few seconds. The tubes are raised above the surface of the bath where a temperature of about −10°C is maintained, and evacuation is carried out by means of a vacuum pump. Best results are obtained with a vacuum between 200-500 μm of mercury. When the pellets appear dry, evacuation is continued at room temperature for half an hour to insure thorough desiccation. The tubes are then sealed off under vacuum with a gas-oxygen torch. The freeze-dried preparations are stored at a refrigeration temperature of approximately 4°C.

Haskins and Anastasiou [44] compared the NRRL method with what they refer to as the PRL (Prairie Regional Laboratory) method, which is similar to the double-vial "batch" method used at the American Type Culture Collection (ATCC), as described by Weiss [87]. There was no significant difference in results from the two methods.

The batch-type technique currently employed by the ATCC is a two-step procedure that involves slow freezing of the spore suspensions followed by primary drying at low temperatures and secondary drying at room temperature, and then sealing off under vacuum on a manifold.

In the ATCC procedure, the fungi are grown on agar medium to the point of optimum sporulation. The mature spores are harvested by flooding the culture with 20% (w/v) solution of skim milk (Difco 0032) which has been sterilized at 116°C for 20 min. Over-heating may cause carmelization of the milk. The spores are gently scraped from the surface of the culture to yield a suspension containing at least 10^6 spores per ml. The spores of cultures grown in broth medium are centrifuged and resuspended in a solution containing 12% sucrose plus one-half strength fresh growth medium. The sucrose is prepared as a 24% solution, sterilized by autoclaving at 120°C for 20 min. An amount of 0.2 ml of the spore suspension is pipetted into sterile, cotton-plugged 11 × 35-mm freeze-drying shell vials (VWR Scientific No. 27921-015) that have been prelabeled with a bake-on ink. The filled vials are immediately refrigerated at 4°C to prevent germination of the spores for a period not to exceed 2 h.

Vials containing samples are first packed upright in a stainless steel container that is placed on the bottom of a mechanical refrigerator at −79°C for 1 h. The container with the frozen samples is then quickly attached to an Atmo-vac plate (Refrigeration for Science, Inc., 51 Alabama Avenue, Island Park, New York) connected to a dry ice/ethyl cellosolve-chilled condenser and a vacuum pump. Crushed dry ice is placed around the container and drying proceeds under a vacuum of 20-30 μm of mercury (Fig. 1). The dry ice completely dissipates within 2 h after the start of run, and drying continues at ambient temperature overnight. Following drying, the cotton-plugged shell vials are inserted into 14 × 85-mm glass shell ampoules (VWR Scientific No. 27921-015)

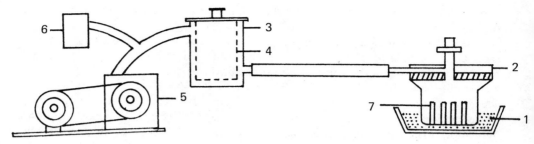

Figure 1 ATCC freeze-drying apparatus, "batch-type" system. 1. Dry ice snow. 2. Atmo-vac plate. 3. Virtis condensor. 4. Reservoir filled with dry-ice snow and ethyl cellosolve. 5. Vacuum pump. 6. Vacuum gauge. 7. Specimen.

containing a few granules of moisture-indicating silica gel and a small wad of cotton cushion (Fig. 2). Two layers of glass fiber paper GF 82 (H. Reeve Angel & Co., Clifton, New Jersey) are packed over the inner vial and the outer ampoule is constricted with an air-gas torch to a narrow capillary. The shell ampoules are then placed on a manifold, evacuated to 50 μm or less, and hermetically sealed with a two-way air-gas burner, after which the freeze-dried preparations are stored at 4°C.

To rehydrate freeze-dried material, 0.4 ml of sterile distilled water is added to the contents of the vial, mixed well, and transferred to a test tube containing 5.6 ml of sterile distilled water. This suspension is allowed to rehydrate for 1 h before being transferred to plates or slants of solid media.

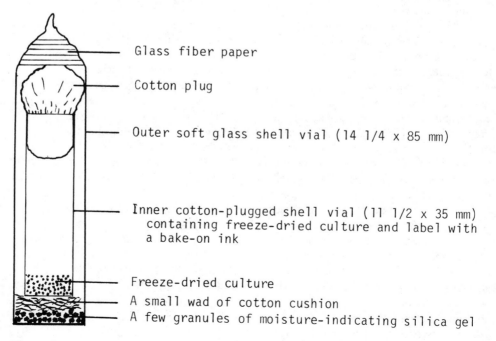

Figure 2 A freeze-dried preparation with the ATCC batch-type method.

At the ATCC, the viability of reconstituted freeze-dried material is evaluated by placing three drops of the hydrated suspension on a plate containing an appropriate agar medium. The plate is tilted, allowing the drops to run across the surface and form three streaks. When growth is visible, the colonies in each streak are counted and evaluated as follows:

Heavy confluent growth	Excellent	(E)
Colonies of 50-100/streak	Good	(G)
Colonies of 10-50/streak	Fair+	(F+)
Colonies of 5-10/streak	Fair	(F)
Ten or less colonies/plate	Poor	(P)
Growth in broth only	Broth only	(BO)
No growth on agar or broth	None	(O)

Preparations giving a rating of less than F are considered unsatisfactory and are not made available for distribution in the freeze-dried state.

Quantitative survivals of fungi after freeze-drying have been reported by Buell [15], Weston [89], Atkin et al. [3], Mazur [58], Graham [38], Haskins [43], and Pedersen [67]. Studies of viability after storage for a period of time have been carried out by Wickerham and Flickinger [91], Haynes et al. [45], Mehrotra and Hesseltine [59], Hesseltine et al. [46], Davis [29], Ellis and Roberson [33], and Schipper and Bekker-Holtman [77]. Effects of storage for 10 years on freeze-dried strains of pathogenic fungi have been reported by Rhoades [76] and Bosmans [12], respectively. The ATCC has employed freeze-drying as a means for preserving pathogenic fungi since 1942 [17].

G. Freezing and Storing in Liquid Nitrogen

Considerable success has been achieved in preserving living fungi through the application of cryogenics. The cryogenic storage temperatures now commonly used are those of liquid nitrogen ($-196°C$) and liquid nitrogen vapor ($-150°C$ and below). Cryoprotective agents that have been found useful in this process include 10% (v/v) glycerol and 5% (v/v) dimethyl-sulfoxide (DMSO) in distilled water [17,47,51]. Apparently Udelnova [84] was the first to use liquid nitrogen for freezing fungi, and the American Type Culture Collection (ATCC) was the first to apply it on a large scale for conservation of a wide variety of fungi [49,50]. Description of the apparatus and explanations of the procedures of liquid nitrogen refrigeration have been reported by Jong [52] and may be briefly summarized.

Both sporulating and nonsporulating fungi can be preserved by this method, and are grown as previously described for freeze-drying. The spores or mycelial fragments are harvested by flooding the slants or plates with 10% glycerol or 5% DMSO and gently scraping the surface of the cultures. An amount of 0.5 ml suspension is pipetted into sterile cotton-plugged, prescored borosilicate ampoules (T. C. Wheaton Co., Milville, New Jersey) or 2.0 ml screw-cap polypropylene vials (Vangard International, Neptune, New Jersey). The polypropylene vials have proved to be superior to the borosilicate ampoules for freezing some strains of fungi [18]. Cultures producing only mycelia are grown on plates containing an appropriate medium and three plugs of the advancing edge of the colony are removed with a 5-mm sterile cork borer and suspended in 0.4 ml of cryoprotective additive per vial or ampoule. Strains yielding colonies in liquid culture small enough to be pipetted are grown in flasks containing a suitable broth, either stationary or on a Gyrotory Shaker model G-10 (New Brunswick Scientific Co., New Brunswick, New Jersey). Cultures in broth are fragmented in a sterile Waring Blendor and suspended in equal parts of 20% glycerol and growth medium or equal parts of 10% DMSO and growth medium to give a final concentration of 10% glycerol or 5% DMSO, respectively. Some strains must be concentrated by centrifugation to obtain sufficient material for freezing. Pathogenic strains are not macerated in a mechanical blender because of the hazard of aerosol dispersion.

Glass ampoules containing fungi pathogenic for humans and animals are always maintained in the vapor-phase of a liquid nitrogen refrigerator. They are not sealed so as to: (1) eliminate the dangers involved in handling pathogenic fungi in the sealing process, (2) prevent the possibility of explosion during thawing, and (3) prevent the possibility of self-inoculation on opening the ampoules. Most of the nonpathogenic fungi are stored in the liquid-phase of a liquid nitrogen refrigerator. It is therefore essential that the ampoules be completely sealed. An improperly sealed ampoule immersed in liquid nitrogen will permit entry of liquid and will explode at the time of thawing due to the sudden expansion of the nitrogen into gas, thus creating a serious hazard. The operator should wear a face mask for safety to avoid danger from exploded ampoules.

The filled vials or ampoules are placed onto pre-labeled aluminum canes (Nasco #A545, Fort Atkinson, Wisconsin) in metal cannisters which are then placed into the freezing chamber of a programmed freezer (Cryo-Med, 49659 Leona Drive, Mt. Clemens, Michigan). The initial cooling is carried out at a rate of $1°C/min$ from room temperature to $-35°C$; subsequent cooling to below $-100°C$ is rapid and uncontrolled. The cooling rate is monitored by a Honeywell Brown Electronik temperature recorder. Then the ampoules are immediately transferred to storage in liquid nitrogen at $-196°C$ or liquid nitrogen vapor storage at a temperature range of about $-150°C$-$180°C$. All strains of pathogenic fungi are stored in the vapor phase of an LN refrigerator and handled with care. At the ATCC an inoculation hood 40032-2 (S. Blickman, Inc., Weehawken, New Jersey) is used for agents of systemic mycoses.

The level of liquid nitrogen in each refrigerator is maintained by an automatic filling controller that regulates the entry of nitrogen from a 1500-gallon storage tank located outside the building for ease of delivery of nitrogen by the manufacturer. The storage tank is self-pressurizing and the refrigerators are filled by means of a vacuum-insulated feed pipe into the laboratory. The flow of liquid nitrogen is controlled by the opening and closing of the solenoid valve in the system and is determined electronically by heat-sensitive thermistors. If the level of liquid in a refrigerator becomes dangerously low, a thermistor becomes sensitized by the thermal change and actuates alarm systems that are transmitted to a 24-h answering service.

For recovery of the fungous cultures frozen in liquid nitrogen, the frozen ampoules or vials are thawed rapidly in 37°C water bath until the last trace of ice is dissipated. This usually takes about 40-60 s for the borosilicate ampoules with moderately vigorous agitation. The polypropylene vials require 60-120 s for the contents to thaw completely. The culture samples are aseptically transferred to an appropriate growth medium.

The major disadvantages of liquid nitrogen refrigeration are the relatively high cost of the apparatus and the liquid nitrogen, the space requirement for refrigeration units, and the need for constant surveillance. At the ATCC, this technique is used as a back-up system for all the seed stocks and for the fungi that cannot be preserved by the freeze-drying technique. The major advantages of the freeze-drying technique are relative economy of time and apparatus, elimination of the need for constant surveillance, and ease of dispatch of cultures. However, both techniques appear to have many advantages in common. There is a reduction in culture variability, saving in time, expense, and labor over handling living stocks, elimination of the need for repeated pathogenicity tests, prevention of loss due to contamination, and assurance of long-term availability of cultures. These two techniques are therefore considered to be the most effective methods for long-term conservation of living fungi in the culture collection.

III. CULTURE COLLECTIONS

For many years throughout the world, there has been a recognized need for facilities where cultures may be deposited, maintained, and conserved for further investigation in such a way that their unaltered identities are assured. Culture collections fulfill these requirements. Several of the larger fungous collections are the American Type Culture Collection (ATCC) at Rockville, Maryland; the Centraalbureau voor Schimmelcultures (CBS) at Baarn, the Netherlands; the Commonwealth Mycological Institute (CMI) at Kew, England; the Institute for Fermentation (IFO) at Osaka, Japan; the Northern Regional Research Center, formerly the Northern Regional Research Laboratory (cited as NRRL) at Peoria, Illinois; and the University of Alberta Mold Herbarium and Culture Collection (UAMH), Alberta, Canada. Many other important collections belonging to industrial concerns as well as specialized government departments exist in the United States and in numerous other countries. The American Type Culture Collection is used as an example to present one way in which a culture collection may develop, and the operation and management involved in the maintenance, preservation, documentation, and distribution of cultures.

A. American Type Culture Collection

The American Type Culture Collection (ATCC) is a unique nationally and internationally recognized resource dedicated to the collection, conservation, documentation, and distribution of authentic cultures of living microorganisms, animal cells, and viruses. Research efforts are focused on comparative microbiology, microbial systematics, and improved methods of characterization, identification, and preservation of cultures. The Collection also provides technical information within the field of microbiology. The ATCC plays a vital role in biosciences, teaching, and industry through service, research, and education [14,26,48]. Table 1 presents available strains of fungi pathogenic for man and animals, and names of depositors.

B. ATCC Mycological Collection

The ATCC methods and procedures for the mycological collection are well established, and each strain is processed according to the following protocol.

1. Acquisition

The head of the ATCC Mycology Department must be familiar with the current nomenclature, the availabilities of type or reference strains of scientific and/or industrial significance, and the demands or potential demands for cultures. The head also assumes the responsibilities of curatorship, systematically reviews current literature, updates information associated with the strains in the collection, scans for every type culture and other

Table 1   Strains of Pathogenic Fungi Available from the ATCC

Organism	ATCC	Depositor
Absidia corymbifera	14049	C. Emmons
	14058	
	28223	W. Knudtson
	32624	
	32625	
	36512	M. Corbel
	44568	
Acladium castellani	760	A. Castellani
	14241	
Acremoniella lutzi	9462	A. de Area Leao
Acremonium kiliense	4301	T. Benedek
	14489	M. Thirumalacher
	14490	
	34716	CBS
Acremonium recifei	9940	C. Emmons
	36328	A. Padhye
Acremonium spinosum	9471	A. de Area Leao
Actinodendron verticillatum	28726	A. Padhye
Ajellomyces capsulata	22635	J. Kwon-Chung
	22636	
	28536	
Ajellomyces dermatitidis	18187	E. McDonough
	18188	
	36470	
Anixiopsis fulvescens	14527	T. Benedek
var. *stercoraria*	18996	J. Rippon
Apiotrichum humicola	38294	V. Hopsu-Havu
Arthroderma benhamiae	16781	L. Ajello
	16782	
	22778	J. Maniotis
	22779	
	22780	
	22781	
	28060	R. Vanbreuseghem
	28061	
	28062	
	28063	
	28064	
	28065	
	28066	
	28067	
	28068	
	28069	
	28433	P. Stockdale
	28434	
	28435	
	28436	
	28437	

Table 1 (continued)

Organism	ATCC	Depositor
	28438	
Arthroderma benhamiae	28439	
(continued)	28440	
	28441	
	32428	CDC
	32429	
	32430	
	32431	
	32432	
	32433	
	32434	
	32636	R. Vanbreuseghem
Arthroderma simii	18593	J. Rippon
	18610	A. Hasegawa
	26040	A. Londero
	38534	S. Desai
Arthroderma tuberculatum	15507	G. Orr
Arthroderma vanbreuseghemii	24952	R. Vanbreuseghem
	24953	
	24954	
	24955	
	24956	
	24957	
	24958	
	24959	
	24960	
	28145	A. Padhye
	28146	
	28283	
	24133	F. Rush-Munro
	34896	S. Shadomy
	44644	M. Hironaga
	44645	
	44646	
Aspergillus flavus	24133	F. Rush-Munro
	34896	S. Shadomy
Aspergillus fumigatus	13073	H. Hasenclever
	14109	C. Emmons
	14110	
	16424	S. Martin
	24007	M. Baxter
	26430	H. Ikemoto
	26933	J. Taylor
	26934	
	34007	B. Schaeffer
	36607	D. Kerridge
	42202	V. Kurup
	42203	
	42204	

Table 1 (continued)

Organism	ATCC	Depositor
Aspergillus fumigatus	16903	K. Raper
var. *ellipticus*	32820	M. McGinnis
Aspergillus nidulans	26424	El Sheikh Mahgoub
Aspergillus oryzae	34712	M. Gordon
Aspergillus penicilloides	16002	A. Castellani
Aspergillus phialiseptus	26606	J. Kwon-Chung
Aspergillus terreus	26604	L. Milne
	28301	J. Rippon
Aureobasidium mansonii	762	A. Castellani
	14249	
	16621	W. Cook
Aureobasidium pullulans	12535	E. Wynne
Auxarthron reticulatum	18427	G. Orr
Auxarthron zuffianum	15607	G. Orr
Basidiobolus haptosporus	14448	C. Drechslera
	16108	M. Thirumalacher
	16109	
	26112	D. Frey
	34122	A. Kamalam
	36033	H. Gugnani
	32866	Pasteur Institute
Basidiobolus meristosporus	36598	E. Drouhet
	36599	
	36600	
	36601	
Basidiobolus ranarum	11230	F. Lombard
	14052	C. Emmons
	24669	G. Koshi
	24670	
	24671	
	32277	R. Vanbreuseghem
Blastomyces dermatitidis	10225	C. Emmons
	14112	
	24327	D. Howard
	24866	R. Garrison
	26197	R. Cox
	26198	
	26199	
	28305	L. Kaufman
	28306	
	28839	R. Garrison
	32090	A. DiSalvo
	38742	E. Alture-Werber
Candida albicans	752	A. Castellani
	753	
	2091	R. Chodat

Table 1 (continued)

Organism	ATCC	Depositor
Candida albicans	10231	C. Emmons
(continued)	10259	A. de Area Leao
	10261	
	11651	G. Scherr
	14053	C. Emmons
	18527	R. Gordon
	18804	CBS
	24433	Z. McGee
	26426	C. Saltarelli
	26427	
	26428	
	26555	L. Montes
	26790	Z. Polak
	28815	E. Grunberg
	28835	M. Collins
	28836	
	28837	
	28956	S. Ganor
	32089	A. Frisk
	32354	J. Kwon-Chung
	32470	J. Kane
	32552	H. Randhawa
	34133	G. Roberts
	34312	D. Parr
	36082	J. Edwards
	36263	M. Gunsekaran
	36801	J. Kwon-Chung
	36802	
	36803	
	38289	V. Hopsu-Havu
	38483	F. Greatorey
	38696	M. Perrot
	44203	G. Land
	44373	P. Augur
	44374	
	44376	Y. Koch
	44505	F. Odds
	44506	
	44806	T. Mitchell
	44807	
	44808	
	44829	M. Pesti
	44830	
	44831	
Candida benhamiae	18807	CBS
Candida chiropterorum	22291	CBS
Candida guilliermondii	6260	A. Castellani
	9390	A. de Area Leao

Table 1 (continued)

Organism	ATCC	Depositor
Candida guilliermondii	14242	A. Castellani
(continued)	34134	G. Roberts
	38290	V. Hopsu-Havu
Candida kruseii	6258	A. Castellani
	28870	D. Yarrow
	34135	G. Roberts
	38293	V. Hopsu-Havu
Candida parapsilosis	14054	C. Emmons
	34136	G. Roberts
	38291	V. Hopsu-Havu
Candida paratropicalis	42678	J. Baker
Candida pseudotropicalis	4135	CBS
	34137	G. Roberts
	38296	V. Hopsu-Havu
	28838	M. Collins
Candida ravautii	18821	CBS
	42214	W. Crozier
Candida steatolytica	18822	CBS
Candida tropicalis	750	A. Castellani
	14056	C. Emmons
	18526	R. Gordon
	28707	D. Drutz
	34139	G. Roberts
	34313	D. Parr
	38292	V. Hopsu-Havu
Candida viswanathii	22981	S. Meyer
	28269	H. Randhawa
Candida sp.	18895	C. Sonck
	34147	G. Roberts
Cephalosporium falciforme	28173	M. Gordon
Cephalosporium serrae	32628	M. de Albornoz
Cephalosporium sp.	12285	C. Emmons
	28172	M. Gordon
Ceratocystis stenoceras	22433	R. Davidson
	22855	F. Mariat
	22856	
Ceratocystis sp.	22853	F. Mariat
	22854	
Cercospora apii	12246	R. Cox
	14281	C. Emmons

Table 1 (continued)

Organism	ATCC	Depositor
Chmelia slovaca	24279	CBS
Chrysosporium pruinosum	16498	C. Emmons
Cladosporium butyri	36948	CBS
Cladosporium carrionii	16264	L. Georg
	22864	D. Frey
	24099	
	32279	R. Vanbreuseghem
Cladosporium castellani	24788	D. Borelli
	44079	D. Marcano
	44080	
	44081	
Cladosporium cladosporioides	26688	F. Polack
Cladosporium resinae f. *avellaneum*	26227	F. Rush-Munro
Cladosporium sphaerospermum	26228	F. Rush-Munro
Cladosporium trichoides	10958	C. Emmons
	22649	J. Bennett
	24928	J. Reid
	28255	D. Crichlow
	32280	R. Vanbreuseghem
	44217	S. Maheswari
	44223	M. Hironaga
Coccidioides immitis	28088	P. Negroni
	28868	M. Collins
	32092	R. Vanbreuseghem
	34020	M. Collins
	34021	
	34615	S. Sun
	34616	
	38142	M. Huppert
	38143	
	38144	
	38145	
	38146	
	38147	
	38148	
	38149	
	38150	
Cochliobolus spicifer	32792	R. Zapater
Conidiobolus coronatus	24868	D. Frey

Table 1 (continued)

Organism	ATCC	Depositor
Conidiobolus coronatus	32125	A. Kamalan
(continued)	32825	
	32826	
	32827	
	32862	A. Padhye
	32863	
	32864	
	32865	
	32867	H. Fromentin
	36032	H. Gugnani
	36602	E. Drouhet
	36603	
	36604	
	36605	
	42063	A. Sekhon
	42064	
Conidiobolus incongruus	24293	H. Eckert
Coprinus cinereus	24329	D. Speller
Cryptococcus albidus	34140	G. Roberts
	38297	J. Hopsu-Havu
Cryptococcus albidus	10672	NRRL
var. diffluens	34141	G. Roberts
Cryptococcus ater	14247	A. Castellani
	42272	CBS
	42273	
Cryptococcus gastricus	32042	D. Yarrow
Cryptococcus laurentii	34142	G. Roberts
Cryptococcus neoformans	4414	E. Hirsch
	11239	C. Emmons
	11240	
	11241	
	11242	
	13690	M. Littman
	14113	C. Emmons
	14114	
	14115	
	14116	
	14117	
	14248	A. Castellani
	18365	J. Reback
	24064	J. Bennett
	24067	
	28204	A. Bakerspigel
	28205	

Table 1 (continued)

Organism	ATCC	Depositor
Cryptococcus neoformans	28737	S. Shadomy
(continued)	28738	
	28769	T. Kobayashi
	28770	
	28771	
	32045	D. Yarrow
	32264	R. Vanbreuseghem
	32265	
	32267	
	32308	H. Randhawa
	32309	
	32310	
	32551	
	32719	IFO
	32737	D. Swinne-Desgain
	32739	
	32741	
	34144	G. Roberts
	34543	F. Staib
	34664	CCY
	34869	J. Kwon-Chung
	34870	
	34877	
	36069	M. Gordon
	36070	
	36071	
	36556	T. Kozel
	36582	N. Miller
	38897	G. Kobayashi
	44104	H. Saez
	44105	
	44384	K. Nishimura
Cryptococcus terreus	34145	G. Roberts
Cryptococcus uniguttulatus	34143	G. Roberts
	38298	V. Hopsu-Havu
Cryptstroma corticale	14694	D. Emanuel
Curvularia lunata	26425	El Sheikh Mahgoub
Curvularia spicifer	34897	L. Ajello
Diplodia gossypina	28570	A. Restrepo
Drechslera hawaiiensis	26061	CDC
	26062	
	26063	
	26064	
	26065	
	26066	
	26067	
	42186	C. Young

Table 1 (continued)

Organism	ATCC	Depositor
Emmonsia ciferrina	16107	M. Thirumalacher
Emmonsia crescens	13704	C. Emmons
	24951	R. Kodousek
	32539	K. Krivance
	32540	
Emmonsia parva	10784	J. Carmichael
	10785	
	14051	C. Emmons
	32541	K. Krivance
Epidermophyton floccosum	9646	C. Emmons
	10227	
	15693	
	18397	L. Ajello
	32498	J. Kane
	38486	F. Greatorex
	38826	A. Grigoriu
	44685	T. Granade
Epidermophyton floccosum var. *nigricans*	26072	M. Hejtmanek
Eurotium rubrum	22757	F. Rush-Munro
Exophiala jeanselmei	10224	C. Emmons
	18148	J. Reback
	34123	M. McGinnis
Exophiala jeanselmei var. *heteromorpha*	24152	A. DiSalvo
Exophiala mansonii	18657	CBS
Exophiala werneckii	9467	NIH
	18122	C. Emmons
	18123	
	18124	
	18125	
	34099	P. Szaniszlo
	34944	G. Volcan
	36317	M. McGinnis
Filobasidiella neoformans	732	N. Evans
	2505	F. Tanner
	2526	
	4189	CBS
	4413	E. Hirsch
	6352	E. Levin
	7472	G. Foster
	9506	O. Felsenfeld
	10226	C. Emmons
	24065	J. Bennett
	24066	
	28957	J. Kwon-Chung

Table 1 (continued)

Organism	ATCC	Depositor
Filobasidiella neoformans	32266	R. Vanbreuseghem
(continued)	32268	
	32269	
	32608	J. Kwon-Chung
	32609	
	34387	K. Erke
	34388	
	34389	
	34390	
	34391	
	34663	CCY
	34872	J. Kwon-Chung
	34876	
	34878	
	34879	
	34880	
	34883	
	36555	T. Kozel
	42347	G. Bulmer
Filobasidiella uniguttulatum	24227	H. Phaff
	32047	CBS
	32048	
Fonsecaea pedrosoi	9475	A. de Area Leao
	9941	C. Emmons
	10221	
	18826	T. Benedek
	18827	
	18828	
	18829	
	18830	
	18831	
	18832	
	28174	M. Gordon
	32282	R. Vanbreuseghem
	44356	I. Iwatsu
Fusarium dimerum	15621	W. Gordon
	28584	R. Zapater
Fusarium moniliforme	38159	M. Rinaldi
Fusarium oxysporum	26225	F. Rush-Munro
Fusarium solani	32793	R. Zapater
	36031	H. Gugnani
Geotrichum candidum	4798	F. Tanner
	18301	J. Sinclair
	34146	G. Roberts
Geotrichum pseudocandidum	36214	H. Saez
Glenospora lanuginosa	14256	A. Castellani

Table 1   (continued)

Organism	ATCC	Depositor
Hansenula petersonii	16761	NRRL
Haplosporangium sp.	10903	W. Jellison
Hapsidiospora denvera	32080	W. Wang
Hendersonula toruloidea	22190	J. Gentles
	22191	
	22192	
	26226	F. Rush-Munro
	26932	C. Campbell
	42101	G. Van Eijk
Histoplasma capsulatum	8136	T. Benedek
	10230	C. Emmons
	10884	
	11378	G. Scherr
	11407	C. Emmons
	11408	
	11656	CDC
	12700	C. Emmons
	14282	
	16585	
	18496	J. Reback
	24867	R. Garrison
	26027	M. Berliner
	26028	
	26029	
	26030	
	26031	
	26032	
	26033	
	26034	
	26320	L. Pine
	26809	R. Garrison
	28122	D. Howard
	28175	M. Gordon
	28176	
	28177	
	28178	
	28179	
	28308	L. Kaufman
	32682	A. diSalvo
	32683	
	38904	G. Kobayashi
Histoplasma capsulatum	24294	D. Grigoriu
var. *duboisii*	24295	
	32281	R. Vanbreuseghem
Histoplasma farciminosum	28798	G. San-Blas
	32136	A. Padhye
	32137	
	32138	

Table 1   (continued)

Organism	ATCC	Depositor
Histoplasma farciminosum (continued)	32139	
	32140	
	32141	
Hyphopichia burtonii	14257	A. Castellani
	14464	D. Borelli
	14465	
	14466	
Kluyveromyces lactis	38322	V. Hopsu-Havu
Leptosphaeria senegalensis	18262	A. El-Ani
	18263	
	18264	
	18265	
	18282	
Leptosphaeria tompkinsii	16412	A. El-Ani
Madurella grisea	10794	J. Mackinnon
Madurella mycetomatis	13140	C. Emmons
	13141	
	14286	
	14287	
	24531	R. Vanbreuseghem
	32938	A. Kamalam
Microsporum audouinii	9079	C. Emmons
	10008	
	10216	
	10868	T. Benedek
	11347	C. Emmons
	11348	
	12332	IFO
	12333	
	14057	C. Emmons
	24580	D. Grigoriu
	24581	
	24705	
	24706	
	26340	J. Carmichael
	26341	
	26837	D. Grigoriu
	26838	
	32335	
	32509	J. Kane
	32511	
	42558	Y. Clayton
	42561	J. Kwon-Chung
	46100	
Microsporum canis	9084	C. Emmons
	9865	A. Hoerlein

Table 1 (continued)

Organism	ATCC	Depositor
Microsporum canis	10214	C. Emmons
(continued)	11621	M. Littman
	11622	
	14055	C. Emmons
	18615	A. Hasegawa
	24880	A. Pier
	26342	J. Carmichael
	28937	M. English
	32507	J. Kane
	32903	S. Watanabe
	36296	H. Saez
	36299	
	42599	Y. Clayton
	44459	W. Tucker
	44686	T. Granade
Microsporum cookei	22863	D. Frey
	34662	D. Grigoriu
Microsporum distortum	13219	CDC
	13220	
	26224	F. Rush-Munro
Microsporum ferrugineum	11992	IFO
Microsporum gallinae	12108	CDC
	22242	L. Ajello
Microsporum gypseum	9083	C. Emmons
	10215	
	13994	
	22713	M. Connole
	24102	A. Bakerspigel
	24103	
	24881	A. Pier
	32500	J. Kane
	36428	G. Morgan-Jones
	42899	W. Loeffler
	42900	
Microsporum nanum	28951	M. O'Keefe
	28952	
	42129	S. Searls
Microsporum persicolor	26042	A. Londero
Microsporum praecox	38000	I. Weitzman
Microsporum racemosum	32208	V. Daum
	38556	J. Rippon
Monosporium apiospermum	9258	C. Emmons
	9468	A. de Area-Leao
	24048	A. Bakerspigel
	24132	F. Rush-Munro
	28206	A. Bakerspigel

Table 1 (continued)

Organism	ATCC	Depositor
Monosporium apiospermum	28256	
(continued)	28257	
Mortierella wolfsii	24296	M. Baxter
	36820	M. Corbel
Mucor circinelloides	26759	L. Kapica
f. sp. *circinelloides*		
Nannizzia cajetani	14386	CDC
	14387	
	14388	
	22865	A. Padhye
	26344	J. Carmichael
	26345	
	26346	
	26347	
	26348	
	26349	
	26350	
	26351	
	26352	
	26353	
	26354	
Nannizzia fulva	16445	CMI
	16446	
	24883	A. Pier
	26355	J. Carmichael
	26356	
Nannizzi grubyia	14419	CDC
	14420	
	14421	
	14422	
	14423	
Nannizzia gypsea	16428	M. Gordon
	18609	A. Hasegawa
	22925	CMI
	22926	
	24163	M. Gordon
	24164	
Nannizzia incurvata	18611	A. Hasegawa
	18612	
	24005	CMI
	24006	
	24165	M. Gordon
	24166	
	24884	A. Pier
	26357	J. Carmichael
	26358	
Nannizzia obtusa	22465	CMI

Table 1   (continued)

Organism	ATCC	Depositor
Nannizzia obtusa (continued)	26359	J. Carmichael
Nannizzia otae	28327	A. Hawegawa
	28328	
Nannizzia persicolor	22439	CMI
	22440	
	22441	
	22464	
Neotestudina rosatii	24280	CBS
Paecilomyces variotii	24330	S. Jang
	24838	A. Patnaik
Paracoccidioides brasiliensis	10237	M. Upton
	14280	C. Emmons
	14283	
	24015	M. deAlbornoz
	24016	
	24017	
	32069	A. Restrepo
	32070	
	32071	
	32072	
	32073	
	32074	
	32075	
	36324	G. San-Blas
Pectinotrichum llanense	22632	G. Orr
Penicillium diversum var. *aureum*	24100	A. DiSalvo
Penicillium marneffei	18224	D. Fennell
Petriellidium boydii	11961	F. Herrero
	14106	C. Emmons
	34381	M. Carter
	36281	D. Stevens
	36282	
	36283	
	36479	E. Alture-Werber
	38697	A. DiSalvo
	44328	M. Hironaga
	44329	
	44330	
	44331	
	44332	
	44333	
Phialophora gougerotii	10986	R. Benham
Phialophora mutabilis	26223	M. Slifkin

Table 1 (continued)

Organism	ATCC	Depositor
Phialophora parasitica	26366	C. Wang
Phialophora richardsiae	26465	N. Conant
	32129	M. Ulloa-Sosa
	44261	I. Weitzman
	44262	
Phialophora verrucosa	4806	F. Weidman
	10223	C. Emmons
	26689	F. Polack
	28182	M. Gordon
	28304	D. Borelli
	38561	I. Iwatsu
Piedraia hortai	24292	CBS
Pityrosporum ovale	14521	CBS
	24047	A. Bakerspigel
	38593	G. Midgley
Pityrosporum pachydermatis	14522	CBS
	24022	M. Baxter
	42756	M. Gordon
	42757	
Pyrenochaeta romeroi	13735	D. Borelli
Ramichloridium cerophilum	24410	D. Borelli
Rhinocladiella compacta	10222	C. Emmons
	28303	D. Borelli
Rhinocladiella spinifera	18218	H. Nielsen
Rhizomucor pusillus	36606	E. Drouhet
	42780	G. Szakacs
Rhizopus arrhizus	14050	C. Emmons
	32619	W. Knudtson
	32620	
	34965	I. Weitzman
Rhizopus cohnii	24793	P. Fragner
Rhizopus formosaensis	34715	L. Ajello
Rhizopus oryzae	11886	CDC
Rollandina hylinospora	14047	H. Kuehn
Saccharomyces cerevisiae	38324	V. Hopsu-Havu
Saksenaea vasiformis	28740	L. Ajello
Sarcinosporon inkin	34899	L. Ajello
	34900	
	34901	
	34902	
	34904	
	36450	I. Salkin
Scedosporium apiospermum	46173	M. Hironaga

Table 1 (continued)

Organism	ATCC	Depositor
Schizophyllum commune	26679	A. Restrepo
Selenotila peltata	18389	D. Yarrow
	18390	
Sporobolomyces salmonicolor	32311	H. Randhawa
	36402	CBS
Sporopachydermia lactativora	32043	CBS
Sporothrix schenckii	6243	T. Benedek
	7968	J. D'Antoni
	8707	R. Pike
	10212	C. Emmons
	10213	
	10268	A. de Area-Leao
	14096	G. Muller
	14284	C. Emmons
	14285	
	14804	J. Reback
	14805	
	16345	
	24646	C. Park
	26327	F. Staib
	26328	
	26330	
	26331	
	26332	
	26334	
	26335	
	26336	
	26337	
	26338	
	26408	J. Bennett
	28183	M. Gordon
	28184	
	28388	F. Mariat
	28906	F. Rush-Munro
	32283	R. Vanbreuseghem
	32284	
	32885	
	32886	
	32790	T. Nisikawa
	32791	
	34898	R. Garrison
	38104	J. Freeman
	38573	W. Dion
Sporothrix schenckii var. *luriei*	18616	L. Ajello
Sterigmatomyces elviae	18894	C. Sonck

Table 1   (continued)

Organism	ATCC	Depositor
Syringospora albicans	32032	D. Yarrow
	32033	
Syringospora stellatoidea	32077	D. Yarrow
Torulaspora hansenii	38325	V. Hopsu-Havu
Torulopsis glabrata	15545	NRRL
	28226	W. Knudtson
	32312	C. Kauffman
	32554	A. Notowicz
	34138	G. Roberts
	38326	V. Hopsu-Havu
Trichophyton ajelloi	24885	A. Pier
	42892	F. Rush-Munro
Trichophyton balcaneum	763	A. Castellani
Trichophyton batonrougei	11898	A. Castellani
Trichophyton concentricum	9358	N. Conant
	14250	A. Castellani
	14251	
Trichophyton equinum	12544	CDC
	12545	
	12546	
	12547	
	26365	G. deVries
	32512	J. Kane
Trichophyton equinum	22443	CMI
var. *autotrophicum*	42894	F. Rush-Munro
Trichophyton erinacei	22442	CMI
	28446	P. Stockdale
	28447	
	28448	
	28449	
	28450	
	28451	
	28452	
	28453	F. Rush-Munro
Trichophyton megninii	7214	CBS
	11093	CDC
	12106	
	12107	
	34008	J. Kane
	34009	
Trichophyton mentagrophytes	4807	F. Weidman
	4808	
	8125	E. Muskatblit
	8294	F. Weidman
	8757	C. Emmons
	8758	

Table 1   (continued)

Organism	ATCC	Depositor
Trichophyton mentagrophytes	9129	
(continued)	9533	USDA
	9972	C. Emmons
	10270	A. de Area Leao
	10271	
	11480	C. Emmons
	11481	
	13996	
	13997	
	18613	A. Hasegawa
	18748	D. Taplin
	18749	
	18750	
	18751	
	18752	
	22839	Schering Corp.
	24198	W. Merz
	24552	F. Blank
	26323	T. Hashimoto
	28185	M. Gordon
	28186	
	28187	
	28939	M. English
	28940	
	32457	G. deVries
	32499	J. Kane
	32506	
	32510	
	34551	D. Poulain
	36107	E. Beneke
	36215	H. Saez
	36297	
	44687	T. Granade
Trichophyton rubrum	10218	C. Emmons
	10272	A. de Area Leao
	10789	C. Emmons
	11900	A. Castellani
	11990	
	14001	C. Emmons
	18753	D. Taplin
	18754	
	18755	
	18756	
	18757	
	18758	
	18759	
	18760	
	18761	
	18762	

Table 1   (continued)

Organism	ATCC	Depositor
Trichophyton rubrum	18763	
(continued)	22402	CBS
	22785	
	28188	M. Gordon
	28189	
	28190	
	28191	
	28202	K. Marton
	28203	
	28941	M. English
	32501	J. Kane
	36262	H. Saez
	38484	F. Greatorex
	44688	T. Granade
	44697	
	44766	
Trichophyton schoenleinii	4822	F. Weidman
	10397	CBS
	11682	CDC
	11683	
	22775	F. Blank
	22776	
	22777	
	32502	J. Kane
Trichophyton soudanense	11723	J. Wood
	22862	D. Frey
	24582	D. Grigoriu
	24583	
	24869	D. Frey
	24870	
	23871	
	24872	
	24873	
Trichophyton terrestre	28572	A. Bakerspigel
	28573	
	42897	F. Rush-Munro
	32505	J. Kane
Trichophyton tonsurans	9292	C. Emmons
	10217	
	10220	
	14000	
	14002	
	24929	R. Bandoni
	28942	M. English
	32504	J. Kane
	44689	T. Granade
	44690	
Trichophyton verrucosum	28943	M. English

Table 1   (continued)

Organism	ATCC	Depositor
Trichophyton verrucosum	32508	J. Kane
(continued)	34469	M. Wawrzkiewicz
	34470	
	34471	
	38485	F. Greatorex
	38535	K. Wawrzkiewicz
	38536	
	42898	F. Rush-Munro
Trichophyton verrucosum var. *album*	10694	L. Georg
Trichophyton verrucosum var. *autotrophicum*	36058	D. Scott
Trichophyton verrucosum var. *discoides*	10695	L. Georg
	26196	G. Pepin
Trichophyton verrucosum var. *ochraceum*	10696	L. Georg
Trichophyton violaceum	8376	C. Emmons
	11902	A. Castellani
	24787	A. Bakerspigel
	28944	M. English
Trichophyton yaoundei	13946	CDC
	13947	
	13948	
Trichosporon beigelii	4155	F. Weidman
	22375	H. Saez
	28592	CBS
	34148	G. Roberts
	38300	V. Hopsu-Havu
Trichosporon capitatum	36553	G. Grunder
Tritirachium roseum	22524	T. Ranakrishnan
	22538	C. La Touche
Tritirachium shiotae	22567	CBS
Wangiella dermatitidis	14488	M. Thirumalacher
	28869	CBS
	34100	P. Szaniszlo

valuable strains that are currently being used by the scientific, industrial, and educational communities and requests reprints of publications related to these cultures.

After reviewing the literature, requests for cultures are made to investigators in the field to deposit their cultures in the ATCC. As a national and international resource of living microorganisms, all acquisitions must be well documented, preferably described in the literature, and acquired from reputable investigators. Major efforts have been made to provide extensive holdings of type cultures; plant, animal and human pathogens; spoilage organisms; food fungi; bioassay strains; cultures used in industrial processing; antibiotic-and mycotoxin-producing strains; genetic stock cultures, and mutant strains of industrial significance.

All reprints concerning the ATCC cultures are included in the ATCC reprint collection. The reprints are indexed by author(s), subject(s), and cross-referenced for easy retrieval, and are microfilmed for convenient storage.

2. Accession

Before a strain is accessioned and catalogued, it is subjected to a series of tests by the scientific staff at the ATCC to check the viability, purity, identity, preferred temperature and media for growth and/or sporulation, and methods of preservation. After being properly preserved, purity and viability are rechecked. Pertinent references relating to each accession are reviewed, and records of definitive information relating to each strain are maintained on microfilm.

3. Preservation

The ATCC fungi are preserved by freeze-drying (lyophilization) and/or storage in liquid nitrogen. When each culture is accepted for deposition, a number of ampoules are prepared for long-term preservation to be set apart as "seed stock," and additional ampoules are designated "order stock" for distribution. When order stock becomes depleted, an ampoule of seed stock is opened, new culture specimens are prepared from it and are refreeze-dried or refrozen as new order stock. The seed stock is always the closest material available to the original deposit. Because cryogenic storage in liquid nitrogen is the most satisfactory method to date for long-term conservation of living fungi, at present at least three ampoules of each strain in the Collection are stored in this state and set aside as reference seed stocks.

In addition, two ampoules of each freeze-dried strain and one of each frozen strain are placed in duplicate repositories established by the ATCC at the Virginia Polytechnic Institute and State University in Blacksburg, Virginia, and the Frederick Cancer Research Center, Frederick, Maryland, respectively. This step is taken to prevent loss of the materials in the event of extensive damage to the ATCC facility.

The ATCC also maintains preservation cards for each strain in the Collection. This record includes the binomial name, ATCC accession number, date preserved, culture age and medium used, growth conditions, protective solution, material preserved (i.e., sexual, asexual spores, or mycelia), results of viability check, and inventory. A set of index cards is on file with reference to the position of each culture stored in the liquid nitrogen refrigerator and the number of ampoules per cane. The top of each cane is properly coded. Each refrigerator has its own coding system. Every ampoule withdrawn from the refrigerator is subtracted from the inventory on the index card, and the number of ampoules in each refrigerator is known at all times. Computerization of these data is now being undertaken.

4. Culture Data and Retrieval

Appropriate literature references relating to each acquisition are reviewed. The master card prepared includes the scientific name, history and host, packing group, availability (in freeze-dried, frozen, or living state), recommendations for growth and sporulation, source of species description for the type, and special applications (e.g., uses for production of antibiotics, mycotoxins, enzymes, vitamins, etc.) with the pertinent references. Data on the strains are retrievable by species name, special use, ATCC accession number, strain and culture designations, and hosts. Data are stored on microfilm. Records are kept of the number of requests made for each strain to help determine the present demand for the strains.

5. Catalogue

If the culture received forms the perfect (sexual) state, it is catalogued under the name of the perfect state. The name of the imperfect (asexual) state, if available, is also designated following the perfect name. However, some of the fungi isolated from the perfect state in nature have never produced perfect states in culture. Therefore, if a culture is received under the perfect name, but forms an imperfect state only, a statement "imperfect state" is made in the main entry of such a strain.

Under each scientific name, the ATCC strain numbers are listed in numerical order. The ATCC accession number is followed by the depositor's name and his strain number or other identifying designation. Next appears the original source of isolation, use, and/or unusual characteristics of the strain, literature citations, and finally the preferred medium and growth temperature [53]. Nomenclature and pertinent references relating to each ATCC fungous culture are kept up-to-date by reviewing the literature.

The catalogues are typed on computer tapes using a computerized text-editing system that allows easy up-dating and provides a photocomposed type-set of copy for use by the printer.

6. Deacquisition

ATCC periodically examines its fungous cultures for relevancy to the scientific community. The identity and value of each strain maintained is reevaluated by the ATCC mycology staff at the time of distribution and reprocessing for preservation. The strains that are atypical and of little scientific or historical significance as judged by the documentation data, distribution rate, and other pertinent criteria are put on a permanent hold for distribution. The reasons for holding are recorded on the ATCC Laboratory Report. The department office keeps a list of these strains. When the list reaches 50 in number, a copy of this list is forwarded to the Professional Services Department, which determines the extent of requests for the cultures. This information is reviewed by the department head. With the Director's approval, candidates for discard are published in various scientific newsletters. If there is no objection from science and society communities, the culture is physically discarded from the collection 1 year after the publication, and associated records are then placed in a discard file.

7. Patent Deposition

The ATCC has acquired the status of international depositary authority for strains of microorganisms and cell cultures to meet requirements of patent procedures [13,30].

An international treaty has been drafted under the auspices of the World Intellectual Property Organization (WIPO) for recognition of international deposit of microorganisms for the purposes of patent procedure. It is called the "Budapest Treaty" and consists of 20 articles followed by 15 rules with the following headings:

Rule 1. Abbreviated Expressions and Interpretation of the Word "Signature"
Rule 2. International Depositary Authorities
Rule 3. Acquisition of the Status of International Depositary Authority
Rule 4. Termination or Limitation of the Status of International Depository Authority
Rule 5. Defaults by the International Depositary Authority
Rule 6. Making the Original Deposit or New Deposit
Rule 7. Receipt
Rule 8. Later Indication or Amendment of the Scientific Description or Proposed Taxonomic Designation or Both
Rule 9. Storage of Microorganisms
Rule 10. Viability Test and Statement
Rule 11. Furnishing of Samples
Rule 12. Fees
Rule 13. Publication by the International Bureau
Rule 14. Expenses of Delegations
Rule 15. Absence of Quorum in the Assembly

Contracting countries include Bulgaria, France, Federal Republic of Germany, Hungary, Japan, Spain, United Kingdom, and the United States of America. Denmark, Finland, India, Indonesia, Italy, Luxembourg, the Netherlands, Norway, Soviet Union, Sweden, Switzerland, Turkey, and Zaire are expected to become contracting countries in the future. The ATCC is also formally designated as an official depository for cultures in connection with patent applications under the European Patent Organization (EPO).

IV. DISTRIBUTION OF CULTURES

Distribution of living fungi within the United States may fall under the jurisdiction of one or more of the following agencies: the Department of Agriculture (both state and national), U.S. Public Health Service, or the U.S. Department of Transportation. International shipments must also be concerned with the rules and regulations of the U.S. Department of Treasury (Customs Service) and the U.S. Department of Commerce.

A. Permit Requirements for Shipping

Movement of all plant pathogens and mycotoxin-producing strains across interstate or international boundaries is restricted by the U.S. Department of Agriculture (USDA) and requires a permit from the Plant Protection and Quarantine Programs (PPQ) and Animal and Plant Health Inspection Service (APHIS). The USDA Application Form #PPQ-526, "Application and Permit to Move Live Plant Pests," is completed by the investigator who will receive the culture and submitted to the plant regulatory official of the state in which the culture will be used. The state in turn mails the form to PPQ for approval. However, the states of Hawaii and Nebraska require a USDA permit for every fungous culture shipped into their respective states.

Highly infectious pathogens and disease vectors of animals and humans that represent a potential hazard to the public health and/or to agriculture require a permit either from the USDA or the Public Health Service (PHS) or both before shipment can be made within the nation. To obtain a permit for animal pathogens, USDA Application Form #VS 16-3 must be completed and submitted to the Organisms and Vectors International and Domestic Control, U.S. Department of Agriculture, Animal Health Division, Federal Center Building, Hyattsville, Maryland 20782 for consideration. For certain agents or vectors of human diseases, PHS Application Form #HSM 13.39 must be completed and sent to the U.S. Public Health Service, Foreign Quarantine Program, Centers for Disease Control, Atlanta, Georgia 30333. If both PHS and USDA permits are required, only one application is made and sent to the Centers for Disease Control who, after taking action, will forward it to USDA.

The Canadian Department of Agriculture requires an annual import permit for all fungous cultures shipped into Canada. In special cases, a "single entry" permit also may be required. Application on Form HA 359 is made to the Chief of Veterinary Biologics, Canada Department of Agriculture, Health of Animals Branch, S.B.I. Building, 2323 Riverside Drive, Ottawa, Ontario K1A OY9, Canada.

Under the Export Administration Regulations, an export license is required from the U.S. Department of Commerce for export of most fungous cultures to all countries except Canada. The license may be obtained from the U.S. Department of Commerce, Bureau of International Commerce, Office of Export Control, Washington, D.C. 20230. A certificate may be needed for certain countries for importation of fungous cultures. For example, an original Swiss Blue Import Certificate or Yugoslavian END-USE Certificate must be accompanied with the application for an export license from U.S. Department of Commerce. This certificate may be obtained from the Swiss Federal Department of Public Economy, Division of Commerce, Import and Export Control or the Yugoslav Chamber of Economy in Belgrade.

B. Shipping Regulations

Culture collections and individuals working with pathogenic fungi and concerned with shipping cultures, either nationally or internationally, must be cognizant of the shipping regulations pertaining to etiologic agents and other biomedical materials. It is mandatory that the shipper comply with the requirements that cultures be prepared and packaged in accordance with specific standards set forth by the Public Health Service (PHS), the International Air Transport Association (IATA), and the U.S. Department of Transportation (DOT).

C. Classification of Etiologic Agents

A fungous culture is considered to be an "etiologic agent" if it conforms to the definition issued by the Public Health Service as a "viable microorganism or its toxin which causes or may cause disease" [42CFR 72.25(c)]. The fungous agents listed in 42CFR 72.25(c) include *Blastomyces dermatitidis, Coccidioides immitis, Cryptococcus neoformans, Histoplasma capsulatum,* and *Paracoccidioides brasiliensis*. In addition to these strains, *Histoplasma capsulatum* var. *duboisii* is listed in the "Classification of Etiologic Agents on the Basis of Hazard", 4th Edition, July 1974, published by the U.S. Department of Health, Education and Welfare, Public Health Service, Center for Disease Control, Office of Biosafety, Atlanta, Georgia 30333.

D. Growth and Packaging of Cultures for Shipping

Cultures for shipping may be prepared as freeze-dried material, agar slants, or broth cultures and the volume limited to 50 ml. If the volume exceeds 50 ml, more stringent packaging requirements are imposed and shipment is permitted by cargo aircraft only (DOT 49CFR 173.387).

Packaging of cultures of 50 ml or less requires enclosing the material in a watertight primary container such as a vial or test tube. This primary container must be enclosed in a secondary container that is both watertight and durable. More than one primary container may be enclosed in the secondary container if the total volume of material does not exceed 50 ml. The primary container or containers must be surrounded by enough absorbent material within the secondary container to absorb the total volume of the etiologic agent in case of leakage or breakage. The secondary container must then be enclosed in an outer shipping container made of cardboard or any material of equal or greater strength.

International shipments must be sent as air mail "letter packages." Some countries do not permit perishable biological material to be sent through the mail (Postal Service Publication 42) and an alternative method of shipment would be via a freight forwarder. The export license number is included in the address label, the forwarder signs and dates the culture shipment, and the license is returned to the Department of Commerce by the shipper.

The PHS "Biomedical Material" label [42CFR 72.25 (c)4] must be placed on the outside of all packages containing etiologic agents. In addition, international shipments require a shipper's certification in triplicate (DOT 49-CFR, CAB 82).

A green customs label obtained from local U.S. post offices expedites delivery, and a violet label is also required for perishable biological materials and may be obtained only by written application from the Office of Mail Classification, Bureau of Finance and Administration, Post Office Department, Washington, D.C. 20260 [2]. The described regulations regarding permits and shipping are in effect as of February 1982 and may be subject to change in the future.

E. Sources of Labels and Shipping Containers

Etiologic agents labels, shipper's certification labels, and shipping containers required under the authority of the Interstate Quarantine regulations (42 CFR, Section 72.25), are available from representative sources listed below.

1. Labels

Labelmaster
7525 North Wolcott Ave.
Chicago, Illinois 60626

Unz and Co.
190 Baldwin Ave.
Jersey City, New Jersey

2. Shipping Containers

Harold Lindner, Inc.
71 Murray St.
New York, New York
10007

Arthur H. Thomas Company
Vine Street at 3rd
P.O. Box 779
Philadelphia, Pennsylvania
19105

Freund Can Company
155 West 84th Street
Chicago, Illinois
60620

REFERENCES

1. Ajello, L., V. O. Grant, and M. A. Gutzke. 1951. Use of mineral oil in the maintenance of cultures of fungi pathogenic for humans. Arch. Dermatol. Syphilol. *63*:747-749.

2. Alexander, M. T. 1976. International shipments of biological materials. Newsletter U.S. Fed. Cult. Collection *6*:11-12.

3. Atkin, L., W. Moses, and P. P. Gray. 1949. The preservation of yeast cultures by lyophilization. J. Bacteriol. *57*:575-578.

4. Atkinson, R. G. 1954. Quantitative studies on the survival of fungi in five-year-old dried soil cultures. Can. J. Bot. *32*:673-678.

5. Bakerspigel, A. 1953. Soil as a storage medium for fungi. Mycologia *45*:596-604.

6. Bakerspigel, A. 1954. A further report on the soil storage of fungi. Mycologia *46*:680-681.

7. Barratt, R. W., G. B. Johnson, and W. N. Ogata. 1965. Wild-type and mutant stocks of *Aspergillus nidulans*. Genetics *52*:233-246.

8. Bell, J. V., and R. J. Hamalle. 1974. Viability and pathogenicity of entomogenous fungi after prolonged storage on silica gel at −20°C. Can. J. Microbiol. *20*:639-642.

9. Benedek, T. 1962. Fragmenta mycologica. II. On Castellani's "water cultures" and Benedek's "mycotheca" in chlorallactophenol. Mycopathol. Mycol. Appl. *17*:255-260.

10. Boesewinkel, H. J. 1976. Storage of fungal cultures in water. Trans. Br. Mycol. Soc. *66*:183-185.

11. Booth, C. 1971. *The Genus Fusarium,* Commonwealth Mycological Institute, Kew.

12. Bosmans, J. 1974. Ten years lyophilization of pathogenic fungi. Mycopathol. Mycol. Appl. *3*:13-23.

13. Brandon, B. A. 1978. Culture deposits at the American Type Culture Collection. Develop. Indust. Microbiol. *19*:169-171.

14. Buchanan, R. E. 1966. Symposium on stability in dynamic microbial systems. III. History and development of the American Type Culture Collection. Q. Rev. Biol. *41*:101-104.

15. Buell, C. B. 1948. Studies on the effect of the lyophil process on fungous spores. M. A. Thesis, Wellesley College, Wellesley, Mass.

16. Buell, C. B., and W. H. Weston. 1947. Application of the mineral oil conservation method to maintaining collections of fungous cultures. Am. J. Bot. *34*:555-561.

17. Butterfield, W., S. C. Jong, and M. T. Alexander. 1974. Preservation of living fungi pathogenic for man and animals. Can. J. Microbiol. *20*:1665-1673.

18. Butterfield, W., S. C. Jong, and M. T. Alexander. 1978. Polypropylene vials for preserving fungi in liquid nitrogen. Mycologia *70*:1122-1124.

19. Carmichael, J. W. 1956. Frozen storage for stock cultures of fungi. Mycologia *48*:378-381.

20. Carmichael, J. W. 1962. Viability of mold cultures stored at −20°C. Mycologia *54*:432-436.

21. Castellani, A. 1939. Viability of some pathogenic fungi in distilled water. J. Trop. Med. Hyg. *42*:225.

22. Castellani, A. 1960. A brief note on the viability of some pathogenic fungi in sterile distilled water. Imprensa Medica *24*:1-3.

23. Castellani, A. 1962. Long viability (more than 12 months) of many pathogenic fungi in sterile distilled water, suggesting a simple method of maintaining fungal strains in mycological collections while apparently preventing pleomorphism of dermatophytes. Ann. N.Y. Acad. Sci. *93*:152-155.

24. Castellani, A. 1963. Further researches on the long viability and growth of many pathogenic fungi and some bacteria in sterile distilled water. Mycopathol. Mycol. Appl. *20*:1-6.

25. Castellani, A. 1967. Maintenance and cultivation of the common pathogenic fungi of man in sterile distilled water. Further researches. J. Trop. Med. Hyg. *70*:181-184.

26. Clark, W. A., and D. H. Geary. 1974. The story of the American Type Culture Collection—its history and development (1899-1973). Adv. Appl. Microbiol. *17*: 295-309.

27. Ciferri, R., and P. Redaelli. 1948. Mancata formazione di forme ascofore e conservazione di culture di funghi patogeni in substrati naturali. Mycopathologia *4*:131-136.

28. Cormack, M. W. 1951. Variation in the cultural characteristics and pathogenicity of *Fusarium avenaceum* and *Fusarium arthrosporioides*. Can. J. Bot. *29*:32-45.

29. Davis, R. J. 1963. Viability and behavior of lyophilized cultures after storage for twenty-one years. J. Bacteriol. *85*:486-487.

30. Donovick, R. 1978. Procedures presently employed at the ATCC in handling cultures deposited for patent purposes. Newsletter U.S. Fed. Cult. Collect. *8*: 6-13.

31. Edwards, G. A., C. B. Buell, and W. H. Weston. 1947. The influence of mineral oil upon the oxygen consumption of *Sordaria fimicola*. Am. J. Bot. *34*:551-555.

32. Elliott, R. F. 1975. Viability of fungous cultures dried and stored over silica gel. New Zealand J. Sci. *18*:577-583.

33. Ellis, J. J., and J. A. Roberson. 1968. Viability of fungous cultures prepared by lyophilization. Mycologia *60*:399-405.

34. Elser, W. J., R. A. Thomas, and G. I. Steffen. 1935. The desiccation of sera and other biological products (including microorganisms) in the frozen state with preservation of the original qualities of products so treated. J. Immunol. *28*: 433-473.

35. Fennell, D. I. 1960. Conservation of fungous cultures. Bot. Rev. *26*:79-141.

36. Fennell, D. I., K. B. Raper, and M. H. Flickinger. 1950. Further investigations on the preservation of mold cultures. Mycologia *42*:135-147.

37. Gordon, W. L. 1952. The occurrence of *Fusarium* species in Canada. II. Prevalence and taxonomy of *Fusarium* species in cereal seed. Can. J. Bot. *30*: 209-251.

38. Graham, S. O. 1956. Germination responses of *Ustilago tritici* (Pers.) Rostr. teliospores in relation to lyophilization. I. Some factors affecting mortality before and after sublimation. Res. Stud. Wash. State Univ. *24*:307-317.

39. Greene, H. C., and E. B. Fred. 1934. Maintenance of vigorous mold stock cultures. Ind. Eng. Chem. *26*:1297-1298.

40. Grivell, A. R., and J. F. Jackson. 1969. Microbial culture preservation with silica gel. J. Gen. Microbiol. *58*:423-425.

41. Guida, V. O., and J. F. doAmaral. 1949-50. Tecnica de conservacao de fungos em areia esteril (Technique of conservation of fungi in sterile sand). Arg. Inst. Biol. S. Paolo *19*:203-206.

42. Hartsell, S. E. 1956. Maintenance of cultures under paraffin oil. Appl. Microbiol. *4*:350-355.

43. Haskins, R. H. 1957. Factors affecting survival of lyophilized fungal spores and cells. Can. J. Microbiol. *3*:477-485.

44. Haskins, R. H., and J. Anastasiou. 1953. Comparisons of the survivals of *Aspergillus niger* spores lyophilized by various methods. Mycologia *45*:523-532.

45. Haynes, W. C., L. J. Wickerham, and C. W. Hesseltine. 1955. Maintenance of cultures of industrially important microorganisms. Appl. Microbiol. *3*:361-368.

46. Hesseltine, C. W., B. J. Bradle, and C. R. Benjamin. 1960. Further investigations on the preservation of molds. Mycologia *52*:762-774.

47. Hubálek, Z., and A. Kocková-Kratochvilová. 1978. Liquid nitrogen storage of yeast cultures. I. Survival, and literature review of the preservation of fungi at ultralow temperatures. Antonie Leeuwenhoek. J. Microbiol. Serol. *44*:229-241.

48. Huppert, M., L. Ajello, S. Bartnicki-Garcia, J. E. Bennett, J. Cazin, Jr., J. E. Domer, J. R. Graybill, H. O. Halvorson, H. W. Larsh, G. Medoff, and M. Puziss (Working Committee). 1978. Proceedings and recommendations of the workshop on medical mycology research and training, national needs and problems. National Institute of Allergy and Infectious Diseases, National Institutes of Health.

49. Hwang, S. W. 1960. Effects of ultra-low temperature on the viability of selected fungus strains. Mycologia *52*:527-529.

50. Hwang, S. W. 1966. Long-term preservation of fungus cultures with liquid nitrogen refrigeration. Appl. Microbiol. *14*:784-788.

51. Hwang, S. W., W. F. Kwolek, and W. C. Haynes. 1976. Investigation of ultralow temperature for fungal cultures. III. Viability and growth rate of mycelial cultures following cryogenic storage. Mycologia *68*:377-387.

52. Jong, S. C. 1978. Conservation of cultures. In S. T. Chang and W. A. Hays (Eds.), The Biology and Cultivation of Edible Mushrooms, Academic Press, London, pp. 119-135.

53. Jong, S. C. 1982. Fungi and mycoviruses. In *Catalogue of Strains I.* 15th edition. American Type Culture Collection, Rockville, Maryland, pp. 261-544.

54. Langeron, M., and R. Vanbreuseghem. 1952. *Precis de Mycologie,* Masson et Cie, Editeurs.

55. Little, G. N., and M. A. Gordon. 1967. Survival of fungus cultures maintained under mineral oil for twelve years. Mycologia *59*:733-736.

56. Marx, D. H., and W. J. Daniel. 1976. Maintaining cultures of ectomycorrhizal and plant pathogenic fungi in sterile water cold storage. Can. J. Microbiol. *22*: 338-341.

57. Mayne, R. Y., J. W. Bennett, and J. Tallant. 1971. Instability of an aflatoxin-producing strain of *Aspergillus parasiticus.* Mycologia *63*:644-648.

58. Mazur, P. 1953. Studies on the effects of low temperatures and dehydration on the viability of fungous spores. Ph.D. Thesis, Harvard Univ., Cambridge, Mass.

59. Mehrotra, B. S., and C. W. Hesseltine. 1958. Further evaluation of the lyophil process for the preservation of Aspergilli and Penicillia. Appl. Microbiol. *6*:179-183.

60. McGinnis, M. R., A. A. Padhye, and L. Ajello. 1974. Storage of stock cultures of filamentous fungi, yeasts and some aerobic actinomycetes in sterile distilled water. Appl. Microbiol. *28*:218-222.

61. Miller, J. J. 1945. Studies on the *Fusarium* of muskmelon wilt. I. Pathogenic and cultural studies with particular reference to the cause and nature of variation in the causal organism. Can. J. Res. *23C*:16-43.

62. Mizrahi, A. and G. Miller. 1968. Long-term preservation of a non-sporulating strain of *Claviceps paspali.* Appl. Microbiol. *16*:1100-1101.

63. Norris, D. 1944. Preservation of tube cultures of fungi and bacteria with liquid paraffin. J. Aust. Inst. Agric. Sci. *10*:77.

64. Ogata, W. N. 1962. Preservation of *Neurospora* stock cultures with anhydrous silica gel. Neurospora Newsletter *1*:13.

65. Onions, A. H. S. 1971. Preservation of fungi. In C. Booth (Ed.), *Methods in Microbiology,* Vol. 4, Academic Press, New York, pp. 113-151.

66. Parina, O. V., V. V. Patrikeev, and S. V. Lysenko. 1972. Investigation of the survival and physiological activity of some yeast strains after long storage in silica gel. Microbiologiya *41*:164.

67. Pedersen, T. A. 1965. Factors affecting viable cell counts of freeze-dried *Cryptococcus terricolus* cells. Antonie Van Leeuwenhoek J. Microbiol. Serol. *31*:232-240.

68. Perkins, D. D. 1962. Preservation of *Neurospora* stock cultures with anhydrous silica gel. Can. J. Microbiol. *8*:591-594.

69. Perkins, D. D. 1977. Details for preparing silica gel stocks. Neurospora Newsletter *24*:16-17.

70. Puhalla, J. E. 1968. Compatibility reactions on solid medium and interstrain inhibition of *Ustilago maydis*. Genetics *60*:461-474.

71. Puhalla, J. E., and S. L. Anagnostakis. 1971. Genetics and nutritional requirements of *Endothia parasitica*. Phytopathology *61*:169-173.

72. Raper, K. B., and D. F. Alexander. 1945. Preservation of molds by the lyophil process. Mycologia *37*:499-525.

73. Raper, K. B., and D. I. Fennell. 1965. *The Genus Aspergillus*, Williams & Wilkins, Baltimore.

74. Raper, K. B., and C. Thom. 1949. *A Manual of the Penicillia*, Williams & Wilkins, Baltimore.

75. Reinhardt, D. J. 1966. Silica gel as a preserving agent for the cellular slime mould *Acrasis rosea*. J. Protozool. *13*:225.

76. Rhoades, H. E. 1958. The effect of storage on viability of lyophilized cultures of bacteria, viruses, yeasts and molds. Am. J. Vet. Res. *19*:765-768.

77. Schipper, M. A. A., and J. Bekker-Holtman. 1976. Viability of lyophilized fungal cultures. Antonie Leeuwenhoek J. Microbiol. Serol. *42*:325-328.

78. Sherf, A. F. 1943. A method for maintaining *Phytomonas sepedonia* in culture for long periods without transfer. Phytopathology *33*:330-332.

79. Sleesman, J. P., P. O. Larsen, and J. Safford. 1974. Maintenance of stock cultures of *Helminthosporium maydis* (races T and O). Plant Dis. Reptr. *58*:334-336.

80. Takashio, M. 1972. Sexual reproduction of some *Arthroderma* and *Nannizzia* on diluted Sabouraud agar with or without salts. Mykosen *15*:11-17.

81. Takashio, M., and R. Vanbreuseghem. 1966. Rajeunissement de cultures de champignons pathogènes. Ann. Soc. Belge Med. Trop. *46*:421-432.

82. Toussoun, T. A., and P. E. Nelson. 1968. *A Pictorial Guide to the Identification of Fusarium Species According to the Taxonomic System of Snyder & Hansen*. Pennsylvania State Univ. Press, University Park.

83. Trollope, D. R. 1975. The preservation of bacteria and fungi on anhydrous silica gel: an assessment of survival over four years. J. Appl. Bacteriol. Tech. Ser. *38*:115-120.

84. Udelnova, I. M. 1957. O tsito-fiziologicheskikh osobennostyakh drozhzhevykh organizmov posle glubokogo okhlazhdenia i ottaivania. Zhurnal Obshchei Biol. *18*:395-401.

85. Vanbreuseghem, R., and M. Van Brussel. 1952. Cultures de dermatophytes sur terre et sur milieu a base de terre. C. R. Soc. Biol. *146*:796-798.

86. Watts, D. J., and J. M. Ashworth. 1970. Growth of myxamoebae of the cellular slime mould *Dictyostelium discoideum* in axenic culture. Biochem. J. *119*:171.

87. Weiss, F. A. 1957. Maintenance and preservation of cultures. In *Manual of Microbiological Methods*. Edited by the Society of American Bacteriologists, McGraw-Hill Book Co., Inc., New York, pp. 99-119.

88. Wernham, C. C. 1946. Mineral oil as a fungus culture preservative. Mycologia *38*:691-692.

89. Weston, W. H., Jr. 1949. Influence of the several steps of the lyophile process on survival of fungous spores. Am. J. Bot. *36*:816-817.

90. Wickerham, L. J., and A. A. Andreasen. 1942. The lyophil process: its use in the preservation of yeasts. Wallerstein Lab. Commun. 5:165-169.
91. Wickerham, L. J., and M. H. Flickinger. 1946. Viability of yeasts preserved two years by the lyophil process. Brewers Dig. 21:55-65.

6

Epidemiology of the Mycoses

Nancy K. Hall / University of Oklahoma Health Sciences Center, Oklahoma City, Oklahoma

Howard W. Larsh / University of Oklahoma, Norman, Oklahoma

I. INTRODUCTION

Epidemiology is the study of the distribution of a disease in a population and factors that influence that distribution. Interactions among an organism, the host, and the environment determine the natural course of any infectious disease. The interplay of these three factors forms the basis for the dynamics of the disease process. The study of the distribution, frequency of occurrence, and etiologic agents of diseases is essential in gathering epidemiologic data.

Historically, many mycotic diseases were treated as parasitological or dermatological disorders because their etiologic agents were not properly identified. The development of more precise diagnostic procedures and laboratory techniques has led to a greater awareness of human mycoses. The incidence of the mycoses is increasing, but whether this increase is due to improved methodology or is a reflection of true environmental changes is unknown. It is certainly possible that the increase in incidence of the mycoses is a combination of both factors. Information on the epidemiologic characteristics of the mycoses in humans is still fragmentary and incomplete since they are not notifiable diseases. It is to be anticipated that data on incidence, prevalence, morbidity, and mortality will become more readily accumulated as health authorities recognize the importance of the mycoses. A resolution made in 1975 by the World Health Organization requested assistance in gathering epidemiologic information on fungal diseases [279]. The accumulation of such material, together with increased awareness of the opportunistic mycotic diseases, will greatly expand current knowledge about the mycoses.

The Committee on Reporting the Frequency of Mycoses reported in May, 1979, that the incidence of aspergillosis, actinomycosis, cryptococcosis, and coccidioidomycosis was markedly increased [89]. These increases were partially traced to the larger number of patients on immunosuppressive therapy, aging, and movement of individuals to endemic areas.

A. Geographic Distribution

The geographic distribution of fungi is dependent on an environment where the organisms can successfully compete with other microbes. Requirements for growth of the fungi include proper nutrition (see Chap. 1, this volume), oxygen for respiration, the presence or absence of light, moisture, salinity, acidity, and appropriate temperatures. Fungi are abundant in soil and water and are frequently associated with decaying vegetable matter, such as leaves or wood.

B. Environmental Factors

The fungi vary widely in their tolerance of temperature extremes, exhibiting a wide range of thermal death points. Many forms are killed by brief exposure to temperatures of 50°C, whereas some of the more thermophilic fungi can survive composting conditions in excess of that temperature. The lower temperature limits are dependent on humidity and time of exposure, but spores of most fungi survive prolonged low-temperature exposure. Temperature is also important in governing the morphologic expression of several species of fungi. Thus, certain fungi exist either as hyphal molds or as yeasts in a specified environment (i.e., in the tissues of a host or in nature), and this dimorphism can be experimentally controlled by temperature and nutritional factors (see Chap. 10, Part A, of this series). Many of the zoopathogenic fungi are dimorphic.

The distribution of fungi is determined by the fact that their spores become airborne and thus seed available sites. The ubiquity of potentially pathogenic fungi and the comparatively low incidence of mycoses suggest that susceptible hosts are usually remarkably resistant to or easily immunized by their encounter with fungi.

The interaction between fungi and their hosts is often quite various. For example, *Microsporum audouinii*, an anthropophilic dermatophyte, produces a comparatively mild noninflammatory infection in man whereas the zoophilic species, *Microsporum canis*, causes an acute, highly inflammatory disease that may result in serious scarring and loss of hair [146]. The reasons for this disparate behavior are not clear.

The maintenance of fungi in special environmental niches generally does not depend on reseeding from infected animals. Exceptions include the commensal *Candida albicans*, an important pathogen frequently associated with man but not generally found in the environment, and the dermatophytes that may persist in keratinaceous debris for a time in soil. Saprophytic existence and growth in the environment are generally characteristics of zoopathogenic fungi.

C. Clinical Manifestations

It is useful to divide diseases caused by fungi into three separate groups relative to their involvement of tissue in the disease process: (1) the superficial, cutaneous mycoses involving skin, hair, and nails, i.e., the uppermost layer of the epidermis, (2) the subcutaneous mycoses involving tissue below the epidermis, (3) the systemic or deep mycoses usually involving many different tissues that may disseminate via the blood or the lymphatic system.

The superficial mycoses are localized to the skin and its appendages. These cutaneous mycoses are caused by organisms that are frequently associated with obligate parasitism of man and animals and are transmitted by direct contact or by sloughed infected hair and skin scales. Among the dermatophytes encountered in tinea infections, only

Microsporum gypseum has been isolated with frequency from the soil. The cutaneous mycoses are often chronic and may cause only a mild inflammatory response. The degree of involvement is often trivial, but more serious allergic responses may be seen.

The subcutaneous mycoses are initiated by the direct implantation of soil or vegetation into the tissues of a susceptible individual. Because of this mechanism of infection, these diseases are not infrequently found in rural or tropical regions.

The deep or systemic mycoses are also caused by organisms acquired from saprophytic sources. During wind storms or periods of relatively low humidity, the fungi which cause systemic disease release spores into the air that are inhaled by individuals. The primary lesion in susceptible individuals is pulmonary and usually is an acute, self-limiting, inflammatory disease. These diseases sometimes progress into a chronic granulomatous state. Rarely the disease may spread hematogenously to other organ systems.

The epidemiological data in this chapter will include the geographic distribution of the etiologic agents, the sources of infection, the incidence and prevalence of disease, and the identification of susceptible individuals within a population with regard to race, age, sex, and occupation.

II. ASPERGILLOSIS

Only invasive forms of aspergillosis are considered in this section. Mycotoxicoses caused by *Aspergillus* spp. are considered in Part B:I of this series.

Aspergillosis in its various manifestations, i.e., pulmonary, disseminated, ocular, and cutaneous, is caused by many different species of the genus *Aspergillus*. The most common pathogenic species in the United States is *Aspergillus fumigatus* [247]. *Aspergillus niger* is found less frequently and is more commonly associated with infections of the external auditory canal [265]. Most of the species are considered opportunistic and are associated with several predisposing factors [5,24,102,159,261]. The increased incidence (four times the number of recognized cases between 1964 and 1971) of aspergillosis suggests that more serious attention needs to be given to this pathogen [188].

A. Ecology

The organism is acquired exogenously and grows luxuriantly on decaying vegetation. The organism will proliferate on grain, compost heaps, organic matter [198], hay or straw [76], soil [218], feathers, and animal fur [211]. The ubiquity of the organism is a reflection of its ability to flourish in temperature extremes [211], to grow in soil of differing salinity and sand composition [20], and to be dispersed by air currents [274]. Many factors influence the distribution of the spores in the air, including humidity, rainfall, wind, sun, and seasonal variation [130,195,202]. It is thought that 8% of all spores inhaled daily (based on an active male breathing 5.7 times 10^7 spores per day) would be aspergilli [20,247]. The percentage increases in an area of high spore load (barns or grass cutting areas). In normal individuals, this spore content would not usually create a problem or initiate a disease process even though the smaller spores (2.0-3.0 μm) would penetrate to the acinar level in the lungs [197]. Experimental models of aspergillosis in mice do not demonstrate lung lesions in animals injected intravenously with *Aspergillus* spores [87]. Any open cavity in the lung associated with a nutrient supply with high amount of free oxygen favors the growth of the organism. Broncho-ciliary cleaning responses may not eliminate the spores. Since aspergilli are so prevalent and the incidence of infection so low, the concept that nearly all patients with aspergil-losis have an underlying primary disease, are undergoing hormone treatment [79], or are on immunosuppressive therapy gains support [241].

B. Geographic Distribution

The worldwide distribution of the organism has been defined with case reports from England [19,215], Germany, Italy, Canada [259], Portugal [270], France (first report by Virchow in 1856), Ireland [111], Belgium, India [117], Australia, North and South America [263], and Africa [134]. The organism also infects plants, insects, birds [3,20, 278], and domestic animals [4].

Seasonal variation is a consideration in that heat and humidity are important in the establishment of the disease [53]. Decreased occurrence of aspergillosis is associated with late summer and autumn in tropical countries.

C. Predisposing Factors

1. Occupation

Aspergillosis is well documented in several occupations, e.g., wig manufacturers and cleaners in France [79], farmers in the United States [263], and pigeon stuffers in Europe [215]. Patterns of occurrence are difficult to establish because of incomplete data. However, in a report of 30 cases where the occupation was defined, 9 of the 30 were housewives [3 of 9 were city dwellers], 5 were farmers, 2 were office workers, and the rest were individual occurrences in varied positions such as a dock worker, a leather cutter, a gardener, and a seamstress [111]. Although occupation may be pre-disposing for the disease, it evidently is not an important factor. Persons having out-door occupations are more frequently exposed, but other situations are no doubt also important in promoting infection.

2. Age, Race, and Sex

Aspergillosis does not seem to have age, race, or sex predilections. In a study of 35 cases of aspergillosis, 100% of the cases occurred in individuals over 40 years of age. Due to the opportunistic nature of the organism, the relationship possibly develops in older hosts who have been immunologically compromised by age. It is felt that im-munological debilitation is a much more important predisposing factor than the influence of age.

There is a disagreement in the literature as to whether males are more susceptible to aspergillosis than females. Hormonal influences have been demonstrated, e.g., estrogen nonspecifically stimulates the reticuloendothelial (RE) system and testosterone shows no effect on the phagocytic mechanism of the RE system [194]. Assays that evaluate the hormonal effects on the in vitro growth of *Aspergillus* showed no measurable effect of progesterone and testosterone, but a marked suppression of growth by estrogen [247]. In a separate study of 35 cases, 68.6% were male and 32% were female. Rather than a true male predilection, however, this information was interpreted to show greater degree of outdoor exposure in the male [111].

3. Other Factors

The possibility of infection by aerosols of *Aspergillus* is enhanced by preexisting disease, trauma [118], lower host resistance, surgical procedures, and chemotherapy [240, 260]. In experimental murine models of aspergillosis, an increase in mortality was observed in animals pretreated with corticosteroids and exposed to various species of *Aspergillus* [228]. Studies in another model involving the pathogenesis of aspergillosis in leukemic chickens suggested that the decrease in normal mature leukocytes may influence the invasiveness of the organism [187]. This influence has also been suggested in patients with acute leukemia [189].

Many debilitating conditions or diseases have been associated with aspergillosis, particularly the pulmonary manifestation of the disease. These include tuberculosis [146,233], leukemia [127,189], other neoplastic disease [188], fungal diseases such as histoplasmosis [209], malnutrition and alcoholism [14], lung damage (chronic obstructive pulmonary disease, empyema, emphysema, bronchiectasis, pneumoconiosis, abscess formation, cystic fibrosis), viral disease, and immunologically mediated diseases such as rheumatoid arthritis, Wegener's granulomatosis, and lupus erythematosus [14,18,111, 189,225].

III. BLASTOMYCOSIS

Blastomyces dermatitidis is the etiologic agent of blastomycosis (synonyms include North American blastomycosis and Gilchrist's disease). The disease manifests itself in two quite different forms, i.e., a pulmonary disease and a progressive disseminated form. The dimorphic fungus is unique among those that cause the systemic mycoses in that so little is known about its location in nature. Lack of a suitable skin test reagent has prevented proper assessment of the incidence of primary pulmonary infection or the frequency of disseminated disease. No conclusive evidence exists to show that *B. dermatitidis* can be transmitted from human to human or from animals to humans. Only one report exists of a presumed human-to-human transmission [208].

A. Ecology

The natural habitat of *B. dermatitidis* remains unknown. Although the infection must be acquired exogenously, the environmental factors that influence the growth of the fungus are unknown. *Blastomyces dermatitidis* has only rarely been isolated from the environment, but it has been repeatedly isolated from infected humans and dogs. Soil is the most likely reservoir for the organism, but the mycelial phase does not survive long when inoculated into unsterilized soil. It is probable that the microbial competition in the soil limits the growth of *B. dermatitidis* in nature. The organism can be grown on tree bark under special laboratory conditions [76]. Factors influencing the survival of the organism in the environment have been reviewed by Ajello [8].

B. Geographic Distribution

In general, cases of blastomycosis are clustered in areas of high annual rainfall. In an overview by Greer of cases in the United States since 1937, the highest incidence occurred in Louisiana, then in descending order: North Carolina, Wisconsin, Illinois, Tennessee, Kentucky, Ohio, District of Columbia, Minnesota, Indiana, Michigan, and

Iowa [111]. A profile of favorable climatic and environmental conditions include annual rainfalls of 45 in, red sand and clay soils, and fertile plains and prairies. The average elevation of the five states showing the highest incidence is 1450 ft. These conditions correspond well with the states bordering the Mississippi River.

In addition to those from the United States, there are numerous reports of blastomycosis from Canada [101,252,275] and scattered reports from Africa [268], Latin America [8], and England [67]. Many other reports exist in the literature showing cases in Japan [31] and South America [61], but the validity of these cases has been questioned. Cases occurring outside the endemic area are to be viewed with skepticism unless a travel history makes possible the acquisition in an endemic area and subsequent travel to a nonendemic area. Epidemiologic information has been limited by the lack of specific skin test antigens and, until recently, of antigens suitable for serologic studies (see Chapter 5, Part B:I of this series).

C. Predisposing Factors

1. Occupation

Historically, blastomycosis was frequently associated with damp conditions [256] and was seen in laborers, farmers, construction workers, and others exposed to dust [47, 123,232,254]. However, indoor activities may show a greater correlation with disease than outdoor occupations [46,140]. In a survey of 106 patients, 61% worked predominantly indoors and 39% had outside occupations [111]. Casual or recreational outdoor exposure (hiking, gardening, etc.) should be considered in those patients with indoor occupations.

2. Age, Race, and Sex

The literature citation of blastomycosis includes reports of patients 6 months of age [250] to 89 years [230]. Although the disease may occur in any age group, a greater incidence is noted between 30 to 60 years of age [46,177,230,254]. This is in contrast to some of the other mycoses such as histoplasmosis where the disease is associated with older, debilitated age groups or the very young.

Racial distribution of blastomycosis must be viewed cautiously with attention given to the locale of the report. Overall distribution seems to favor white-to-nonwhite occurrence by 3:1. Regional studies show 86-93% white preponderance in northern United States [46,140,230] and 60% black predominance in the South [46]. The racial occurrence of blastomycosis appears to reflect the general population distribution.

There is a male preponderance of cases of blastomycosis in the United States. Reports vary from 9 males:1 female [46,177,230] to 6 males:1 female [111]. Although males are exposed to more varied environments, this does not explain the difference in occurrence. The number of cases in the male population also varies with the disease manifestion, e.g., 5 males:1 female in disseminated systemic blastomycosis and 10 males:1 female in disseminated cutaneous cases [46]. These ratios are similarly reflected in canine cases [93].

3. Other Factors

Other disease conditions frequently appear concomitantly with blastomycosis. Such associations include tuberculosis [46,255,264], diabetes [46,119,253], cardiovascular problems [2,46], and neoplasms [2], particularly squamous cell carcinomas [171]. Linn [149] has described a close association between the pseudoepitheliomatous lesions in blastomycosis and squamous cell carcinoma.

IV. CANDIDIASIS

Candida infections have assumed a prominence today that is undoubtedly a reflection both of increased recognition and increased occurrence. The introduction of antibiotic therapy, with the attendant alteration of normal flora of a patient, the widespread use of corticosteroids, and the newer cytotoxic drugs, have increased the incidence of opportunistic infections caused by *Candida* (often *Candida albicans*). Other species involved in opportunistic disease include *C. pseudotropicalis*, *C. tropicalis*, *C. stellatoidea*, *C. parapsilosis*, *C. guilliermondii*, and *C. krusei* [223]. The disease process often involves the skin and mucous membranes but may also become systemic and be found in the lungs [111], viscera [51], and central nervous system [111]. Readers should be aware of an additional reference on the topic of this section, which appeared after the initial construction of this chapter: Odds, F. S. 1979. *Candida and Candidosis*. University Park Press, Baltimore.

A. Ecology

As part of the normal flora of humans, *C. albicans* is found in the mouth, throat, gastrointestinal tract, and vagina [203]. International records show the incidence of *Candida* spp. in the vagina to be 35%, in the sputum to be up to 77%, and in the gut to be 85% [279]. Environments that are moist, warm, unexposed to light, and with an acidic pH favor the growth of the yeast. There are also certain relationships that may exist with other organisms such as fungi and the pyogenic cocci [64]. The organisms are widespread, may exist as saprobes, and have been isolated from the air [50,114].

Direct contact from person to person, or indirect contact via the clothing, may transfer *C. albicans*. Newborns become infected during passage through the birth canal, during nursing, or by contaminated feeding bottles [282] and hand cream. Animal-to-man transmission has not been documented; however, man-to-animals transmission has been noted [282]. Hospitals record a particularly high incidence of *Candida* infections in patients with organ transplantation [283], malignancies [135], and immunologic disorders [234].

B. Geographic Distribution

Largely because of its usually endogenous acquisition, this disease is not limited in distribution by geographic factors [111]. Some reports suggest that infection with *C. albicans* occurs more frequently in tropical climates, but the disease seems to be rather evenly distributed across the United States.

C. Predisposing Factors

Since candidiasis is an opportunistic pathogen, there is no occupational association with infection, nor is race considered a contributing factor. The preponderance of females having genital candidiasis and the greater number of reports in the literature of female *Candida* infections is reflected in the literature on the relative susceptibility of males and females. For example, Greer [111] made a survey of 252 cases and found a female-to-male distribution of 188 to 64, a fact that reflects the common vulvar and vaginal manifestations of the disease.

The development of candidiasis is affected by a number of predisposing factors, e.g., trauma, pregnancy, obesity, hormonal imbalances, antibiotic therapy, tuberculosis, and neoplasms [57,60]. The predisposing influence of drug therapy is apparent in many of these cases [284]. The overall immunological debilitation of patients in these various circumstances undoubtedly leads to complicating candidal infection [129].

Oral contraceptives [45], the use of radiation, and steroid therapy may result in depressed immunologic competence of the host and these factors have been associated with candidiasis.

V. CHROMOMYCOSIS

The names of etiologic agents of chromomycosis are subject to dispute (see Chap. 7, Part A). Since such nomenclature does not figure prominently in the authors' discussion, the names given are those used in a standard reference [79]. However, other opinions on the matter have been expressed. In parentheses are given names suggested by some. There is also some disagreement of the inclusion of *Wangiella* (*Exophiala*) *dermatitidis* among agents of chromomycosis, and a new agent of the disease has been recorded, *Rhinocladiella aquaspersa*. However, the agents listed are the ones recorded in the literature herewith reviewed. A comprehensive list of the pathogenic, dematiacious fungi and the general sorts of diseases for which they may be responsible was presented by Dr. L. Ajello (Centers for Disease Control, Atlanta, Georgia) at a workshop of the American Society for Microbiology/Medical Mycological Society of the Americas in Dallas, Texas, March 1, 1981.

Chromomycosis (chromoblastomycosis or verrucose dermatitis) is a chronic, localized mycotic infection of skin and subcutaneous tissue. It is characterized by lesions which can be nodular, verrucoid, and sometimes ulcerative. The principal etiologic agents are *Fonsecaea compacta*, *F. pedrosoi*, *Wangiella* (*Exophiala*) *dermatitidis*, *Phialophora verrucosa*, and *Cladosporium carrionii*. These fungi produce abundant spores which are capable of causing infection.

A. Ecology

The organisms causing chromomycosis are saprobic, existing in soil and on decaying wood or vegetation [52]. Any soil type appears to support the growth of the various species. The fact that endemic areas are usually moist and in tropical climates may be a reflection of the environmental conditions favoring growth of plants which these fungi parasitize. The spores of these fungi are resistant to temperature extremes and withstand abrupt environmental changes well [190]. The organisms have been isolated from thorns, dirt-contaminated utensils, and decaying vegetable material [217]. Chromomycosis is not considered a contagious disease. Instead it is acquired from the environment from infected plants and soil [216].

Phialophora verrucosa has a predilection for wood and wood products and causes blue discoloration of wood pulp [52]. Gezuela [100] reviewed sources of *F. pedrosoi* and found the organism frequently associated with decaying palm wood. Other aspects of the distribution of the etiologic agents of chromomycosis have been reviewed by Al-Doory [14].

B. Geographic Distribution

As stated above, the etiologic agents of chromomycosis occur worldwide, favoring tropical over temperate climates. Its greatest incidence is in tropical and subtropical zones between 30°N and 30°S [190], although the disease has been reported from every continent.

Highest incidence in the Americas is in Brazil, followed closely by Costa Rica [251], and Cuba [190]. In Africa, there is concentration of reports from Madagascar [38].

C. Predisposing Factors

Since the disease is acquired from the environment by some type of primary injury to the dermis, the occurrence of the disease is higher in regions of the world where shoes are not worn. Occupation is a primary consideration and a higher incidence is observed in agricultural workers.

Chromomycosis is more frequently found in males than in females [222,251]. Age is not critical with reports of cases in patients 14-70 years of age [251]. Although most cases have been diagnosed in Caucasians 25-50 years of age, all races are thought to be equally at risk [190].

VI. COCCIDIOIDOMYCOSIS

Three types of infection may be caused by *Coccidioides immitis*: (1) a rare form of the disease involving a primary cutaneous lesion, (2) the common form of primary pulmonary disease which usually is self-limiting [29], and (3) disseminated coccidioidomycosis affecting the pulmonary system [22], bone [30], viscera, skin [137], and meninges [33]. The disease produces granulomatous inflammation and detectable humoral responses. Complement fixation, precipitin, and gel-diffusion assays are available in addition to a skin test [201,249].

Coccidioidomycosis was first described by Posadas in 1892 in Argentina [206] and by Rixford in 1894 in the United States [219]. In 1957, a compilation of cases in California was based on 450 reports in that state alone. The endemic areas of California, Arizona, Texas, and New Mexico are well-recognized [7]. The disease also occurs in cattle [23,207], wild rodents, dogs [168,213], monkeys [55], rabbits, and mice. A monographic treatment of coccidioidomycosis appeared after the initial construction of this chapter [Stevens, D. A. (ed.). 1980. *Coccidioidomycosis*. Plenum Publishing Corp., New York].

A. Ecology

Coccidioides immitis exists in nature as a mycelium comprised of septate hyphae that form arthroconidia [205]. The fungus has been isolated from soil [70,74] and exists best in areas of high temperatures where the surface of the soil becomes arid and competitive organisms are not abundant [72,167]. The organism can also grow in decaying vegetable matter and sandy soils [73,74,81]. The fungus may lie dormant 5-10 cm below the soil surface, and it has been suggested that rainfall may stimulate its growth [169].

Introduction of *C. immitis* into the tissues is accompanied by the development of the parasitic, endosporulating form of growth of the organism. Variation in colonial morphology among isolates from human material is not infrequent. Huppert et al. [125] have described over 70 colonial variants of this sort. Such cultural variations remain consistent and are typical of given isolates. Therefore, colonial variants can be used as epidemiological markers.

Aerosolization and inhalation of the spores of the organism are the mechanism of infection. The arthroconidia are easily carried on dust particles which disseminate these infectious spores. The recent California outbreak of over 550 cases well demonstrates the fact that the organism is readily spread [86].

B. Geographic Distribution

In the United States, the occurrence of coccidioidomycosis is concentrated in the San Joaquin Valley [71], northern California [157,277], and, more generally, in the western and southwestern states of Arizona, Nevada, Texas, New Mexico, and Utah. Endemic regions in the Americas include Venezuela [41] and Mexico [107,170]. The first reported case by Posadas in 1892 was in Argentina [206]. Establishment of the confines of the disease is difficult because subclinical cases are frequent and are not recognized. Estimates of the occurrence in California alone range in excess of 30,000 cases per year [29]. The occurrence of cases outside the endemic area is well documented; these cases arise either from spores that contaminate materials shipped from the endemic area or by travel of an infected individual to a nonendemic area before disease is manifested. Numerous reports between 1912 and 1964 outline the sorts of episodes that have occurred: a 1916 case in Missouri [150], a case report from Chicago [120], the summary of cases by Kritzer [139], cases reported in Texas and Hawaii [83], and episodes with several cases have also been reported from Colorado, North Carolina, Pennsylvania, Massachusetts, Maryland, Illinois, New Jersey, New York, Georgia, Ohio, West Virginia, Washington, and Wisconsin [111]. Association of the disease with military training facilities in endemic areas underlines the importance of controlling the environmental exposure of recruits.

Similar studies have been conducted in Central and South America. Endemic area information is available from Argentina and in the state of Sonora, Mexico [170]. Utilization of skin-testing procedures has assisted in outlining the extent of exposure to *C. immitis* [197]. A thorough survey by Mayorga [179] revealed over 25% of the population tested in Zacapa and Gualan had positive skin tests. But Greer reported [111] that Guzman tested almost 20,000 Hondurans and showed a very low percentage of positive individuals (0.2%).

C. Predisposing Factors

1. Occupation

The method by which *C. immitis* becomes airborne, is inhaled, and finally establishes infection allows for extensive exposure regardless of an individual's occupation [131, 147]. Any person exposed to dust or soil clouds in an endemic area may come in contact with the organism. A review of 614 cases by Greer [111] identified 90% of the individuals as having indoor occupations. Military recruits who are brought into a training camp within an endemic area are extremely susceptible because they lack any previous exposure to the organism [27]. This no doubt explains the larger number of cases in military personnel than among the native population in a given area.

2. Age, Race, and Sex

Although coccidioidomycosis may occur in infants and in older adults [281], the highest incidence is reported in those between 20 and 50 years of age. The age span is markedly influenced by the types of groups included in epidemiological studies.

Careful analysis of cases in endemic areas shows a predilection of dark-skinned races to disseminated forms of disease, a fact reflecting a susceptibility difference in the populations [97,124,242]. Disseminated disease is more likely to occur in dark-skinned individuals, e.g., Blacks, Mexicans, and Filipinos [97]. Another important factor in the virulence of the organism apart from race is associated with hormonal balance, especially in pregnant women. Prognosis is guarded when coccidioidomycosis occurs during a pregnancy [248].

The male-to-female distribution shows a greater frequency of occurrence in males in primary pulmonary disease. In a review of 600 cases of coccidioidomycosis, the distribution was 488 males and 112 females. In prepubescent males and females, the occurrence is approximately equal. Females show a greater tendency to develop the allergic response of erythema nodosum. Dissemination of the disease occurs more frequently in males.

3. Other Factors

The frequency of exposure to *Coccidioides immitis* together with the rarity of progressive, disseminated disease suggests that the immunological response of the host is crucial to the outcome in coccidioidomycosis. But the immunological deficiency governing disseminated disease has not yet been identified.

Other factors predisposing to more severe disease include primary neoplasms (e.g., lymphosarcoma) with coccidioidomycosis acting as a secondary invader [34]; prolonged prednisone therapy [44] associated with myelofibrosis and miliary coccidioidomycosis; and tuberculosis [59,84,132].

VII. CRYPTOCOCCOSIS

In its most commonly recognized clinical form, cryptococcosis involves the central nervous system. Clinical manifestations of the disease, therefore, include meningitis or cerebral abscess. The fungus *Cryptococcus neoformans* enters a susceptible host by the respiratory tract and may establish a primary pulmonary infection that seemingly often goes undetected. In fact, the central nervous system invasion is thought to be a rare, malignant manifestation of what is a common and ordinarily benign disease [40]. Cutaneous disease has been recorded but is a manifestation of dissemination, not of primary inoculation [37]. The central nervous system disease is generally chronic in progression.

The disease has been recognized since the turn of the century and has several synonyms including European blastomycosis, torulosis, and Busse-Buschke's disease [56]. Reports through 1946 discussed the clinical manifestations and the pathology of the lesions [257]. The early literature contains reports of cases and reviews [239, 262,271]. Better recognition of the clinical manifestations and more efficient laboratory techniques have improved the detection of cryptococcosis [193].

The disease is not thought to be contagious and occurs sporadically in both man and animals [111]. Many animals other than humans are susceptible to *C. neoformans* (e.g., cattle, monkeys, dogs, cats, sheep, horses, mice, guinea pigs, and foxes) [111, 245,271,276].

A. Ecology

Cryptococcus neoformans exists as a saprophyte in nature and has been isolated from pigeon excreta, from the throat and skin of normal individuals [212], from raw milk [43], and from the urine, sputum, or spinal fluid of patients [77]. Because of this distribution, Evans and Harrell [80] suggested that the disease may be acquired either endogenously or exogenously. Current thought is that all pathogenic strains of cryptococci are from exogenous sources [79]. Some exceptions do exist as reviewed by Howard [121]. He documents that the isolation of *C. neoformans* from fecal, sputum, or saliva specimens is rare, but that the organism may be found to colonize transiently the pulmonary systems of individuals with primary disease of various sorts.

Soil isolates of the organism are also common [192,237,243], particularly in soil contaminated with pigeon excreta. The organism was originally cultured from peach juice [121]. There are well-established reservoirs of the fungus, but there is some difficulty in associating a particular case with a given exogenous site of acquisition [192].

Four serotypes of the encapsulated yeast can be distinguished. The most prevalent serotype isolated from patients in the United States is serotype A [25], with infrequent isolations of serotypes B or C, except in southern California where these serotypes comprise about half the isolates. However, the B and C serotypes have not been isolated from natural sources in southern California. Indeed, the location of these serotypes in nature is still largely unknown [274,280].

B. Geographic Distribution

Cryptococcus neoformans is distributed throughout the world but occurs most frequently in the United States and Australia. There are no established endemic areas, and it is felt that there are random distributions of the disease.

In the United States, the greatest incidence occurs in states on the eastern, southern, and western borders. Cases have also been reported in the Great Lakes and the Mississippi River Valley. Again, this random pattern reinforces the unusual distribution of the organism. In a survey of 67 cases outside the United States, 30 occurred in Australia, 9 in South America, 8 in China, 7 in South Africa, and 7 in Europe [111].

C. Predisposing Factors

1. Occupation

Cryptococcosis does not have an association with any particular occupation. It is felt that most normal people have cellular defenses that are capable of spontaneously handling the disease.

2. Age, Race, and Sex

The disease can occur in any age or racial group, and in either sex. About two-thirds of patients are males between 30 and 50 years of age [152]. In smaller studies where race was designated, Caucasian patients were in the majority [111].

3. Other Factors

The opportunistic nature of this disease is well-established [273]. The compromised host is open to infection by the organism. Association of cryptococcosis has been established in patients with deficiencies in cellular immunology [98,110,152,158], with Hodgkin's disease [151], with other lymphoproliferative diseases [127], and with long-term steroid therapy [26].

VIII. DERMATOPHYTOSES

Infections of the epidermis, hair, and nails are caused predominantly by fungi belonging to the genera *Epidermophyton, Microsporum,* and *Trichophyton.* Classification of the diseases is based on the portion of the body affected. The general term for these sorts of afflictions is tinea to which is added an adjective indicating the area involved, e.g., tinea capitis, tinea barbae, tinea corporis, etc. Two infections caused by *Trichophyton* spp. are quite distinctive in their clinical presentations: (1) favus (*T. schoenleinii*), and (2) tinea imbricata (*T. concentricum*).

There are several review articles available updating the species of fungi known to cause dermatophytoses: one in 1957 by Georg on nutritional and morphologic characteristics [99] and another by Ajello [9] enumerating 20 species of *Trichophyton,* 14 of *Microsporum,* and one of *Epidermophyton,* together with a consideration of their perfect states (see Chap. 6, Part A, of this series).

A. Ecology

The dermatophytoses may be acquired from soil or by direct contact with infected materials from humans or animals. The natural habitat of *M. gypseum, M. fulvum,* and *M. cookei* is the soil where keratinous debris supports the growth. Baiting of soil with hair, skin, or wool is the common technique for the retrieval of such organisms [176,266]. Although other organisms have been isolated from the soil (*T. ajelloi* and *T. terrestre*), it is not an important source of infection for the most part [62].

The causative agents of tinea capitis are usually transmitted by infected, sloughed, epithelial cells and/or infected hair. Transmission occurs frequently by contact with furniture and clothing contaminated with fallen hair, or with brushes and combs that are contaminated with dermatophyte incitants of tinea capitis, e.g., *M. audouinii, T. tonsurans,* and *T. violaceum* [161].

Trichophyton mentagrophytes can occur transiently in the soil but is more frequently transmitted directly from person to person or from animal to humans. Animals are a source of infection for humans, e.g., *T. equinum* from horses, *T. verrucosum* from cattle, *T. simii* from monkeys, and *M. gallinae* from the chickens [62].

B. Geographic Distribution

There are dynamic changes in the occurrence of species throughout the world [42,153,154, 169]. In the United States in the early 1940s, the frequency of tinea capitis caused by

M. audouinii increased markedly [79]. Fluctuations in regional occurrence of certain species can also be a reflection of people's economic status, their personal hygiene, and personal habits. Certain species do remain localized, e.g., *M. ferrugineum* is found in Far Eastern countries such as Japan, whereas favus is endemic to Africa and southeastern Europe [79].

C. Predisposing Factors

Predisposing factors such as occupation, race, or sex have little influence on the distribution and frequency of the dermatophytoses. The decrease in immune competency with increasing age may increase the occurrence of infection in older individuals. Immunosuppressive therapy could affect resistance.

IX. HISTOPLASMOSIS

Inhalation of infectious conidiospores of *Histoplasma capsulatum* generally results only in inapparent, subclinical disease, the only manifestation of which is conversion of the skin test with histoplasmin from negative to positive. In a small percentage of episodes, a more or less acute, primary pulmonary infection occurs and this disease sometimes becomes chronic. Rarely a progressive, malignant, disseminated form of the disease occurs among those who manifest any illness. Symptomatic disease of the acute, chronic, and disseminated form occurs in the United States at a rate of approximately 200,000 new cases annually. The nonreportability of the disease may disguise the true morbidity and mortality [24] and the skin test reactivity in endemic areas is very high [14]. A monograph on histoplasmosis has recently appeared (Schwarz, J. 1981. *Histoplasmosis*. Praeger, New York.)

A. Ecology

Histoplasma capsulatum is widespread in nature. The principal reservoir is the soil [48, 75]. Dispersion of the organism is associated with the excreta of blackbirds (especially starlings), chickens, and bats [92,144]. Whereas the birds act as passive carriers, bats have a gastrointestinal infection [65,138,238]. The organism has been isolated from dogs [63,180] and other domestic and wild animals [79,186], but there is no evidence that the disease may be transmitted directly from animal to humans, from human to human, or from humans to animal [143,184,185,231]. The role of birds in the ecology of the organism may be to enrich the soil by producing increased nitrogen supplies [111] or to act passively in distribution of spores. Competition by the normal flora of soil has been reported to affect the growth of *H. capsulatum* and alter the ability of the organism to survive [66].

B. Geographic Distribution

Although histoplasmosis is a disease that occurs worldwide, the preponderance of reported cases are in the continental United States [91]. In one study of 103 reported cases outside the United States, 46% were from South America (predominantly Argentina), 19% from Africa, 15% from Europe, 5% from the East Indies Archipelago, 5% from Central America, and the remaining cases (10%) from Asia, Cuba, Canada, Hawaii, and Mexico [111]. Important reviews reporting incidence of histoplasmosis in different geographic areas include the report of 27 patients in Russia [254a] and a report of the first case of histoplasmosis in Greece [270a].

Within the United States, histoplasmosis occurs to the greatest extent in Arkansas, Ohio, Missouri, Kansas, and Colorado [94]. Thirty-one states in the continental United States have been shown to be endemic areas for this pathogen. It has been suggested that climatic and environmental conditions that favor the growth of the organism are restricted, and this explains why there are only sporadic cases reported in some geographic regions. Diagnosed cases of histoplasmosis are poorly documented in some regions, and it is probable that the disease is more prevalent than previously thought [28]. Histoplasmosis skin sensitivity is a good measure of prior exposure to the fungus [69]. This information has been extensively reviewed by Ajello [11], Edwards and Billings [68], and Larsh [143].

C. Predisposing Factors

1. Occupation

The occupations of patients show little in common except outdoor activities and extensive exposure to soil, dust, or bat guano. Five hundred and fifty-six cases were evaluated on the basis of occupation. The results showed over four-fifths of the patients were exposed out-of-doors in such diversified activities as maneuvers of soldiers, farmers, construction workers, and school children. Acquisition of the disease is frequently associated with the cleaning of chicken houses, gardening, or dusty environments [14]. This information reinforces the concepts of the aerosol route of infection and the natural occurrence of the organism in the soil.

2. Age, Race, and Sex

Persons of any age may become infected with the organism. Certain clinical presentations are found more frequently in limited age groups, e.g., extrapulmonary histoplasmosis occurs most frequently in the very young or the very old [53].

Racial susceptibility is not generally recognized as a factor in this disease. Larsh [143], however, has reported that the pulmonary manifestations affect primarily the white male showing a white-over-black patient ratio of 24 to 1 and a low incidence in females.

3. Other Factors

There is a significant association of the occurrence of histoplasmosis with other diseases, in particular tuberculosis [272], malignant lymphoma [220], and sarcoidosis [128]. The associations appear to be a reflection of a compromised or debilitated host of which *H. capsulatum* takes opportunistic advantage, though a more specific relation has on occasion been suggested. For example, the clinical manifestations of sarcoidosis have been linked to interaction with antigens from the fungus [204]. Those cases of patients with culturally proven histoplasmosis and underlying sarcoidosis died of caseous necrosis of the adrenals. The investigators theorized that the symptoms of sarcoidosis were produced by the fungal antigens. Sarcoidosis remains idiopathic and *H. capsulatum* is simply one of several etiologic agents that have been suggested over the years.

A cause and effect relationship between malignant lymphoma and invasion by *H. capsulatum* is impossible to establish [220]. Some patients with histoplasmosis develop a pseudoleukemic condition, while others exhibit a true leukemia resulting in lowered resistance to infection by *H. capsulatum*. Disseminated histoplasmosis may occur in Hodgkin's disease, but there is no special relation between the two diseases [204]. In general, the literature confirms that lymphomas are immunocompromising and that

H. caosykatyn is simply one of several microorganisms that may take advantage of such compromising situations.

X. MYCETOMAS

Mycetomas are localized, tumor-like lesions located in the subcutaneous tissue, fascia, and bone. A monographic consideration of this disease is available: Magoub, E. S. and I. G. Murray. 1973. *Mycetoma.* William Heinemann Medical Books, London. Histopathologically, the lesions are granulomatous and can form draining abscesses. The lesions are usually located on an extremity, commonly a hand or foot. Two kinds of mycetomas are recognized: actinomycetomas, whose etiologic agents include *Nocardia brasiliensis, N. asteroides, N. caviae, Actinomadura pelletieri, A. madurae,* and *Streptomyces somaliensis,* and the eumycetomas, some of whose etiologic agents are *Madurella mycetomatis, M. grisea, Pseudallescheria boydii, Exophiala jeanselmei, Acremonium recifei, A. falciforme, A. kiliense, Curvularia lunata, C. geniculata, Pyrenochaeta romeroi, Leptosphaeria senegalensis, Fusarium solani,* and *Aspergillus nidulans* [78,106,162,164,166,235].

A. Ecology

Neither type of mycetoma is contagious [176]. Humans are infected by subcutaneous inoculation of the etiologic agents from the environment [172].

In contrast to the relatively low frequency of mycetoma is the commonness of some of the etiologic agents in the environment, e.g., *P. boydii.* The various agents are found in nature and can be isolated from soil and vegetable material [6,181]. Both *N. asteroides* and *N. brasiliensis* have been isolated from soil [108,109]. *Actinomadura pelletieri* was isolated by Segretain and Mariat in Africa in 1968 [236]. Ajello isolated *Pseudallescheria boydii* in 1952 in the United States [6]. Although some of the etiologic agents are frequently isolated from the soil in the United States, mycetomas are rarely seen in this country.

B. Geographic Distribution

Some of the agents of both the eumycetomas and those of the actinomycetomas are found worldwide with greatest occurrence in tropical and subtropical regions. There is some inconsistency in the frequency of occurrence of the disease in that similar climates do not have the same incidence of mycetomas. Perhaps this inconsistency reflects a disparate distribution of the organisms in the soil.

The organisms are considered endemic in an area between the Tropic of Cancer and the Tropic of Capricorn. Although the greatest concentration of cases reviewed by Abbott occurred in Africa, there is an unevenness of distribution [1]. For example, 3265 new cases were reported from 1961-1962 in Sudan [78], whereas Vanbreuseghem reported only rare occurrence in the Congo [267].

Mycetomas are very important in Mexico. The most common agent is *N. brasiliensis* [103,104]. Again, there are regional differences with an endemic zone located in Morelos, Mexico.

C. Predisposing Factors

Mycetomas are more commonly found in males. This is probably a result of greater exposure of the male workers of a culture rather than a true predisposition of the organism for men. However, it has been suggested that a female's normal hormonal levels are protective and that there may be increased incidence of mycetomas during pregnancy [145].

Although no age group is spared, mycetomas are most frequently seen in young adults 15-40 years of age [108]. Race is not an important factor except as it relates to regional residence, and occupation (farming) appears to be the most important consideration.

XI. PARACOCCIDIOIDOMYCOSIS

Recognition of paracoccidioidomycosis came in 1908 when Lutz reported two cases in Brazil. He described a chronic, granulomatous, mucocutaneous disease and isolated a slow-growing white mold from the lesions. The etiologic agent, *Paracoccidioides brasiliensis,* has also been reported in the United States [111] in 1954, but most of the patients had lived for long periods in endemic areas. Nearly all of the research on this disease has been done by South American investigators. The organism has an affinity for lymph glands and mucous membranes, but it may affect any organ. There are a few reports that the disease may be a benign, self-limiting infection, but this situation is not yet established [95]. However, paracoccidioidomycosis is more commonly observed to be a progressive, chronic disease often ending in death. Epidemiologic studies using skin test material (paracoccidioidin) have outlined endemic areas and have demonstrated hypersensitive individuals [54,124]. The occurrence of subclinical disease is, therefore, difficult to establish [16,17].

A. Ecology

The pathogenesis of *Paracoccidioides brasiliensis* is still speculative, and the exact source of the organism has never been found. Early reports of isolation of the organism from soil were mistaken. However, there have been several recent reports of successful isolation of *P. brasiliensis* from soil [13]. Many other investigators have failed to isolate the organism from soil, guano, and plant material [221].

It is believed that *P. brasiliensis* is an exogenously acquired organism and probably resides in vegetation. It is possible that the saprophytic stage may exist in nature in an alternate morphologic form (perhaps a sexual form) difficult to recover [199]. The organism has been isolated from the gastrointestinal tract of bats [116] and humans, and it has been found in diseased peridontal tissue and carious teeth.

Although the disease has not been associated with animals, it is conceivable that some animals may serve as a reservoir [32]. There is no evidence of man-to-man transmission nor of animal-to-man transmission, although skin test surveys indicate sensitivity in cows and horses [54].

B. Geographic Distribution

There is a restricted geographic distribution of *P. brasiliensis.* The disease is virtually confined to South America, with the highest incidence in Brazil and in Argentina. This limits the area to 23°N to 34°S latitude. However, paracoccidioidomycosis has not been reported in all areas within these boundaries [14].

There are many documented autochthonous cases in Brazil [142], Argentina [224], and Colombia [111,214]. Cases that have been seen in individuals outside the endemic area have been traced to visits to Latin America or to former residence in the endemic areas. There are a few isolated cases, including one case from Africa [227] and one in the United States that had visited Venezuela [88] briefly.

C. Predisposing Factors

1. Occupation

Since most of the reported cases have been adult males who were commonly agricultural workers, it is assumed that the disease predominates among those engaged in soil-related occupations. However, there are increasing numbers of cases reported in city dwellers, industrial employees, and people of low income (perhaps relating to the state of malnutrition) [111,155,214].

2. Age, Race, and Sex

The disease is usually found in adults with slight variation in the age distribution in different countries [111]. The highest incidence is in the third and fourth decade of life. Rather than reflecting susceptibility, the age occurrence may reflect only the amount of contact with the organism. Since the natural habitat remains obscure, this is only an assumption, but one supported in normal populations by the increasing skin test sensitivity in older people.

There is apparently no racial predilection in paracoccidioidomycosis [16]. Lacaz [142] reported on more than 2000 cases and noted that Caucasian immigrants tended to have a more serious form of the disease than did persons native to the Latin American locale. There is also some evidence that a cellular immune defect may be present and *P. brasiliensis* may be an opportunist [39,54,58,182,183].

The male:female ratio is approximately 13:1 [113]. This could be a reflection of male-related occupational exposure; however, in endemic areas women work in fields as much as men [113]. Skin test sensitivity shows approximately equal sex distribution [112,214]. Experimental data show the possibility of hormonal factors inhibiting the organism's growth [191].

XII. SPOROTRICHOSIS

Sporotrichosis is a chronic, usually subcutaneous mycosis caused by *Sporothrix schenckii* or *S. schenckii* var. *luriei*. In the most commonly observed clinical form of sporotrichosis, the lesions are localized and may ulcerate and suppurate. In rare cases, the disease may be acquired by inhalation to involve the lungs or may disseminate to the central nervous system.

The mode of infection in sporotrichosis seems to be straightforward, i.e., the fungus is a saprobe that is acquired by primary inoculation into subcutaneous tissue [174]. There are also rare reports of primary pulmonary disease acquired by inhalation and of disseminated involvement [79].

A. Ecology

Sporothrix schenckii exists as a saprobe growing on such substrates as wood, straw, thorns, moss, and plant debris. This accounts for the most common types of local infection related to puncture wounds incurred during gardening or farming. There is some variation in the characteristics of isolates newly cultured from nature [10,122,165, 173]; however, the existence of *S. schenckii* in association with plant debris is well-established. A review of this problem is reported by Mackinnon [163].

There is a puzzling relationship between *S. schenckii* and *Ceratocystis stenoceras* in that the only morphologic criterion separating the two genera is the hyaline state of *Ceratocystis* conidia and the hyaline and dark-walled conidia of *Sporothrix*. In addition, *C. stenoceras* has been shown to be pathogenic for animals [175].

Sporotrichosis occurs in domestic animals with several reports from Latin America. The animals include cats [90], dogs [156], and mules [12,226]. Animals are not considered reservoirs; however, there are a few instances related to bites of insects and animals, but such cases have not been rigorously documented [14]. The occurrence of multiple cases in a family or group are traced not to human-to-human transmission, but to external sources [244].

B. Geographic Distribution

Several review articles have summarized 275 cases occurring in the United States up to 1952 [246] and 75 additional cases through 1964 [229]. These reports are not a true reflection of the incidence of the disease because not all cases are reported or published.

A high incidence of the disease occurs in South America, in particular Brazil, e.g., São Paulo [15] and Rio de Janeiro [200], in Uruguay [163], in Columbia [108a], and less frequently in Mexico [105,210]. The percentages reported in other portions of the world are much lower, e.g., Spain [96] and Canada [85].

C. Predisposing Factors

There is no evidence of differential susceptibility to sporotrichosis based on age or sex of an individual. Any apparent differences are usually related to common exposure and/or occupational factors.

There are reports of sporotrichosis occurring not as a primary process, but secondary to other diseases such as sarcoidosis [82]. Sporotrichosis has also been reported in patients with hematologic malignancy who have been on steroid therapy or on administered antitumor chemotherapy [160].

XIII. ZYGOMYCOSES AND OOMYCOSES

The zygomycoses and oomycoses are a diverse collection of fungal diseases caused by members of the subdivisions Zygomycotina and Mastigomycotina. A frequently used though no longer accurate synonym for these diseases is phycomycoses which includes: (1) mucormycosis (caused by the genera *Absidia, Cunninghamella, Mortierella, Mucor,* and *Rhizopus* among others); (2) entomophthoramycoses (caused by fungi belonging to the order Entomophthorales); and (3) oomycoses (including members of the class Oomycetes) [79,196]. These diseases are relatively rare, occurring predominantly as a syndrome involving the nasal, orbital, lymphatic, and central nervous systems [115,133,258].

A. Ecology

The zygomycoses and oomycoses are not considered contagious: man and animals are exposed to the spores from the environment. The organisms are found on plant material, fruit, vegetation, and on animal dung. Higher temperatures in decaying material favors the growth of those Mucoraceae that are thermophilic.

Basidiobolus haptosporus resides in the intestinal tract of frogs and toads without causing disease. Other etiologic agents of zygomycoses do cause disease in animals, e.g., *Mucor* and *Absidia* induce abortion in swine and cattle [19], *Entomophthora* causes insect diseases, *Saprolegnia* infects fish, and *Hyphomyces* infects horses.

B. Geographic Distribution

The organisms mentioned above are widely distributed throughout the world. *Basidiobolus* was first isolated from man in Indonesia and is widely distributed in Africa and southeast Asia [148]. Other agents of entomophthoramycoses are found in tropical areas of the Americas, Africa, and Asia. A review of these diseases and their appropriate classification is presented by Clark [49] (See also Chap. 3, Part A, of this series).

In African countries, these mycoses have been reported in Nigeria, Brazil, Colombia, and the Congo [35]. Bras et al. [35] reported the first human case from the West Indies. Baker [21] has also reviewed 255 human cases of mucormycosis.

In the United States, mycotic nasal polyps were reported by Bridges and co-workers [36]. The first deep entomophthoraceous infection in man was reported by King [136].

C. Predisposing Factors

In general, there are no differences in occurrence of zygomycoses in males and females or in different races. Martinson and Clark [178], however, have reported 11 cases of entomophthoramycoses from Nigeria showing a male-to-female ratio of 10:1. These cases are generally found in young adults under 20 years of age.

The zygomycoses are more often considered opportunistic rather than primary diseases. Predisposing factors in order of importance are: (1) diabetes mellitus, (2) blood dyscrasias [141], (3) corticosteroid therapy, (4) endocrine imbalances, and (5) malnutrition [21]. Immunosuppression during cancer therapy has also been a predisposing factor in mucormycosis [126].

COMMENTS

This chapter was intended as a general survey rather than a comprehensive review. It should be noted that the subject of the epidemiology of the mycoses received lengthy consideration a few years ago (see Ref. 14). A change in scheduling for this three-volume set on *Fungi Pathogenic for Humans and Animals* has led to some delay in the appearance of this chapter after its original drafting. In a few instances, more recent coverage is suggested.

REFERENCES

1. Abbott, P. 1956. Mycetoma in the Sudan. Trans. R. Soc. Trop. Med. Hyg. *50*:11-30.

2. Abraham, A., and H. F. Luddecke. 1956. North American blastomycosis and bronchial carcinoma. Dis. Chest. *28*:687.

3. Ainsworth, G. C., and P. K. C. Austwick. 1959. *Fungal Diseases of Animals.* Commonwealth Agricultural Bureaux, Farnham Royal, Slough, England.

4. Ainsworth, G. C., and R. E. Rewel. 1949. The incidence of aspergillosis in captive and wild birds. J. Comp. Pathol. Ther. *59*:213-224.

5. Aisner, J., S. C. Schimpff, J. E. Bennett, V. M. Young, and P. H. Wiernik. 1976. *Aspergillus* infections in cancer patients. Association with fireproofing in a new hospital. *JAMA 235*:411-412.

6. Ajello, L. 1952. The isolation of *Allescheria boydii,* an etiologic agent of mycetomas, from soil. Am. J. Trop. Med. *1*:227-238.

7. Ajello, L. 1957. *Coccidioides immitis*: isolation procedures and diagnostic criteria. In *Proceedings of Symposium on Coccidioidomycosis,* Public Health Service Publ. No. 575, pp. 47-52.

8. Ajello, L. 1967. Comparative ecology of respiratory mycotic disease agents. Bacteriol. Rev. *31*:6-24.

9. Ajello, L. 1968. A taxonomic review of the dermatophytes and related species. Sabouraudia *6*:147-159.

10. Ajello, L., and W. Kaplan. 1969. A new variant of *Sporothrix schenckii.* Mykosen *12*:633-644.

11. Ajello, L. 1971. Distribution of *Histoplasma capsulatum* in the United States. In L. Ajello, E. W. Chick, and M. L. Furcolow (Eds.), *Histoplasmosis, Proceedings of the Second National Conference,* C. C. Thomas, Springfield, Ill., pp. 103-122.

12. Albornoz, J. E. 1945. Primer caso de esporotricosis equina comprobado en el pais. Rev. Med. Vet. Bogota *14*:33-42.

13. Albornoz, M. 1971. Isolation of *P. brasiliensis* from rural soil in Venezuela. Sabouraudia *9*:248-253.

14. Al-Doory, Y. (Ed.). 1975. *The Epidemiology of Human Mycotic Diseases.* C. C. Thomas, Springfield, Ill.

15. Almeida, F. P., S. A. Sampaio, C. S. Lacaz, and J. Castro-Fernandes. 1955. Dados estatisticos sobre a esporotricose. An. Bras. Dermatol. *30*:9-12.

16. Angulo-Ortega, A., and L. Pollak. 1970. Paracoccidioidomycosis. In R. D. Baker (Ed.), *Human Infections with Fungi, Actinomycetes and Algae.* Springer-Verlag, Berlin, pp. 507-576.

17. Angulo-Ortega, A. 1972. Calcifications in paracoccidioidomycosis: are they the morphological manifestation of subclinical infections? In *Paracoccidioidomycosis, Proceedings of the First Pan American Symposium,* Pan Am. Health Organ. Sci. Publ. No. 254, Washington, D.C., pp. 129-133.

18. Aslam, P. A., C. E. Eastridge, and F. A. Hughes. 1971. Aspergillosis of the lung-an eighteen year experience. Chest *59*:28-32.

19. Austwick, P. K. C., and J. A. J. Venn. 1961. Mycotic abortion in England and Wales 1954-1960. In *Proceedings of the Fourth International Congress on Animal Reproduction.* The Hague, pp. 562-568.

20. Austwick, P. K. C. 1965. Pathogenicity. In K. B. Raper and D. I. Fennell (Eds.), *The Genus Aspergillus,* Williams & Wilkins, Baltimore, pp. 82-126.

21. Baker, R. D. 1971. *Human Infection with Fungi, Actinomycetes and Algae.* Springer-Verlag, Berlin.

22. Bass, H. E., S. I. Kooperstein, M. M. Friedman, and G. H. Kastlin, 1946. Pulmonary coccidioidomycosis. Dis. Chest *12*:371-386.

23. Beck, M. D. 1931. *Epidemiology.* California State Dept. Public Health Special Bull. No. 57, pp. 16-25.

24. Beneke, E. S. 1978. Geographic distribution and epidemiology of mycoses. In *Medical Mycology. Suppl. No. 1, Mykosen, Proceedings of the International Cilag-Chemic Symposium,* Grosse, Berlin, pp. 17-23.

25. Bennett, J. E., K. J. Kwon-Chung, and D. H. Howard. 1977. Epidemiologic differences among serotypes of *Cryptococcus neoformans*. Am. J. Epidemiol. *105*:582-586.

26. Bennington, J. L., S. L. Haber, and N. L. Morgenstern. 1964. Increased susceptibility to cryptococcosis following steroid therapy. Dis. Chest *45*:262-263.

27. Bernstein, I. L., and J. Scharz. 1948. Results of skin testing in military personnel. Ann. Intern. Med. *48*:791-796.

28. Bezjak, V., and S. J. Farsley. 1970. Prevalence of skin sensitivity to histoplasmin and coccidioidin in various Ugandan populations. Am. J. Trop. Med. Hyg. *19*:664-669.

29. Birsner, J. W. 1954. The roentgen aspects of five hundred cases of pulmonary coccidioidomycosis. Am. J. Roentgenol., Radium Ther. Nucl. Med. *72*:556-573.

30. Birsner, J. W., and S. Smart. 1956. Osseous coccidioidomycosis: a chronic form of dissemination. Am. J. Roentgenol., Radium Ther. Nucl. Med. *76*:1052-1060.

31. Bonoff, C. P. 1950. Acute primary pulmonary blastomycosis. Radiology *54*:157-164.

32. Borelli, D. 1971. Algunos aspectos ecologicos de la paracoccidioidomicosis. Dermatol. Venez. *13*:1190-1192.

33. Boshes, L. D., I. C. Sherman, C. J. Hesser, A. Milyer, and H. MacLean. 1956. Fungus infections of the central nervous system. Arch. Neurol. Psychiatry *75*:175-197.

34. Bower, G. C. 1958. Pulmonary lymphosarcoma with alveolar capillary block and associated coccidioidomycosis. Am. Rev. Tuberc. *78*:468-473.

35. Bras, G., C. C. Gordon, C. W. Emmons, K. M. Pendegast, and M. Sugar. 1965. A case of phycomycosis observed in Jamaica, infection with *Entomophthora coronata*. Am. J. Trop. Med. Hyg., *14*:141-145.

36. Bridges, C. H., and C. W. Emmons. 1961. A phycomycosis of horses caused by *Hyphomyces destruens*. J. Am. Vet. Med. Assoc. *138*:579-589.

37. Brier, R. L., M. Coleman, and J. Stone. 1957. Cutaneous cryptococcosis. Presentation of a case and a review of previously reported cases. Arch. Dermatol. *75*:262-263.

38. Brygoo, E. R., and G. Segretain. 1960. Etude clinique epidemiologique et mycologique de la chromoblastomycose a Madagascar. Bull. Soc. Pathol. Exot. *53*:443-475.

39. Campbell, C. C. 1972. The "pilot wheel": a change in course. In *Paracoccidioidomycosis, Proceedings of the First Pan American Symposium*, Pan Am. Health Organ. Sci. Publ. No. 254, Washington, D.C., pp. 306-312.

40. Campbell, G. D. 1966. Primary pulmonary cryptococcosis. Am. Rev. Respir. Dis. *94*:236-243.

41. Campins, H. 1967. Coccidioidomycosis in Venezuela. In L. Ajello (Ed.), *Coccidioidomycosis*. Papers from the Second Symposium on Coccidioidomycosis, University of Arizona Press, Tucson, pp. 279-287.

42. Carrion, A. L. 1965. Dermatomycoses in Puerto Rico. Arch. Dermatol. (Chicago) *91*:431-437.

43. Carter, H. S., and J. L. Young. 1950. Note on the isolation of *Cryptococcus neoformans* from a sample of milk. J. Pathol. Bacteriol. *62*:271-273.

44. Castellot, J. J., R. L. Creveling, and F. W. Pitts. 1960. Fatal miliary *coccidioidomycosis* complicating prolonged prednisone therapy in a patient with myelofibrosis. Ann. Intern. Med. *52*:254-258.

45. Catterall, R. D. 1971. Influence of gestogenic contraceptive pills on vaginal candidosis. Br. J. Vener. Dis. *47*:45-47.

46. Cherniss, E. I., and B. A. Waiskren. 1956. North American blastomycosis: a clinical study of forty cases. Ann. Intern. Med. *44*:105-123.

47. Chick, E. W., W. D. Sutliff, J. H. Rakich, and M. L. Furcolow. 1956. Epidemiological aspects of cases of blastomycosis admitted to Memphis, Tennessee, hospitals during the period of 1922-1954. A review of eighty-six cases. Am. J. Med. Sci. *231*: 253-262.
48. Christie, A. 1950. Histoplasmosis and pulmonary calcification—geographic distribution. Ann. N.Y. Acad. Sci. *50*:1283-1298.
49. Clark, B. M. 1968. Epidemiology of phycomycosis. In G. E. W. Wolstenholme and R. Porter (Eds.), *Systemic mycoses*, J. & A. Churchill, London, pp. 179-205.
50. Clayton, Y. M., and W. C. Noble. 1966. Observations on the epidemiology of *Candida albicans*. J. Clin. Pathol. *19*:76-78.
51. Climie, A. R. W., and R. Rachmaniff. 1965. Fungal (*Candida*) endocarditis following open heart surgery. J. Thorac. Cardiovasc. Surg. *50*:431-437.
52. Conant, N. F. 1937. The occurrence of a human pathogenic fungus as a saprophyte in nature. Mycologia *29*:597-598.
53. Conant, N. F., D. T. Smith, R. D. Baker, and J. L. Callaway. 1971. *Manual of Clinical Mycology*. Saunders, Toronto, Canada.
54. Conti-Diaz, I. A. 1972. Skin tests with paracoccidioidin and their importance. In *Paracoccidioidomycosis, Proceedings of the First Pan American Symposium*, Pan Am. Health Organ. Sci. Publ. No. 254, Washington, D.C., pp. 197-202.
55. Converse, J. L., R. E. Reed, H. W. Kuller, R. J. Trautman, E. M. Snyder, and J. G. Ray, Jr. 1967. Experimental epidemiology of coccidioidomycosis. I. Epizootiology of naturally exposed monkeys and dogs. In L. Ajello (Ed.), *Coccidioidomycosis*, Papers from the Second Symposium on Coccidioidomycosis, University of Arizona Press, Tucson, pp. 397-402.
56. Cook, A. W. 1951. *Cryptococcus* (torula) meningitis. Report of two cases. JAMA *146*:1105-1107.
57. Cooper, T., A. G. Morrow, W. C. Roberts, and L. G. Herman. 1961. Postoperative endocarditis due to *Candida*: clinical observation and the experimental production of the lesion. Surgery *50*:341-346.
58. Correa, A., and R. Giraldo. 1972. Study of immune mechanisms in paracoccidioidomycosis. I. Changes in immunoglobulins (IgG, IgM, and IgA). In *Paracoccidioidomycosis, Proceedings of the First Pan American Symposium*, Pan Am. Health Organ. Sci. Publ. No. 254, Washington, D.C., pp. 245-250.
59. Cotton, B. H., J. R. R. Penido, J. W. Birsner, and C. E. Babcock. 1954. Coexisting pulmonary coccidioidomycosis and tuberculosis. Am. Rev. Tuberc. *70*:109-120.
60. Craig, J. M., L. H. Schiff, and J. E. Boone. 1955. Chronic moniliasis associated with Addison's disease. Am. J. Dis. Child. *89*:669-684.
61. DaFonseca, O. 1955. Deep skin and pulmonary mycoses in Brazil. In T. N. Sternberg and V. D. Newcomer (Eds.), *Therapy of Fungus Diseases*, Little, Brown, Boston, pp. 56-57.
62. Dawson, C. O. 1968. Ringworm in animals. Rev. Med. Vet. Mycol. 6:223-233.
63. De Monbreun, W. A. 1939. The dog as a natural host of *Histoplasma capsulatum*. Am. J. Trop. Med. *19*:565-587.
64. DePape, A. J. 1959. Moniliasis associated with staphylococcal infection after antibiotic therapy. Can. Med. Assoc. J. *80*:205-207.
65. DiSalvo, A. F. 1971. The role of bats in the ecology of *Histoplasma capsulatum*. In L. Ajello, E. W. Chick, and M. L. Furcolow (Eds.), *Histoplasmosis, Proceedings of the Second National Conference*, C. C. Thomas, Springfield, Ill., pp. 149-161.
66. Dobbs, C. G., and W. H. Hinson. 1953. A widespread fungistasis in soils. Nature (Lond.) *172*:197-199.
67. Dowling, G. B., and R. R. Elworthy. 1976. Case of blastomycetic dermatitidis (gilchrist). Proc. R. Soc. Med. *19*:4-10.

68. Edwards, P. Q., and E. L. Billings. 1970. Worldwide pattern of skin sensitivity to histoplasmin. Am. J. Trop. Med. Hyg. *20*:288-319.

69. Edwards, P. Q., and J. H. Klaer. 1956. World-wide geographic distribution of histoplasmosis and histoplasmin sensitivity. Am. J. Trop. Med. Hyg. *5*:235-257.

70. Egeberg, R. O., A. E. Elconin, and M. C. Egeberg. 1964. Effects of salinity and temperature of *Coccidioides immitis* and three antagonistic soil saprophytes. J. Bacteriol. *88*:473-476.

71. Egeberg, R. O., and A. F. Ely. 1956. *Coccidioides immitis* in the soil of the southern San Joaquin Valley. Am. J. M. Sci. *231*:151-154.

72. Elconin, A. E., R. O. Egeberg, and M. C. Egeberg. 1964. Significance of soil salinity on the ecology of *Coccidioides immitis*. J. Bacteriol. *87*:500-503.

73. Elconin, A. E., R. O. Egeberg, and R. Lubarsky. 1957. Growth patterns of *Coccidioides immitis* in the soil of an endemic area. In *Proceedings of Symposium on Coccidioidomycosis*, U.S. Public Health Service Publ., No. 575, pp. 168-170.

74. Emmons, C. W. 1942. Isolation of *Coccidioides* from soil and rodents. Public Health Rep. *57*:109-111.

75. Emmons, C. W. 1949. Isolation of *Histoplasma capsulatum* from soil. Public Health Rep. *64*:892-896.

76. Emmons, C. W. 1951. Isolation from soil of fungi which cause disease in man. Trans. N.Y. Acad. Sci. *14*:51-54.

77. Emmons, C. W. 1955. Saprophytic sources of *Cryptococcus neoformans* associated with the pigeon (*Columbia Livia*). Am. J. Hyg. *62*:227-232.

78. Emmons, C. W. 1965. Report of a survey of mycoses in Africa. WHO. Mycoses/Inf. *66*:5-23.

79. Emmons, C. W., C. H. Binford, J. P. Utz, and K. J. Kwon-Chung. 1977. *Medical Mycology*, 3rd ed., Lea & Febiger, Philadelphia.

80. Evans, E. E., and E. R. Harrell, Jr. 1952. Cryptococcosis (torulosis): a review of recent cases. Univ. Mich. Med. Bull. *18*:43-63.

81. Evenson, A. E., and J. W. Lamb. 1964. Slime flux of mesquite as a new saprophytic source of *Cryptococcus neoformans*. J. Bacteriol. *88*:542.

82. Falcone, M. W., and V. F. Garagusi. 1969. Sporotrichosis and nocardiosis in a patient with Boeck's sarcoid. Sth. Med. J. *62*:315-318.

83. Fennel, E. A. 1935. Coccidioidal granuloma in Hawaii. Proc. Staff Meet. Clin., Honolulu, *6*:1-6.

84. Firestone, G. M., and E. S. Benson. 1949. Coexisting disseminated coccidioidomycosis and tuberculosis. Am. Rev. Tuberc. *59*:415-428.

85. Fischer, J. B., and M. V. Markkanen. 1951. Sporotrichosis. Can. Med. Assoc. J. *65*:49-50.

86. Flynn, N. M., P. D. Hoeprich, M. M. Kawachi, K. K. Lee, R. M. Lawrence, E. Goldstein, G. W. Jordan, R. S. Kundargi, and G. A. Wong. 1979. An unusual outbreak of windborne coccidioidomycosis. N. Engl. J. Med. *301*(7):358-361.

87. Ford, S., and L. Friedman. 1967. Experimental study of the pathogenicity of aspergilli for mice. J. Bacteriol. *94*:928-933.

88. Fountain, F. F., and W. D. Sutliff. 1969. Paracoccidioidomycosis in the United States. Am. Rev. Respir. Dis. *99*:89-93.

89. Fraser, D., J. Ward, L. Ajello, and B. Plikaytis. 1979. Aspergillosis and other systemic mycoses. JAMA *242*:1631-1635.

90. Freitas, D. C., G. Moreno, J. A. Bottino, E. N. Mos, and A. M. Saliba. 1965. Esporotricose em caes e gatos. Rev. Fac. Med. Vet. Zootec. Univ. São Paulo 7:381-387.

91. Furcolow, M. L. 1958. Recent studies on the epidemiology of histoplasmosis. Ann. N.Y. Acad. Sci. *72*:127-163.

92. Furcolow, M. L. 1960. *Epidemiology of Histoplasmosis.* C. C. Thomas, Springfield, Ill.

93. Furcolow, M. L., E. W. Chick, J. F. Busey, and R. W. Menges. 1970. Prevalence and incidence studies of human and canine blastomycosis. I. Case in the United States. 1885-1968. Am. Rev. Respir. Dis. *102*:60-67.

94. Furcolow, M. L., and J. Sitterley. 1951. Further studies of the geography of histoplasmin sensitivity in Kansas and Missouri. J. Kans. Med. Soc. *52*:584-589.

95. Furtado, T. 1972. Infection vs. disease in paracoccidioidomycosis. In *Paracoccidioidomycosis, Proceedings of the First Pan American Symposium,* Pan Am. Health Organ. Sci. Publ. No. 254, Washington, D.C., pp. 271-277.

96. Gay Prieto, J. 1963. Esporotricosis. In *Actas Finales, fifth congress Iber. Latinoamer. Dermatol.,* Buenos Aires, p. 316.

97. Geller, R. D. 1973. Coccidioidin sensitivity among southwestern American Indians. Am. Rev. Respir. Dis. *107*:301-302.

98. Gentry, L. O., and J. S. Remington. 1971. Resistance against *Cryptococcus* conferred by intracellular bacteria and protozoa. J. Infect. Dis. *123*:22-31.

99. Georg, L. 1957. *Dermatophytes, New Methods in Classification.* Communicable Disease Center, Atlanta, Ga.

100. Gezuele, E., J. E. Mackinnon, and I. A. Conti-Diaz. 1972. The frequent isolation of *Phialophora verrucosa* and *Phialophora pedrosoi* from natural sources. Sabouraudia *10*:266-273.

101. Gilles, M. 1933. A case of blastomycosis. Can. Med. Assoc. J. *29*:183-185.

102. Gonzalez-Mendoza, A. 1970. Opportunistic mycosis. In *Proceedings of the First International Symposium on the Mycoses,* Pan Am. Health Organ. Sci. Publ. No. 205, Washington, D.C., pp. 16-25.

103. Gonzalez-Ochoa, A., and A. Gonzalez-Mendoza. 1960. La micolo gia medica en Mexico. Mycopathologia *13*:56.

104. Gonzalez-Ochoa, A., and M. de los Angeles-Sandoval. 1960. Aislamiento de *Nocardia brasiliensis* y *asteroides* a partir de suelos. Rev. Inst. Salubr. Enferm. Trop. *20*: 147-149.

105. Gonzalez-Ochoa, A. 1965. Contribuciones recientes al conocimiento de la esporotricosis. Gac. Med. Mex. *95*:463-474.

106. Gonzalez-Ochoa, A. 1966. Micetoma por *Nocardia brasiliensis.* Mem I Reunion Mex-Centroamer Dermatol. Mexico, D. F., pp. 152-158.

107. Gonzalez-Ochoa, A. 1967. Coccidioidomycosis in Mexico. In L. Ajello (Ed.), *Coccidioidomycosis,* Papers from the Second Symposium on Coccidioidomycosis. University of Arizona Press, Tucson, pp. 293-299.

108. Gonzales-Ochoa, A. 1975. Mycetomas. In E. W. Chick, A. Balows, and M. L. Furcolow (Eds.), *Opportunistic Fungal Infections, Proceedings of the Second International Conference,* C. C. Thomas, Springfield, Ill., pp. 177-192.

108a. Gonzalo-Calle, V. and A. Restrepo-M. 1961. Esporotricosia. Antioquia Med. *11*:4444-4447.

109. Gordon, R. E., and W. A. Hagan. 1936. A study of some acid-fast actinomycetes from soil, with special reference to pathogenicity for animals. J. Infect. Dis. *59*: 200-206.

110. Goren, M. B. 1967. Experimental murine cryptococcosis: effect of hyperimmunization to capsular polysaccharide. J. Immunol. *98*:914-922.

111. Greer, A. E. 1962. *Fungus Diseases of the Lung.* C. C. Thomas, Springfield, Ill.

112. Greer, D. L., D. Estrada, and L. Trejos. 1974. Dermal sensitivity to paracoccidioidin and histoplasmin in family members of patients with paracoccidioidomycosis. Am. J. Trop. Med. Hyg. *23*:87-98.

113. Greer, D. L., and A. Restrepo. 1975. The epidemiology of paracoccidioidomycosis.

In Y. Al-Doory (Ed.), *The Epidemiology of Human Mycotic Diseases,* C. C. Thomas, Springfield, Ill., pp. 117-141.

114. Gregory, P. H. 1973. *Microbiology of the Atmosphere,* 2nd ed., Leonard Hill Books, Aylesbury, England.

115. Gregory, J. E., A. Golden, and W. Haymaker. 1943. Mucormycosis of the central nervous system. Report of three cases. Bull. Johns Hopkins Hosp. *73*:405-419.

116. Grose, E., and J. R. Tramsett. 1965. *P. brasiliensis* recovered from the intestinal tract of three bats (*A. lituratus*) in Columbia, S. A. Sabouraudia *4*:124-125.

117. Grover, S., B. S. Chaubey, M. Nawag, and M. K. Sonsati. 1977. Pulmonary aspergillosis. J. Assoc. Physicians India *25*:541-545.

118. Haley, L. D. 1950. Etiology of otomycosis. III. Arch. Otolaryngol. *52*:214-219.

119. Harrell, E. R., F. C. Bobco, and A. C. Curtis. 1955. A study of North American blastomycosis and its treatment with stilbamidine and 2-hydroxy-stilbamidine. Ann. Intern. Med. *43*:1076-1091.

120. Hirsch, E. F. 1923. Introduction of coccidioidal granuloma in Chicago. JAMA *81*:375-377.

121. Howard, D. H. 1973. The commensalism of *Cryptococcus neoformans.* Sabouraudia *11*:171-174.

122. Howard, D. H., and G. F. Orr. 1963. Comparison of strains of *Sporotrichum schenckii* isolated from nature. J. Bacteriol. *85*:816-821.

123. Howles, J. K., and C. I. Black. 1953. Cutaneous blastomycosis. A report of 58 unpublished cases. J. La. State Med. Soc. *105*:72-78.

124. Huntington, R. W., Jr. 1959. Morphology and racial distribution of fatal coccidioidomycosis. Report of a ten-year autopsy series in an endemic area. JAMA *169*:115-118.

125. Huppert, M., S. H. Sun, and J. W. Bailey. 1967. Natural variability in *Coccidioides immitis.* In L. Ajello (Ed.), *Coccidioidomycosis,* Papers from the Second Symposium on Coccidioidomycosis, University of Arizona Press, Tucson, pp. 323-328.

126. Hutter, R. V. P. 1959. Phycomycetous infection (mucormycosis) in cancer patients. Cancer *12*:330-350.

127. Hutter, R. V. P., and H. S. Collins. 1962. The occurrence of opportunistic fungus infections in a cancer hospital. Lab. Invest. *11*:1035-1045.

128. Israel, H. L., E. DeLamater, M. Sones, W. D. Willis, and A. Mirmelstein. 1952. Chronic disseminated histoplasmosis: an investigation of its relationship to sarcoidosis. Am. J. Med. *12*:252-253.

129. Jensen, H. K., P. A. Hansen, and J. Blom. 1970. Incidence of *C. albicans* in women using oral contraceptives. Acta Obstet. Gynecol. Scand. *49*:293-296.

130. Jillson, O. F., and M. Adami. 1955. Allergic dermatitis produced by inhalant molds. Arch. Dermatol. *72*:411-419.

131. Joffe, B. 1960. An epidemic of coccidioidomycosis probably related to soil. N. Engl. J. Med. *262*:720-722.

132. Kahn, M. 1950. Primary coccidioidomycosis and concomitant tuberculosis. Am. Rev. Tuberc. *61*:887-891.

133. Kamalam, A., and A. S. Thambiah. 1975. Basidiobolomycosis with lymph node involvement. Sabouraudia *13*:44-48.

134. Kane, P. A., A. M. Sarr, J. L. Courbil, J. C. Derrien, D. Coly, B. Diop, A. Nadio, and M. Sankal'e. 1976. Pulmonary aspergillosis. The first case in Dakar. Bull. Soc. Med. Afr. Noire Lang. Fr. *21*:157-160.

135. Kaufman, H. J. 1970. *Candida* oesophagitis in children with malignant disorders. Ann. Radiol. *13*:157-162.

136. King, D. S., and S. C. Jong. 1976. Identity of the etiological agent of the first deep entomophthoraceous infection of man in the United States. Mycologia *68*:181-183.

137. Kirshbaum, J. D. 1950. Disseminated coccidioidomycosis with severe cutaneous manifestations. Ill. Med. J. *97*:157-160.

138. Klite, P. D., and F. H. Diercks. 1965. *Histoplasma capsulatum* in fecal contents of bats in the Canal Zone. Am. J. Trop. Med. *14*:433-439.

139. Kritzer, M. D., M. Biddle, and J. F. Kessel. 1950. An outbreak of primary pulmonary coccidioidomycosis in Los Angeles, California. Ann. Intern. Med. *33*:960-990.

140. Kunkel, W. M., Jr., L. A. Weeds, J. R. McDonald, and O. T. Clagett. 1954. Collective review: North American blastomycosis-Gilchrist's disease; a clinicopathologic study of ninety cases. Int. Abstr. Surg. *99*:1-26.

141. Kwon-Chung, K. J., R. C. Young, and M. Orlando. 1975. Pulmonary mucormycosis caused by *Cunninghamella elegans* in a patient with myelogenous leukemia. Am. J. Clin. Pathol. *64*:540-544.

142. Lacaz, C. S. 1967. Compendio de Micologia Médica. Sarvier, São Paulo.

143. Larsh, H. W. 1975. The epidemiology of histoplasmosis. In Y. Al-Doory (Ed.), *The Epidemiology of Human Mycotic Diseases,* C. C. Thomas, Springfield, Ill., pp. 52-73.

144. Larsh, H. W., A. Hinton, and G. C. Cozad. 1956. Natural reservoir of *Histoplasma capsulatum.* Am. J. Hyg. *63*:18-27.

145. Lavalle, P. 1971. Epidemiologia del micetoma y de la esporotricosis. Presented at XIII Jornadas Acad. Nal. Med. Mex. Puebla, Pue, Jan.

146. Le Riche, W. H., and J. Milner. 1971. *Epidemiology as Medical Ecology,* Longman, London.

147. Levan, N. E. 1954. Occupational aspects of coccidioidomycosis. Calif. Med. *80*:294-298.

148. Joe, L. K., N-I. T. Eng, S. Tjokronegoro, and C. W. Emmons. 1960. Phycomycosis (mucormycosis) in Indonesia—description of a case affecting the subcutaneous tissue. Am. J. Trop. Med. *9*:143-148.

149. Linn, J. E. 1958. Pseudo-epitheliomatous perirectal tissue: report of a case of squamous epithelioma due to blastomycosis. Sth Med. J. *51*:1101-1104.

150. Lipsitz, S. H. 1916. Systemic blastomycosis and coccidioidal granuloma with a description of the first case of coccidioidal granuloma reported in Missouri. J. Mo. State Med. Assoc. *13*:534-536.

151. Littman, M. L., and L. E. Zimmerman. 1956. *Cryptococcosis. Torulosis or European blastomycosis,* Grune & Stratton, New York.

152. Littman, M. L., and J. E. Walter. 1968. Cryptococcosis: current status. Am. J. Med. *45*:922-932.

153. Londero, A. T. 1964. Dermatomycosis in the hinterland of Rio Grande do Sul (Brazil). Dermatol. Int. *3*:64-68.

154. Londero, A. T. 1970. Prevalence of cutaneous mycoses in Latin America. In *Proceedings of the First International Symposium on the Mycoses.* Pan. Am. Health Organ. Sci. Publ. No. 205, Washington, D.C., pp. 13-17.

155. Londero, A. T. 1972. Paracoccidioidomycosis; a clinical and mycological study of 41 cases observed in Santa Maria, R. S. Brazil. Am. J. Med. *52*:771-775.

156. Londero, A. T., R. M. de Castro, and O. Fischman. 1964. Two cases of sporotrichosis in dogs in Brazil. Sabouraudia *3*:273-274.

157. Loofbourow, J. C., D. Pappagianis, and T. Y. Cooper. 1969. Endemic coccidioidomycosis in northern California: an outbreak in the Capay Valley of Yolo County. Calif. Med. *111*:5-9.

158. Louria, D. B., T. Kaminski, and G. Finkel. 1963. Further studies on immunity in experimental cryptococcosis. J. Exp. Med. *117*:509-520.

159. Louridas, G. 1976. Bronchopulmonary aspergillus. An epidemiological study in a hospital population. Respiration *33*:281-288.

160. Lynch, P. J., J. J. Voorhees, and E. R. Harrell. 1970. Systemic sporotrichosis. Ann. Intern. Med. *73*:23-30.

161. Mackenzie, D. W. R. 1963. "Hairbrush diagnosis" in detection and eradication of non-fluorescent scalp ringworm. Br. Med. J. *2*:363-365.

162. Mackinnon, J. E. 1954. A contribution to the study of the causal organisms of maduromycosis. Trans. R. Soc. Trop. Med. Hyg. *48*:470-480.

163. Mackinnon, J. E. 1970. Ecology and epidemiology of sporotrichosis. In *Proceedings of the First International Symposium on the Mycoses,* Pan Am. Health Organ. Sci. Publ. No. 205, Washington, D.C., pp. 169-181.

164. Mackinnon, J. E., and R. C. Artaganeytia Allende. 1956. The main species of pathogenic aerobic actinomycetes causing mycetomas. Trans. R. Soc. Trop. Med. Hyg. *50*:31-40.

165. Mackinnon, J. E., I. A. Conti-Diaz, E. Gezuele, E. Civila, and S. da Luz. 1969. Isolation of *Sporothrix schenckii* from nature and considerations on its pathogenicity and ecology. Sabouraudia *7*:38-45.

166. Macotela-Ruiz, E. 1970. Epidemiology and ecology of mycetomas. In *Proceedings of the First International Symposium on the Mycoses,* Pan Am. Health Organ. Sci. Publ. No. 205, Washington, D.C., pp. 185-194.

167. Maddy, K. T. 1957. Ecological factors possibly relating to the geographic distribution of *Coccidioides immitis.* In *Proceedings of Symposium on Coccidioidomycosis,* U.S. Public Health Service Publ. No. 575, pp. 144-157.

168. Maddy, K. T. 1957. A study of one hundred cases of disseminated coccidioidomycosis in the dog. In *Proceedings of Symposium on Coccidioidomycosis,* U.S. Public Health Service Publ. No. 575, pp. 107-118.

169. Maddy, K. T. 1965. Observations on *Coccidioides immitis* found growing naturally in soil. Ariz. Med. *22*:261-288.

170. Madrid, G. S. 1950. Coccidioidomycosis en el Estado de Sonora. Prensa Med. (Hermasillo) *10*(3).

171. Manwaring, John H. 1949. Unusual forms of *Blastomyces dermatitidis* in human tissues. Arch. Pathol. *48*:421-425.

172. Mariat, F. 1967. Notes epidemiologiques a propos des mycetomes. In *Recent Progress in Microbiology,* Univ. of Toronto Press, Toronto, pp. 668-684.

173. Mariat, F. 1968. The epidemiology of sporotricosis. In G. E. W. Wolstenholme, and R. Porter (Eds.), *Systemic Mycoses.* J. & A. Churchill, London, pp. 144-159.

174. Mariat, F. 1968. The epidemiology of the mycoses; some comments in relation to a particular case of sporotrichosis. In Ciba Fdn. Symposium, *Systemic Mycoses,* Churchill, London, pp. 144-163.

175. Mariat, F. 1971. Adaptation de Ceratocytis a la vie parasitaire chez l'animal. Sabouraudia *9*:191-205.

176. Mariat, F. and C. Adan-Campos. 1967. La technique du carre tapis, methode simple de prelevement dan les mycoses superficielles. Ann. Inst. Pasteur. *113*: 666-668.

177. Martin, D. S., D. T. Smith. 1939. Blastomycosis (American blastomycosis, Gilchrist's disease). II. A report of thirteen new cases. Am. Rev. Tuberc. *39*: 275-304.

178. Martinson, F. D., and B. M. Clark. 1967. Rhinophycomycosis entomophthorae in Nigeria. Am. J. Trop. Med. Hyg. *16*:40-47.

179. Mayorga, P. R. 1967. Coccidioidomycosis in Central America. In L. Ajello (Ed.), *Coccidioidomycosis,* Papers from the Second Symposium on Coccidioidomycosis, University of Arizona Press, Tucson, pp. 287-291.

180. McClellan, J. T. 1951. Histoplasmosis with brief reference to two cases from Kentucky, one in a dog. J. Kans. Med. Assoc. *49*:210-213.

181. McClung, N. M. 1960. Isolation of *Nocardia asteroides* from soils. Mycologia *52*:154-156.

182. Mendes, N. F., C. C. Musatti, C. Leao, E. Mendes, and C. K. Naspits. 1971. Lymphocyte cultures and skin allograft survival in patients with South American blastomycosis. J. Allergy Clin. Immun. *48*:40-45.

183. Mendes, E., and A. Raphael. 1971. Impaired delayed hypersensitivity in patients with South American blastomycosis. J. Allergy Clin. Immunol. *47*:17-22.

184. Menges, R. W. 1971. Clinical manifestations of animal histoplasmosis, In L. Ajello, E. W. Chick, and M. L. Furcolow (Eds), *Histoplasmosis, Proceedings of the Second National Conference*, C. C. Thomas, Springfield, Ill., pp. 162-169.

185. Menges, R. W., M. L. Furcolow, and A. Hinton. 1954. The role of animals in the epidemiology of histoplasmosis. Am. J. Hyg. *59*:113-118.

186. Menges, R. W., R. T. Habermann, L. A. Selby, H. R. Ellis, R. F. Behlow, and C. D. Smith. 1963. A review and recent findings on histoplasmosis in animals. Vet. Med. *58*:331-338.

187. Merkow, L. P., S. M. Epstein, H. Sidransky, E. Verney, and M. Pardo. 1971. The pathogenesis of experimental pulmonary aspergillosis. Am. J. Pathol. *62*:57-74.

188. Meyer, R. D., L. S. Young, D. Armstrong, and B. Yu. 1973. Aspergillosis complicating neoplastic disease. Am. J. Med. *54*:6-15.

189. Mirsky, H. S., and J. Cuttner. 1972. Fungal infection in acute leukemia. Cancer *30*:348-352.

190. Montero-Gei, F. 1970. Ecology and epidemiology of chromomycosis. In *Proceedings of the First International Symposium on the Mycoses*, Pan Am. Health Organ. Sci. Publ. No. 205, Washington, D.C., pp. 182-184.

191. Muchmore, H. G., B. A. McKown, and J. A. Mohr. 1972. Effect of steroid hormones on the growth of *P. brasiliensis*. In *Paracoccidioidomycosis, Proceedings of the First Pan American Symposium*, Pan Am. Health Organ. Sci. Publ. No. 254, Washington, D.C., pp. 300-304.

192. Muchmore, H. G., E. R. Rhoades, G. E. Nix, F. G. Felton, and R. E. Carpenter. 1963. Occurrence of *Cryptococcus neoformans* in the environment of three geographically associated cases of cryptococcal meningitis. N. Engl. J. Med. *268*: 1112-1114.

193. Newberry, W. M., Jr., J. E. Walter, J. W. Chandler, Jr., and F. E. Tosh. 1967. Epidemiologic study of *Cryptococcus neoformans*. Ann. Intern. Med. *67*:724-732.

194. Nicol, T., B. Vernon-Roberts, and D. C. Quantock. 1965. The influence of various hormones on the reticulo-endothelial system: endocrine control of body defence. J. Endocrinol. *33*:365-383.

195. Noble, W. C., and Y. M. Clayton. 1963. Fungi in the air of hospital wards. J. Gen. Microbiol. *32*:397-402.

196. Nottebrock, H., H. J. Scholer, and M. Wall. 1974. Taxonomy and identification of mucormycosis-causing fungi. I. Synonymy of *Absidia ramosa* with *A. corymbifera*. Sabouraudia *12*:64-74.

197. Orie, N. G., G. A. DeVries, and A. Kikstra. 1960. Growth of aspergillus in human lung. Am. Rev. Respir. Dis. *82*:649-662.

198. Ortiz, Y. 1966. Dermatologia y geografia en Mexico. Dermatol. Rev. Mex. *10*: 343-408.

199. Padilha-Goncalves, A. 1972. Epidemiological factors in paracoccidioidomycosis. In *Paracoccidioidomycosis, Proceedings of the First Pan American Symposium*, Pan Am. Health Organ. Sci. Publ. No. 254, Washington, D.C., pp. 53-58.

200. Padilha-Goncalves, A., and D. Peryassu. 1954. A esporotricose no Rio de Janeiro (1936-1953). Hospital (Rio) *46*:10-22.

201. Pappagianis, D., C. E. Smith, and M. T. Saito. 1957. Preparation and property of a complement fixing antigen from mycelia of *Coccidioides immitis*. In *Proceedings of Symposium on Coccidioidomycosis*, U.S. Public Health Publ. No. 575, pp. 57-63.

202. Pepys, J., R. W. Riddell, K. M. Citron, Y. M. Clayton, and E. I. Short. 1959. Clinical and immunologic significance of *Aspergillus fumigatus* in the sputum. Am. Rev. Respir. Dis. *80*:167-180.

203. Perl, G., A. F. Guttmacher, and H. Jakubowicz. 1955. Vaginal candidiasis. Obstet. Gynecol. *5*:640-648.

204. Pinkerton, H., and L. Uvernon. 1952. Histoplasmosis. Arch. Intern. Med. *90*: 456-467.

205. Plunkett, O. A., and F. E. Swatek. 1957. Ecological studies of *Coccidioides immitis*, In *Proceedings of Symposium on Coccidioidomycosis*, Public Health Service Publ. No. 575, pp. 158-160.

206. Posadas, A. 1892. Un nuevo caso de micosis fungordea con psorospermias. An. Circ. Med. Argent. *15*:585-597.

207. Prachal, C. J. 1957. Coccidioidomycosis in Arizona cattle. In *Proceedings of Symposium on Coccidioidomycosis*, Public Health Service Publ. No. 575, pp. 105-106.

208. Procknow, J. J. 1966. Disseminated blastomycosis treated successfully with the polypeptide antifungal agent X-5079C. Evidence for human to human transmission. Am. Rev. Respir. Dis. *94*:761-772.

209. Procknow, J. J., and D. F. Loewen. 1960. Pulmonary aspergillosis with cavitation secondary to histoplasmosis. Am. Rev. Respir. Dis. *82*:101-111.

210. Ramirez, J. 1960. Esporotricosis: algunos datos estadisticos a proposito del estudio de un caso. Dermatologia (Mexico City) *4*:120-127.

211. Raper, K. B., and D. I. Fennell. 1965. *The Genus Aspergillus*. Williams & Wilkins, Baltimore.

212. Ravits, H. G. 1949. Cutaneous cryptococcosis. A survey of cryptococcus on normal and pathologic skin. J. Invest. Dermatol. *12*:271-284.

213. Reed, R. E. 1957. Nonfatal coccidioidomycosis of dogs. In *Proceedings of Symposium on Coccidioidomycosis*, Public Health Service Publ. No. 575, pp. 101-104.

214. Restrepo. A., M. Robledo, F. Gutierrez, M. Sandement, E. Castaneda, and G. Calle. 1970. Paracoccidioidomycosis (South American blastomycosis): a study of thirty-nine cases observed in Medellin, Columbia. Am. J. Trop. Med. Hyg. *19*: 68-76.

215. Riddell, R. W. 1956. Fungus diseases in Britain. Br. Med. J. *2*:783-786.

216. Ridley, M. F. 1957. The natural habitat of *Cladosporium carrionii*, a cause of chromoblastomycosis in man. Aust. J. Dermatol. *4*: 23-27.

217. Ridley, M. F. 1961. The saprophytic occurrence of fungi causing chromoblastomycosis. *Recent Advances in Botany. IX International Botanical Congress, 1959*, University of Toronto Press, Toronto, pp. 312-316.

218. Rippon, J. W., and M. Soo Hoo. 1973. Aspergillosis: comparative virulence, metabolic rate, growth rate and ubiquinone content of soil and human isolates of *Aspergillus terreus*. Abstr. Annu. Meet. Am. Soc. Microbiol., 1973, Mm 34.

219. Rixford, E. 1894. Case for the diagnosis presented before the San Francisco Medico-Chirurgical Society. March 5, 1894. Occidental Med. Times *8*:326.

220. Rodger, R. C., O. L. Terry, and C. H. Binford. 1951. Histoplasmosis, cryptococcosis and tuberculosis complicating Hodgkin's disease. Am. J. Clin. Pathol. *21*:153-157.

221. Rogers, A. L., and E. S. Beneke. 1964. Human pathogenic fungi recovered from Brazilian soil. Mycopathol. Mycol. Appl. *22*:15-20.

222. Romero, A., and A. Trejos. 1953. La chromoblastomicosis en Costa Rica. Rev. Biol. Trop. *1*:95-115.

223. Rook, G. D., and D. Brand. 1950. *Candida krusei* as a pathogen; case report of an unusual infection of the tonsils. Pediatrics *6*:638-642.

224. Salfelder, K., G. Doehnert, and H. R. Doehnert. 1969. Paracoccidioidomycosis; anatomic study with complete autopsies. Virchows Arch. Pathol. Anat. Physiol. *348*:51-76.

225. Salfelder, K., M. De Mendelovici, and J. Schwarz. 1971. Multiple deep mycoses. In *Proceedings of the Fifth Congress of the International Society for Human and Animal Mycology*, Louis-Jean, Paris.

226. Saliba, A. M., B. Sorenson, and J. S. Marcondes-Veiga. 1963. Esporotricose em muar. Biologico (São Paulo) *29*:209-212.

227. Salles, C. A. 1964. *Blastomyces (Paracoccidioides brasiliensis)* in Africa. Nature (Lond.) *204*:1211-1212.

228. Sandhu, D. K., R. S. Sandhu, V. N. Damodaran, and H. S. Randhawa. 1970. Effect of cortisone on bronchopulmonary aspergillosis in mice exposed to spores of various *Aspergillus* species. Sabouraudia *8*:32-38.

229. Schneidau, J. D., L. M. Lamar, and M. A. Hairston. 1964. Cutaneous hypersensitivity to sporotrichin in Louisiana. JAMA *188*:371-373.

230. Schwarz, J., and G. L. Baum. 1951. Blastomycosis. Am. J. Clin. Pathol. *21*:999-1029.

231. Schwarz, J., and G. L. Baum. 1957. The history of histoplasmosis 1906 to 1956. N. Engl. J. Med. *256*:253-258.

232. Schwarz, J., and L. Goldman. 1955. Epidemiologic study of North American blastomycosis. Arch. Dermatol. Syphilol. *71*:84-88.

233. Seabury, J. H., and M. Samuels. 1963. The pathogenetic spectrum of aspergillosis. Am. J. Clin. Pathol. *40*:21-33.

234. Seelig, M. S. 1966. Mechanisms by which antibiotics increase the incidence and severity of candidiasis and alter the immunological defenses. Bacteriol. Rev. *30*:442-459.

235. Segretain, G., J. Baylet, A. Darasse, and R. Camain. 1959. *Leptosphaeria senegalensis* n. sp. Agent de mycetomes a grain noirs. C. R. Acad. Sci. (D). *248*:3730-3732.

236. Segretain, G., and F. Mariat. 1968. Recherches sur la presence d'agents de mycetomes dans le sol et sur les epineux du Senegal et de la Mauritanie. Bull. Soc. Pathol. Exot. *61*:194-202.

237. Sethi, K. K. 1967. Pigeons and mycoses. N. Engl. J. Med. *276*:62.

238. Shacklette, M. H., F. H. Diercks, and N. B. Gale. 1962. *Histoplasma capsulatum* recovered from bat tissue. Science *135*:1135.

239. Shapiro, L. L., and J. B. Neal. 1925. Torula meningitis. Arch. Neurol. Psychiatry *13*:174-190.

240. Sidransky, H., and L. Friedman. 1959. The effect of cortisone and antibiotic agents on experimental pulmonary aspergillosis. Am. J. Pathol. *35*:169-183.

241. Sidransky, H., and M. A. Pearl. 1961. Pulmonary fungus infections associated with steroid and antibiotic therapy. Dis. Chest. *39*:630-642.

242. Sievers, M. L. 1964. Coccidioidomycosis among southwestern American Indians. Am. Rev. Respir. Dis. *90*:920-926.

243. Silva, M. E., and L. A. Paula. 1963. Isolation of *Cryptococcus neoformans* from excrement and nests of pigeons (*Columbia livia*) in Salvador, Bahia (Brasil). Rev. Inst. Med. Trop. São Paulo. *5*:9-11.

244. Silva, Y. P., and N. A. Guimarals. 1964. Esporotricose familiar epidemica. Hospital (Rio) *66*:573-579.

245. Simon, J., R. E. Nichols, and E. V. Morse. 1953. An outbreak of bovine cryptococcosis. J. Am. Vet. Med. Assoc. *122*:31-35.

246. Singer, J. I., and J. E. Muncie. 1952. Sporotrichosis: etiologic considerations and report of additional cases from New York. New York State J. Med. *52*: 2147-2153.

247. Sinski, J. T., 1975. The epidemiology of aspergillosis. In Y. Al-Doory (Ed.), *The Epidemiology of Human Mycotic Diseases,* C. C. Thomas, Springfield, Ill., pp. 210-226.

248. Smale, L. E., and J. W. Birsner. 1949. Maternal deaths from coccidioidomycosis. JAMA *140*:1152-1154.

249. Smith, C. E., M. T. Saito, and S. A. Simons. 1956. Pattern of 39,500 serologic tests in coccidioidomycosis. JAMA *160*:546-552.

250. Smith, J. G., Jr., J. S. Harris, N. F. Conant, and D. T. Smith. 1955. An epidemic of North American blastomycosis. JAMA *158*:641-646.

251. Solano, E. 1966. Cromomicosis. Acta Med. Costarric. *9*:77-85.

252. Solway, L. J., M. Kohan, and H. G. Pritzker. 1939. A case of disseminated blastomycosis. Can. Med. Assoc. J. *41*:331-336.

253. Staab, W. J., Jr., and H. S. Van Ordstrand. 1958. Pulmonary blastomycosis: a report of a case treated with 2-hydrostilbamidine. Cleveland Clin. Q. *25*:164-168.

254. Starrs, R. A., and M. O. Klotz. 1948. North American blastomycosis (Gilchrist's disease). A study of the disease from a review of the literature. Arch. Intern. Med. *82*:1-53.

254a. Stepanishtcheva, Z. G., A. M. Arievitch, O. B. Minsker, T. B. Soofeyeva. 1971. Investigation of deep mycosis in the USSR. Intern. J. Dermatol. *11*:181-183.

255. Stillians, A. W., and H. E. Klemptner. 1953. Blastomycosis in tuberculosis patient. JAMA *153*:558-561.

256. Stober, A. M. 1914. Systemic blastomycosis. Arch. Intern. Med. *13*:509-556.

257. Stoddard, J. L., and E. C. Cutler. 1916. Torula infection in man. Monographs of the Rockefeller Institute for Medical Research. No. 6. *25*:1.

258. Straatsma, B. R., L. E. Zimmerman, and J. D. M. Gass. 1963. Phycomycosis. A clinical pathologic study of fifty-one cases. Lab. Invest. *11*:963-985.

259. Stuart, E. A., and F. Blank. 1955. Aspergillosis of the ear: a report of 29 cases. Can. Med. Assoc. J. *72*:334-337.

260. Sutliff, W. D., J. C. Larkin, and L. Hyde. 1959. Mycotic diseases of the lung. Med. Clin. North Am. *43*:219-238.

261. Symmers, W. S. C. 1962. Histopathologic aspects of the pathogenesis of some opportunistic fungal infections, as exemplified in the pathology of aspergillosis and the phycomycetoses. Lab. Invest. *11*:1073-1090.

262. Taber, K. W. 1937. Torulosis in man: report of a case. JAMA *108*:1405-1406.

263. Tan, K. K., S. Kenji, and K. L. Tan. 1966. Disseminated aspergillosis, case report and review of the world literature. Am. J. Clin. Pathol. *45*:697-703.

264. Tompkins, V., and J. Schleifstein. 1953. Small forms of *Blastomyces dermatitidis* in human tissues. Arch. Pathol. *55*:432-435.

265. Utz, J. P., J. L. German, D. B. Louria, C. W. Emmons, and F. C. Bartter. 1959. Pulmonary aspergillosis with cavitation. N. Engl. J. Med. *260*:264-268.

266. Vanbreuseghem, R. 1952. Technique biologique pour l'isolement des dermatophytes du sol. Ann. Soc. Belge Med. Trop. *32*:173-178.

267. Vanbreuseghem, R. 1967. Early diagnosis, treatment and epidemiology of mycetoma. Rev. Med. Vet. Mycol. *6*:49-60.

268. Vandepitte, J., and F. Gatti. 1972. La Blastomycose Nord-Americaine en Afrique: Son Existence en Republique de Zaire. In *Proceedings of the Second International Colloquium of Medical Mycology,* Prince Leopold Institute of Tropical Medicine, Antwerp.

269. Velez, G. C., and A. Restrepo. 1966. Tinea capitis. Antioquia Med. *16*:15-30.

270. Villar, J. G., J. C. Pimentel, and R. Avila. 1967. Some aspects of pulmonary aspergilloma in Portugal. Dis. Chest *51*:402-405.

270a. Vlachos, J. D. 1972. First case of histoplasmosis in Greece. Pathol. Europaea. *7*: 289.

271. Voyles, G. Q., and E. M. Beck. 1946. Systemic infection due to *Torula histolytica* (*Cryptococcus hominis*): report of four cases and review of the literature. Arch. Intern. Med. *77*:504-515.

272. Walls, K., M. L. Furcolow, and P. H. Lehan. 1958. Histoplasmosis as a problem in tuberculosis sanitoriums throughout the United States. J. Lab. Clin. Med. *51*: 266-270.

273. Walter, J. E., and R. W. Atchison. 1966. Epidemiological and immunological studies of *Cryptococcus neoformans*. J. Bacteriol. *92*:82-87.

274. Walter, J. E., and E. G. Coffee. 1968. Distribution and epidemiologic significance of the serotypes of *Cryptococcus neoformans*. Am. J. Epidemiol. *87*:167-172.

275. Watson, S. H., S. Moore, and F. Blank. 1958. Generalized North American blastomycosis. Can. Med. Assoc. J. *78*:35-38.

276. Weitzman, I., P. Bonaparte, V. Guevin, and M. Crist. 1973. Cryptococcosis in a field mouse. Sabouraudia *11*:77-79.

277. Werner, S. B., D. Pappagianis, I. Heindl, and A. Michel. 1972. An epidemic of coccidioidomycosis among archeology students in northern California. N. Engl. J. Med. *286*:507-512.

278. White, F. H., D. J. Forrester, and S. A. Nesbitt. 1976. Salmonella and aspergillus in common loons overwintering in Florida. J. Am. Vet. Med. Assoc. *169*:936-937.

279. World Health Organization Official Records. 1975. No. 226:29.

280. Wilson, D. E., J. E. Bennett, and J. W. Bailey. 1968. Serologic grouping of *Cryptococcus neoformans*. Proc. Soc. Exp. Biol. Med. *127*:820-823.

281. Winn, W. A., H. B. Levine, J. E. Broderick, and R. W. Crane. 1963. A localized epidemic of coccidioidal infection. Primary coccidioidomycosis occurring in a group of ten children. N. Engl. J. Med. *268*:867-870.

282. Winner, H. I. 1975. The epidemiology of candidosis. In Y. Al-Doory (Ed.), *The Epidemiology of Human Mycotic Disease*, C. C. Thomas, Springfield, Ill., pp. 152-157.

283. Winner, H. I., and R. Hurley. 1964. *Candida albicans*. J. & A. Churchill, London.

284. Woods, J. W., I. H. Manning, and C. N. Patterson. 1951. Monilial infections complicating the therapeutic use of antibiotics. JAMA *145*:207-211.

7

Detection of Fungi in Tissues

Masahiko Okudaira / Kitasato University, Kangawa, Japan

I. INTRODUCTION

The development and widespread use of a number of new antibiotics have remarkably reduced the threat posed by many infectious diseases. However, most of the bactericidal and bacteriostatic antibiotics are ineffective against the majority of zoopathogenic fungi, and therefore, opportunistic fungous infections have become problems of central importance in modern medicine [3,7,13,32,34,35,74]. The increase in the number of deep mycoses has been emphasized by the results of autopsy surveys, because in many instances these infections are terminal complications in compromised patients and are detected only at autopsy [27,29,44,48]. The increased awareness of fungous infections is based not only upon extensive therapy for malignancies and immunological disorders, but also on the increasing interest in fungous infections and on the recent progress in investigative histopathological methods.

In almost all fungous infections, the parasitic forms of the causative fungi can be detected in the center of the lesion. Therefore, it should be emphasized that the central portion of lesions ought to be examined and that it is always essential to perform cultural examinations along with histopathological studies.

The fungi are ubiquitous in nature and over 50,000 species have been listed in the literature [1,10,14,17,62]. Although only a limited number of fungi are known to be pathogenic for humans, the increasing number of recognized opportunistic fungi [61] augments continually the estimate of potential zoopathogens.

Detection of fungi in tissue is essentially a morphological study, therefore all investigators must prepare materials carefully for microscopic observation. Although fungi within infected tissues show considerable variation not only in form and size, but also in staining features, the investigator should search for specific morphological characteristics that will identify the causative fungus at the generic level. Adequate fixation of pathological specimens, dehydration with alcohol, embedding carefully in paraffin, thin sectioning, and good staining are required for the detection and generic diagnosis of fungi in tissue. It is the author's opinion that one needs to be familiar with a variety of staining methods when intending to search microscopically for fungal elements in tissue.

II. METHODS FOR DETECTION OF FUNGI IN TISSUE

There are many methods for the detection of fungi in tissue. The more common and routine procedures employed in most laboratories will be described in this section.

A. Direct Microscopic Examination

Most mycological specimens may be examined directly in a fluid state, usually after treatment with potassium hydroxide (KOH). A 10% solution of KOH is necessary for the examination of skin scales, hairs, and nail scrapings. Gentle heating of the KOH preparation over a low flame of a Bunsen burner or of an alcohol lamp is helpful in clearing the material and eliminating air bubbles.

Pus, sputum, and exudates from ulcerative lesions are examined by placing a drop of these materials in 10% KOH on a glass slide and gently pressing a coverglass on the preparation to make a thin smear. Spinal, pleural, or peritoneal fluid and urine should first be centrifuged at 2000-3000 rpm for 10-15 min and the sediment then examined in the same way as described for pus, sputum, and exudates.

The selection of proper and adequate material from the patient is very important since an improper selection accounts for many negative findings. It is wise to take plenty of material for direct examination [69]. A mixture of one drop of lactophenol cotton blue solution and one drop of KOH solution provides a method of mounting mycological specimens that stains fungal elements beautifully.

A recipe for lactophenol cotton blue solution is as follows:

Phenol crystals	20 g
Lactic acid, syrup	20 ml
Glycerin	40 ml
Distilled water	20 ml
Cotton blue	0.05 g

The cotton blue should be added after the other materials have been dissolved by gentle heating [21].

In cases of suspected cryptococcal infection, one drop of India ink (diluted 1:3 in distilled water) should be mixed with the material. The ink is repelled by the capsule, and a halo effect around the cryptococcal yeast cells is thereby created.

B. Staining Methods

The purposes of investigating fungous infections histopathologically are to recognize tissue reactions to the infection, to detect fungous elements in the tissue, and to disclose, where possible, those morphological characteristics that serve to identify the fungus. Needless to say, an accurate diagnosis of fungous infections must be based, whenever possible, on both cultural results and histopathological detection of fungal elements in infected foci. With this object in mind, I have evaluated a number of staining methods for the detection of fungi in tissue (Table 1) [48].

The selection of a staining method for the detection of fungal elements in tissue depends to some extent upon the investigator's choice. Investigators often favor a method with which they have acquired the most extensive experience. Obviously, that method will be the best for the detection of fungal elements in their opinion.

Table 1 Evaluation of Staining Methods for Detection of Fungi in Tissue Sections

A. The best stain for the majority of fungous infections
    Grocott's method

B. Valuable for most fungous infections
    Periodic acid Schiff reaction
    Gridley's stain
    Bauer's stain
    Bielschowsky-Pap's silver stain
    Gram's stain
    Hematoxylin and eosin stain

C. Good for study on internal structures of fungous cells
    Mallory's Azan stain
    Heidenhain's iron hematoxylin stain
    Giemsa stain

D. Useful for demonstration and identification of specific fungi
    Mayer's mucicarmin stain for *Cryptococcus neoformans* and *Rhinosporidium seeberi*

E. Poor for fungus detection
    van Gieson's stain
    Methylene blue stain

The principal procedures currently used at the Armed Forces Institute of Pathology, Washington, D.C., [38] for the staining of fungi in tissues are as follows:*

1. Grocott's Method for Fungi (GMS) [23]

  a. Fixation: 10% buffered neutral Formalin (10% Formalin) can be used.

  b. Technique: Cut paraffin sections at 6 μm.

  c. Solutions:

4% Chromic acid solution
Chromic acid   4 g
Distilled water   100 ml

  5% Silver nitrate solution
Silver nitrate   5 g
Distilled water   100 ml

  3% Methenamine solution
Hexamethylenetetramine (methenamine)   3 g
Distilled water   100 ml

  5% Borax solution
Borax   5 g
Distilled water   100 ml

  Methenamine-silver nitrate solution (stock)
Silver nitrate, 5% solution   5 ml
Methenamine, 3% solution   100 ml

A white precipitate forms but immediately dissolves on shaking. Clear solution remains usable for months. Store in a refrigerator.

  Methenamine-silver nitrate solution (working)
Methenamine-silver nitrate solution (stock)   25 ml
Distilled water   25 ml
Borax, 5% solution   2 ml

Make fresh.

  1% Sodium bisulfite solution
Sodium bisulfite   1 g
Distilled water   100 ml

  0.1% Gold chloride solution
Gold chloride, 1% solution   10 ml
Distilled water   90 ml

This solution may be used repeatedly.

  2% Sodium thiosulfate (HYPO) solution
Sodium thiosulfate   2 g
Distilled water   100 ml

*Reprinted with permission from *The Manual of Histologic Staining Methods of the Armed Forces Institute of Pathology,* 3rd ed., L. G. Luna (Ed.), McGraw-Hill Book Company, New York, 1968.

0.2% Light green solution (stock)

Light green, SF (yellow)	0.2 g
Distilled water	100 ml
Glacial acetic acid	0.2 ml

Light green solution (working)

Light green (stock)	10 ml
Distilled water	50 ml

d. *Staining Procedure*: Use a control slide.

1. Deparaffinize and hydrate to distilled water.
2. Oxidize in 4% chromic acid solution for 1 h.
3. Wash in tap water for a few seconds.
4. Sodium bisulfite solution for 1 min to remove residual chromic acid.
5. Wash in running water for 5-10 min.
6. Rinse with three or four changes of distilled water.
7. Place in freshly mixed working methenamine-silver nitrate solution in oven at 58-60°C for 60 min or until sections turn yellowish brown.
8. Rinse in six changes of distilled water.
9. Tone in gold chloride solution for 2-5 min.
10. Rinse in distilled water.
11. Remove unreduced silver with sodium thiosulfate (hypo) solution for 2-5 min.
12. Wash thoroughly in tap water.
13. Counterstain with working light green solution for 30-45 s.
14. Dehydrate in 95% alcohol, absolute alcohol, and clear in xylene, two changes each.
15. Mount with Permount or Histoclad.

e. *Results*:

Fungi—sharply delineated in black
Mucin—taupe to dark gray
Inner parts of hyphae—old rose
Background—pale green

f. *Remarks*: This technique gives to all forms of fungi, as well as to the filaments of *Actinomyces israelii* and *Nocardia asteroides*, a black-brown coloration. Slides previously stained with most other strains may be used by removing coverglasses in xylol and running through alcohols to water. Subsequent chromic acid treatment will remove any remaining stain. Instead of counterstaining with light green, a counterstain of hematoxylin and eosin has been recommended [10], because it stains the background tissue components clearly and thus allows the fungus to be seen and the tissue response to be studied at the same time.

2. MacCallum-Goodpasture Method for Gram-Positive and Gram-Negative Bacteria

a. *Fixation*: Any well-fixed tissue.

b. *Technique*: Cut paraffin sections at 6 μm.

c. *Solutions*:

Goodpasture's solution

Basic fuchsin	0.59 g
Aniline	1 ml
Phenol crystals (melted)	1 ml
Alcohol, 30%	100 ml

Gram's iodine solution

Iodine	1 g
Potassium iodide	2 g
Distilled water	300 ml

Stirling's gentian violet solution

Gentian violet (crystal violet)	5 g
Alcohol, 100%	10 ml
Aniline	2 ml
Distilled water	88 ml

Saturated picric acid solution

Picric acid	2 g
Distilled water	100 ml

d. *Staining Procedure*: Use a control slide.

1. Deparaffinize and hydrate to distilled water.
2. Goodpasture's solution for 10 min.
3. Rinse in distilled water.
4. Differentiate in full-strength Formalin for a few minutes (fixes Goodpasture stain).
5. Wash in running water for 3 min.
6. Saturated picric acid solution for 3-5 min.
7. Rinse in distilled water.
8. Differentiate in 95% alcohol for 30 s.
9. Rinse in distilled water.
10. Stirling's gentian violet solution for 3 min.
11. Rinse in distilled water.
12. Gram's iodine solution for 1 min.
13. Rinse in distilled water. Blot, but leave moist.
14. Differentiate in a solution of equal parts of aniline and xylene; several changes until section appears light purplish red.
15. Xylene, two changes.
16. Mount with Permount or Histoclad.

e. *Results*:

Gram-positive organisms—blue
Gram-negative organisms—red
Other elements—various shades of red to purple

3. McManus' Method for Glycogen (Periodic Acid Schiff—PAS) [43]

a. *Fixation*: 10% buffered neutral Formalin.

b. *Technique*: Cut paraffin sections at 6 μm.

c. *Solutions*:

Normal hydrochloric acid solution

Hydrochloric acid (sp. gr. 1.19)	83.5 ml
Distilled water	916.5 ml

Coleman's Feulgen solution

Dissolve 1 g basic fuchsin in 200 ml hot distilled water. Bring to boiling point. Cool and add 2 g potassium metabisulfite, and 10 ml normal hydrochloric acid. Let bleach for 24 h, then add 0.5 g activated carbon (Norit). Shake for 1 min and filter through coarse filter paper. Repeat filtration until solution is colorless. Store in a refrigerator.

Schiff reagent solution

Dissolve 1 g basic fuchsin in 200 ml hot distilled water. Cool to 50°C. Filter and add 20 ml normal hydrochloric acid. Cool further and add 1 g anhydrous sodium bisulfite or sodium metabisulfite. Keep in the dark for 48 h until solution becomes straw-colored. Store in a refrigerator.

Test for Schiff reagent solution

Pour a few drops of Schiff reagent solution into 10 ml of 37-40% formaldehyde in a watch glass. If the solution turns reddish purple rapidly, it is good. If the reaction is delayed and the resulting color is deep blue-purple, the solution is breaking down.

0.5% Periodic acid solution

Periodic acid	0.5 g
Distilled water	100 ml

0.2% Light green solution (stock)

Light green, SF yellowish	0.2 g
Distilled water	100 ml
Glacial acetic acid	0.2 ml

Light green solution (working)

Light green (stock)	10 ml
Distilled water	50 ml

Harris' hematoxylin solution

Hematoxylin crystals	2 g
Alcohol, 100%	50 ml
Ammonium or potassium alum	100 g
Distilled water	1000 ml
Mercuric oxide (red)	2.5 g

Dissolve the hematoxylin in the alcohol and the alum in the water with the aid of heat. Remove from the heat and mix the two solutions. Bring to a boil as rapidly as possible (limit this heating to less than 1 min and stir often). Remove from the heat and add the mercuric oxide slowly. Reheat to a simmer until it becomes dark purple, remove from the heat immediately and plunge the vessel into a basin of cold water until cool. The stain is ready for use as soon as it cools. Addition of 2-4 ml of acetic acid per 100 ml of solution increases the precision of the nuclear stain. Filter before use.

   d. *Staining Procedure*:

1. Deparaffinize and hydrate to distilled water.
2. Oxidize in periodic acid solution for 5 min.
3. Rinse in distilled water.
4. Coleman's Feulgen or Schiff reagent solution for 15 min.
5. Wash in running water for 10 min for pink color to develop.
6. Harris' hematoxylin for 6 min, or light green counterstain for a few seconds. Light green is recommended for counterstaining sections in which fungi are to be demonstrated. Omit steps 7-11 if light green is used.
7. Wash in running water.
8. Differentiate in 1% (HCl) acid alcohol—three to ten quick dips.
9. Wash in running water.
10. Dip in ammonia water to blue sections.
11. Wash in running water for 10 min.
12. Dehydrate in 95% alcohol, absolute alcohol, and clear in xylene, two changes each.
13. Mount with Permount or Histoclad.

   e. *Results*:

Nuclei—blue
Fungi—red
Background—pale green (with light green counterstaining)

   Note: Glycogen, mucin, reticulum, fibrin or thrombi, colloid droplets, the hyalin of arteriosclerosis, hyalin deposits in glomeruli, granular cells in the renal arterioles where preserved, most basement membranes, the colloid of pituitary stalks and thyroid, and amyloid infiltrations may also give a positive reaction, which is rose to purplish red.

4. Mayer's Mucicarmine Method for Mucin and *Cryptococcus* [42]

   a. *Fixation*: 10% buffered neutral Formalin.

   b. *Technique*: Cut paraffin sections at 6 μm.

   c. *Solutions*:

Weigert's iron hematoxylin solution

   Solution A
Hematoxylin crystals   1 g
Alcohol, 95%   100 ml

   Solution B
Ferric chloride, 29% aqueous   4 ml
Distilled water   95 ml
Hydrochloric acid, concentrated   1 ml

Working solution
Equal parts of Solution A and Solution B.

Mucicarmine solution

Carmine	1 g
Aluminum chloride, anhydrous	0.5 g
Distilled water	2 ml

Mix stain in small evaporating dish. Heat on electric hot plate for 2 min. Liquid becomes black and syrupy. Dilute with 100 ml of 50% alcohol and let stand for 24 h. Filter. Dilute 1 part mucicarmine solution with 4 parts tap water for use.

0.25% Metanil yellow solution

Metanil yellow	0.25 g
Distilled water	100 ml
Glacial acetic acid	0.25 ml

d. Staining Procedure:

1. Deparaffinize and hydrate to distilled water.
2. Working solution of Weigert's hematoxylin for 7 min.
3. Wash in running water for 10 min.
4. Diluted mucicarmine solution for 60 min.
5. Rinse quickly in distilled water.
6. Metanil yellow solution for 1 min.
7. Rinse quickly in distilled water.
8. Dehydrate in 95% alcohol, absolute alcohol, and clear in xylene, two changes each.
9. Mount with Permount or Histoclad.

e. Results:

Mucin—deep rose to red
Capsule of *Cryptococcus*—deep rose to red
Nuclei—black
Other tissue elements—yellow

Note: Carminophilic properties will be obscured if sections are overstained with Weigert's hematoxylin and/or metanil yellow solution.

5. Other Methods

The majority of the fungi can be detected in hematoxylin and eosin-stained sections. However, there are a few notable exceptions. For example, *Sporothrix* is very difficult to find and *Candida* is usually difficult to recognize, especially in old lesions. For practical purposes, specific staining techniques such as Grocott's method or the PAS reaction are required, as shown in Table 1 [48]. Gridley's fungous stain and Bielschowsky-Pap's reticulum stain are also useful for the detection of fungi in tissue. The pigment of the dematiaceous fungi can be observed without special strains, but the Fontana-Masson stain [36] and Schmorl's stain [36] are also useful [40].

The identification of pathogenic fungi in organs already fixed with Formalin or other fixatives depends exclusively on the morphological characteristics and staining behavior of the fungi. Therefore, the detailed morphological description of the appearance of fungal elements in tissue is an important area of study in medical mycology, and the descriptions should be based on standard references.

C. Fluorescent Antibody Techniques

The fluorescent antibody (FA) technique was originated and developed by Coons et al. [15,16] and has been used in the field of medical mycology. The first application of this method in medical mycology was reported by Eveland et al. [18], who used FA techniques for the detection of *Cryptococcus neoformans* and its polysaccharide components in Formalin-fixed tissue. Since then, a number of reports on the use of FA techniques for the detection and identification of fungi in tissue have been made [11,26,30,45]. FA techniques are currently considered to be a valuable adjunct to the histopathological diagnosis of mycotic infections, especially of pathogens involved in opportunistic fungous infections [10,31].

Description of the preparation of the fungous antigens, the production of antisera, the preparation of fluorescent conjugates, and the purification of conjugates can be found in several of the recently published laboratory guide books [10,11,62].

The indirect FA method is much more convenient than the direct method for routine work. In the indirect method, a fluorescein-conjugate directed against the globulins of the animal species producing the initial antibody is used to make the antigen-antibody reaction visible. In the first step, unlabeled antibody serves to detect specific antigens in the tissue. In the second step, the fluorescein-tagged antiglobulin combines with the antigen-antibody complexes and illuminates them.

The FA technique is useful in detecting and identifying fungi in histologic sections that have been previously stained with hematoxylin and eosin, by the Giemsa stain, or by the Gram stain, but sections previously stained by the PAS, Gridley, or Grocott procedures cannot be used for FA, because the oxidation of fungal polysaccharides alters their antigenicity so that they do not react with the antibodies [10]. In contrast, long time storage of Formalin-fixed tissues, either wet or in paraffin blocks, does not seem to affect the antigens of the fungi therein [45].

After staining by the FA technique, fungous elements emit a brilliant greenish fluorescence, while the tissue components show a light bluish autofluorescence providing a relatively beautiful contrast (Fig. 1). It should be noted, however, that the intensity of the specific fluorescence by fungous cells is not equal, i.e., the intensity of staining varies among individual fungal cells within the same focus [45].

D. Miscellaneous Methods

1. Fluorochromic Methods

Fluorochromic methods were originally applied to tissues to detect mucin [25] and acid mucopolysaccharides [72]. Subsequently, these fluorescent stains have been applied to the detection of fungi in tissue [12,60,75,76]. Thirty different fluorochromes have been tested for their usefulness in the detection of fungi in tissue. Thirteen (Table 2) have proven valuable for the detection of fungi in tissue sections [75,76]. Staining methods are very easy and simple, and examples of three such procedures are given here. Formalin fixation or other fixation methods such as Zenker's solution and alcohol

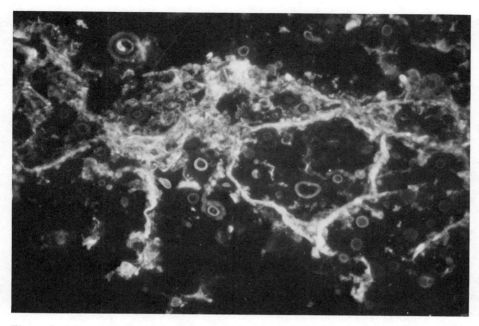

Figure 1 Diagnosis of fungous infections by immunofluorescence. *Cryptococcus neoformans* in a pulmonary lesion of cryptococcosis stained with a specific fluorescent antibody preparation. The cells of *Cryptococcus neoformans* emit a brilliant greenish fluorescence, while the outer zone of the capsular material appears as a chestnut burr-like structure. Fluorescent antibody stain, 528X.

Table 2 Suitable Fluorochromes for the Detection of Fungi in Tissue

Fluorochrome	Concentration (%)	Solvent
Acridingelb (Merck)	0.05	Citrate buffer, pH 2.1
Acridinorange (Gruebler)	0.05	Citrate buffer, pH 2.1
Auramin puriss (Gruebler)	0.01	Distilled water
Aurophosphin (Gruebler)	0.05	Citrate buffer, pH 2.1
Brankophore P (Bayer)	0.05	Distilled water
Congo red (Gruebler)	0.05	Citrate buffer, pH 2.1
Coriphosphin H. K. (Gruebler)	0.05	Citrate buffer, pH 2.1
Coriphosphin O (Gruebler)	0.05	Citrate buffer, pH 2.1
Euchrysin GNX (Gruebler)	0.05	Distilled water
Neutralrot extra (Gruebler)	0.05	Distilled water
Primulin (Gruebler)	0.05	Citrate buffer, pH 2.1
Pyronin (Gruebler)	0.05	Citrate buffer, pH 2.1
Rheonin (Bayer)	1.0	Citrate buffer, pH 2.1
Rhodamin G. D. (Gruebler)	0.1	Distilled water

may be used. Paraffin-embedded materials yield good results. The paraffin section should be cut at 6 μm.

   a. Rheonin Stain for Crytpococcus neoformans [75]:

   (1) Staining Procedure:

1. Deparaffinization with xylene and alcohol to distilled water as usual.
2. Immerse in saturated aqueous solution of aluminum carbonate for 2-3 min.
3. Rinse in running water for 1 min.
4. Blot with filter paper.
5. Stain with 1% rheonin in citrate buffer solution (pH 2.1) for 30-90 s.
6. Rinse in running water for 1 min.
7. Blot and dry.
8. Mount in autofluorescent-free liquid paraffin and cover with a coverglass.

   (2) Results:

Cryptococcus neoformans—bright reddish brown
Amyloid body, cartilage and goblet cells—reddish brown
Other tissue elements—green yellow

   b. Acridine Orange Method for Fungi [12,60]:

   (1) Staining Procedure:

1. Remove the paraffin from sections as usual, hydrate into water.
2. Stain in Weigert's iron hematoxylin for 5 min.
3. Wash in tap water for 3-4 min.
4. Stain in 1:1000 aqueous acridine orange for 2 min.
5. Rinse in tap water or distilled water for 30 s.
6. Dehydrate in 95% alcohol for 1 min.
7. Dehydrate in absolute alcohol and clear in xylol.
8. Mount with nonfluorescing mount medium (XAM-Gurr's or liquid paraffin).

   (2) Results: Most of fungi show yellow-green, green, red to yellow, and/or red secondary fluorescence with ultraviolet light.

   c. Congo Red Stain [76]:

   (1) Staining Procedure:

1. Deparaffinization.
2. Stain in 1% congo red aqueous solution for 10 min.
3. Decolorize in saturated aqueous solution of lithium carbonate.
4. Differentiation in 80% alcohol.
5. Wash in tap water.
6. Blot and dry rapidly (use of an electric dryer is recommended for rapid drying).
7. Mount with liquid paraffin.

   (2) Results: Most fungi emit an orange to red fluorescence. *Candida, Histoplasma,* and *Paracoccidioides* emit a brilliant red fluorescence. With this method, fluorescence

hardly fades at all even after a long period of ultraviolet irradiation. Other tissue components give off a light yellow-green autofluorescence which makes a beautiful contrast with that of the fungal elements.

It has been shown that fungi of the same genus emit the same color of fluorescence after being stained with a given fluorochrome stain [75,76]. It is also known that fungi actively growing in acute lesions emit a strong fluorescence, while those dormant forms in chronic granulomatous lesions emit a much weaker fluorescence [56].

d. Cresyl-Violet Stain: Klatzo et al. [33] reported a method for demonstrating fungi in tissue by means of a polarized light microscope after staining with cresyl-violet.

III. HISTOPATHOLOGY OF FUNGOUS INFECTIONS AND APPEARANCE OF FUNGI IN TISSUES

The tissue changes that accompany fungous infections vary in relation to the following factors: the genus of fungi, the infecting dose of the fungus, metabolic products of the fungi, the organ or tissue involved, the resistance of the host, allergic factors, the age of host, different stages or duration of the infection, and the presence of preexisting or underlying disease. In most of the fungous infections, tissue changes are not specific and the inflammatory reactions to various kinds of fungi tend to be similar, especially in chronic infections caused by fungi of limited pathogenicity. The accurate diagnosis of fungous infections must be based on both cultural and histopathological examinations.

Traditionally, fungous infections are classified as superficial, cutaneous, subcutaneous, or systemic, depending on the predominant anatomic involvement and the degree of invasiveness by the fungus. Accordingly, the tissue changes in fungous diseases will be described in keeping with this sort of approach.

A. Superficial Infections

Superficial or surface mycoses are produced by several unrelated fungi and involve hair and epidermal sites.

Piedra is a fungous infection of the hair shaft caused by *Piedraia hortai* (black piedra) or *Trichosporon beigelii* (white piedra). Black piedra is characterized by the presence of stony hard nodules along the hair shaft. In the nodule, round or elliptical arthroconidia, intertwined hyphae, and elliptical asci are recognizable by microscopic examination. The nodules of white piedra are softer and more easily detached from the hair. The hyphae lie perpendicular to the surface of the hair and segment into oval or rectangular cells (arthroconidia). Budding cells (blastoconidia) are also seen in the mycelial mass which does not contain asci.

Tinea versicolor, caused by *Malassezia furfur* (sometimes referred to as *Pityrosporum orbiculare*) is a chronic, symptomatic, superficial fungous disease characterized by fawn to brown-colored, desquamating macules involving principally the trunk. A large number of round, budding cells (blastoconidia) and hyphal elements are found in the horny layer of the epidermis.

Tinea nigra is a fungous infection of palmer surfaces caused by *Exophiala werneckii*. Brown-colored, short and septate hyphal elements and blastoconidia are found in the horny layer of the epidermis.

In these superficial fungous infections, an inflammatory cell reaction which is compromised simply of a nonspecific, minimal, small, round-cell infiltrate in the upper dermis is observed [14,63].

B. Cutaneous Infections

Most fungous infections are named on the basis of the genus of the etiologic agent, nosology thus reflecting fungal taxonomy. However, the classification of dermatophytoses on an etiologic basis has proven unsatisfactory, because a single species of dermatophyte can cause a variety of clinical and pathologic manifestations, and because similar clinical and pathological pictures can be caused by different species of dermatophytes. Therefore, the descriptive terminology of ringworm infections has been based on the part of the body affected (Table 3).

Dermatophytoses are infections caused by fungi that invade keratinized tissues, e.g., nails, hair, and the horny layer of the epidermis. A broader term dermatomycoses includes any fungous infection of the skin, e.g., those caused by *Candida* species [62].

The dermatophytes are divided into three genera: *Trichophyton, Microsporum,* and *Epidermophyton.* The genus *Trichophyton* infects hair, skin, and nails; *Microsporum* infects hair and skin; and *Epidermophyton* infects skin and nails. The species of these three genera cause identical changes in infected skin or nails. Because the macroconidium, the morphology of which delineates the three genera, is never seen in the infected tissue [6], generic identification can only be made by culture.

The histopathological changes in the skin induced by dermatophytes are nonspecific. Therefore, fungous elements must be demonstrated. Since such elements stain poorly with hematoxylin and eosin, the PAS, Grocott, or Gridley stains are recommended for their detection. The fungal elements that are disclosed in the dermatophytoses consist of hyphae and round structures that lie at the junction of the stratum corneum and the stratum Malpighi of the epidermis or in the walls of intraepidermal vesicles. Fre-

Table 3   A Clinical Classification of the Dermatophytoses

I.	Tinea superficialis
	A. Tinea capitis (*Microsporum* and *Trichophyton* spp.)
	B. Tinea favosa or favus (*Trichophyton schoenlinii*)
	C. Tinea corporis (*Microsporum* and *Trichophyton* spp.)
	D. Tinea barbae (*Trichophyton* spp.)
	E. Tinea imbricata (*Trichophyton concentricum*)
	F. Tinea cruris (*Epidermophyton floccosum* and *Trichophyton* spp.)
	G. Tinea manuum (*Microsporum* and *Trichophyton* spp.)
	H. Tinea pedis (*Microsporum* and *Trichophyton* spp. and *Epidermophyton floccosum*)
	I. Tinea unguium (*Microsporum* and *Trichophyton* spp. and *Epidermophyton floccosum*)
II.	Tinea profunda
	A. Kerion Celsi (*Microsporum canis* and *M. gypseum*)
	B. Sycosis trichophytica (*Microsporum* and *Trichophyton* spp.)
	C. Granuloma trichophyticum (*Trichophyton* spp.)
III.	Dermatophytid (*Trichophyton* spp.)

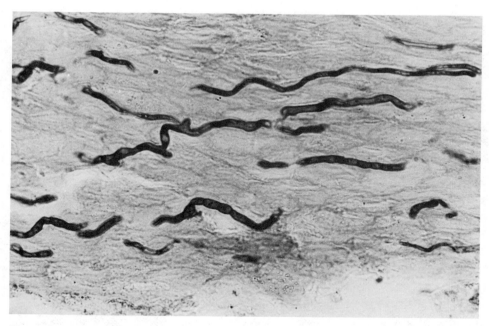

Figure 2 Tinea pedis caused by *Trichophyton mentagrophytes*. Fungal elements in
horny layer of the epidermis. Most of the hyphae run parallel to the skin surface.
Twisted pattern and septation of hyphae are also seen. Periodic acid Schiff stain, 574X.

quently there is little or no inflammatory reaction. The hyphal elements are slender,
tube-like structures with septa. Transverse sections of hyphae are observed as empty
rings and arthroconidia occur as solid, round bodies.

Tinea of the glabrous skin may manifest itself as an acute, subacute, or chronic
dermatitis. Organisms are present in varying numbers in the horny layer. *Trichophyton*
and *Microsporum* infections frequently show only hyphal elements (Fig. 2).
Epidermophyton floccosum infections show both spores and hyphae [58]. Tinea capitis
and tinea barbae present a picture of perifolliculitis, with or without giant cells.

Favus displays perifollicular crusts that consist of hyperkeratotic and parakeratotic
material, fibrin, and inflammatory cells. The crusts contain many hyphae and a few
spores. These fungous elements are present in the adjacent horny layer and within
and around hairs. A dense inflammatory reaction with many plasma cells and occasional
giant cells is present in the dermis. Old lesions show fibrosis and loss of skin appendages.

In cases of tinea profunda, a nodular perifollicular granuloma which is composed of
polymorphonuclear leucocytes, epithelioid cells, multinuclear giant cells of the foreign
body type, plasma cells, and lymphocytes with occasional eosinophils may be found.
Fungal elements are seen in necrotic hairs and the surrounding tissues. Cases of deep
tissue involvement by the dermatophytes show an epithelioid cell reaction accompanied
by plasma cells, lymphocytes, eosinophils, and multinucleated giant cells in fresh foci,
while old lesions have a central caseous necrosis. Fungal elements in granulomas of
deep tissues are remarkably pleomorphic (Fig. 3) [67].

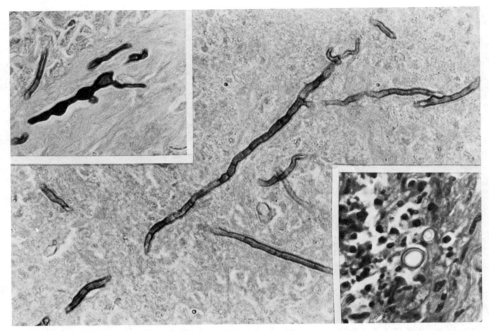

Figure 3   Fungal elements in a granuloma caused by *Trichophyton rubrum*. Upper left: Arthroconidia and hyphae, Gridley's stain, 566X. Center: Septate branching hyphae, Gridley's stain, 566X. Lower right: Large spores surrounded by an inflammatory infiltrate. Such spores are found in lymph nodes with caseation necrosis. Hematoxylin and eosin stain, 566X.

C. Inoculation Mycoses

Cutaneous and subcutaneous mycoses caused by traumatic implantation of a fungus into the skin are customarily considered together as the inoculation mycoses. Sporotrichosis, chromomycosis, and mycetoma are clinically recognizable subdivisions of this category, but a number of subcutaneous abscesses are also acquired by inoculation.

1. Sporotrichosis

Sporotrichosis is a chronic, usually benign, infection caused by *Sporothrix schenckii*. It most commonly involves the skin and subcutaneous tissues, but occasionally the skeletomuscular tissues, mucous membranes, and visceral organs are also affected [39]. Epidemics have been reported among miners [71]. The outstanding characteristics of sporotrichosis include: (1) the cutaneous, lymphatic type of infection that is unique among all fungous infections; (2) the paucity of causative organism in tissue sections; (3) the relative ease of cultural detection of the organism; (4) the occurrence of asteroid bodies in tissue sections; (5) the high incidence of positive sporotrichin skin reaction; and (6) the fact that potassium iodide is effective in the treatment of the disease [20].

Histopathologically, the epidermis shows hyperkeratosis, parakeratosis, and irregular acanthosis which may progress to pseudoepitheliomatous hyperplasia (Fig. 4). Intra-

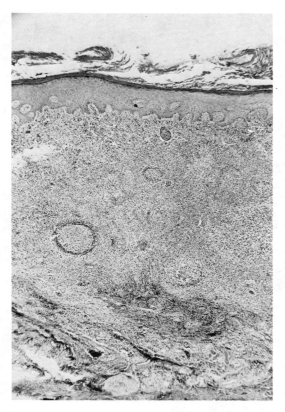

Figure 4 Cutaneous lesion of sporotrichosis. Hyperkeratosis, parakeratosis, and irregular acanthosis of the epidermis with a diffuse and dense inflammatory cell infiltrate. Several microabscesses throughout the dermis are seen. Hematoxylin and eosin stain, 32X.

epidermal microabscesses may be found in some cases. A dense inflammatory reaction, which is a combination of pyogenic and granulomatous components, commonly occurs in the dermis and subcutaneous tissues. The inflammatory reaction consists of polymorphonuclear leukocytes, lymphocytes, plasma cells, epithelioid cells, and multinucleated giant cells. Thus, a remarkable variety of inflammatory cells is characteristically seen in the lesions of sporotrichosis.

Many tissue sections must be examined in order to find *Sporothrix schenckii*. The fungous cells which occur singly or in clusters (Fig. 5) are round, 3-5 μm in diameter, and actively budding in fresh lesions. In cases on long-term steroid therapy, a large number of fungous cells may be seen in the lesions. In the lymphatic, metastatic foci, the tissue reaction tends to be granulomatous and the fungous cells are smaller in number than in the primary lesion. On rare occasions, hyphal elements of the fungus may be observed (Fig. 6) [49]. There is no capsule around the fungous cells.

Asteroid bodies that are considered characteristic of sporotrichosis may also be found in other mycoses. The asteroid body usually appears as a single central spore

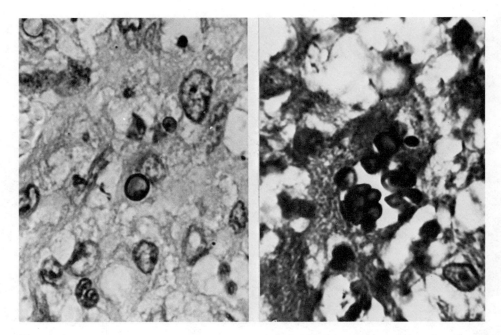

Figure 5 *Sporothrix schenckii* in tissue. On the left in the center of the photograph is a single nonbudding organism. On the right is a grape-like spore cluster, some members of which are budding. Periodic acid Schiff stain, 812X.

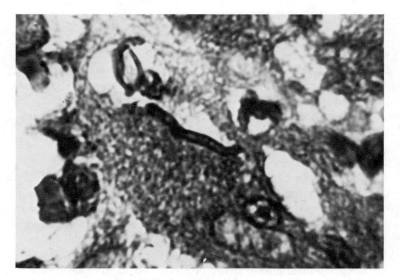

Figure 6 Sporotrichosis. A hyphal element in a giant cell. Periodic acid Schiff stain, 1944X. (From Ref. 49.)

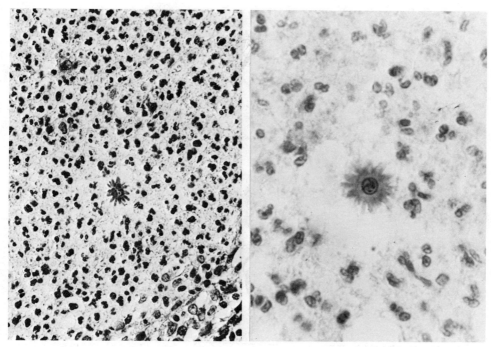

Figure 7   Asteroid bodies in sporotrichosis. Left: An asteroid body in the center
of a microabscess. The asteroid body consists of eosinophilic, stellate material. A
granulomatous reaction around the microabscess occurs in the right lower corner of
the photograph. Hematoxylin and eosin stain, 332X. Right: An asteroid body
which is surrounded by weakly PAS-positive, stellate material. Periodic acid Schiff
stain, 716X.

surrounded by eosinophilic, stellate material in hematoxylin and eosin stain sections
(Fig. 7).

In experimental sporotrichosis of small animals, cigar-shaped fungous cells are the
predominant form (Fig. 8) [50]. Cigar-shaped organisms are rarely seen in human infections.

2. Chromomycosis and Related Dermal Afflictions Caused by Dematiaceous Fungi

A variety of human infections are caused by dematiaceous fungi. Some of these are
listed in Table 4 [10,20,62]. The nomenclature of the group is presently uncertain,
but some commonly employed names together with one or two synonyms are suggested in the Table (see also Ref. 10).

Chromomycosis is a chronic, granulomatous disease caused by certain dematiaceous
fungi. Usually the lesions involve exposed skin surfaces and are remarkably verrucous
(dermatitis verrucosa). Cutaneous infections result from the traumatic implantation
of the causative fungus into the skin [2,9].

Histopathologically, pseudoepitheliomatous hyperplasia of the epidermis, granulomatous changes in the upper and mid-dermis, and the presence of brown pigmented
fungal cells (sclerotic cells) are characteristic findings of chromomycosis. In contrast

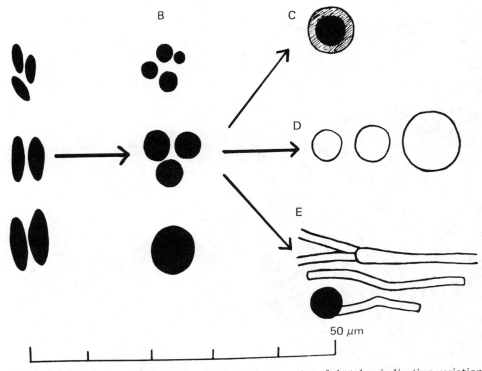

50 μm

Figure 8 *Sporothrix schenckii* in murine tissue. A series of sketches indicating variations in the form of the fungus observed following intraperitoneal inoculation of the yeast phase into mice: A. Cigar bodies. B. Yeast-like round forms. C. Yeast-like round forms with central mass. D. Yeast-like round forms with thin walls. E. Hyphal patterns. (From Ref. 52.)

Table 4 Examples of Mycoses Caused by Dematiaceous Hyphomycetes

Disease	Fungi	Some suggested synonyms in the literature
1. Tinea nigra	*Exophiala werneckii*	—
2. Chromomycosis	*Cladosporium carrionii*	—
	Fonsecaea compactum	*Rhinocladiella compacta*
	Fonsecaea pedrosoi	*Rhinocladiella pedrosoi*
	Phialophora verrucosa	—
	Rhinocladiella aquaspersa	*Acrotheca aquaspersa* and *Ramichloridium cerophilum*
3. Subcutaneous abscesses[a]	*Exophiala jeanselmei*	*Exophiala gougerotii*
	Exophiala spinifera	—
	Phialophora parasitica	—
	Phialophora repens	—
	Phialophora richardsiae	—
	Wangiella dermatitidis	*Exophiala dermatitidis*
4. Mycetoma	*Exophiala jeanselmei*	(see above)
5. Brain abscess	*Cladosporium bantianum*	*Cladosporium trichoides*
	Wangiella dermatitidis	(see above)
	Fonsecaea pedrosoi	(see above)

[a]The number of etiologic agents of lesions of this sort is very large. A few examples of related forms are presented. More extended lists appear in the references [e.g., 10,20,62].
Source: Ref. 20.

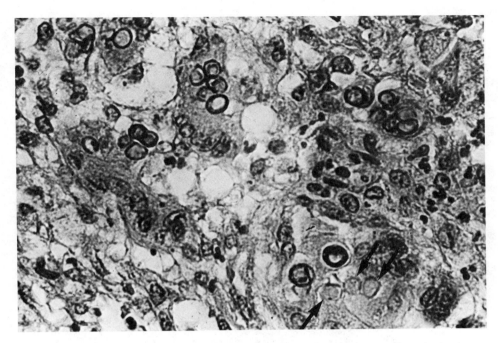

Figure 9 Cutaneous lesion of chromomycosis caused by *Fonsecaea pedrosoi*. A number of sclerotic cells are seen. Some of the sclerotic cells are dark due to abundant brown pigment and are thick-walled. Others (indicated with arrows) are light due to a scanty amount of brown pigment. Tissue reaction is principally epithelioid cell granuloma with multinucleated giant cells. Hematoxylin and eosin stain, 574X.

to sporotrichosis, the cutaneous, granulomatous changes have little tendency to involve the subcutaneous fat [5] and are principally histiocytic reactions consisting of epithelioid cells, multinucleated giant cells, and accompanied by eosinophils, plasma cells, lymphocytes, and neutrophils. Occasionally, minute abscesses may be observed; however, there is no caseous necrosis of the cutaneous lesions.

The sclerotic cells are round or spherical in shape, 5-15 μm in diameter, usually brown in color, have a somewhat thick cell wall, and can be found singly or in clusters (Fig. 9). Sclerotic cells reproduce by fission which can be seen occasionally in sections (Fig. 10). But blastoconidia are not seen in the cutaneous lesions of chromomycosis.

A bird's eye view of a skin lesion of chromomycosis is illustrated in Fig. 11. Skin lesions caused by *Fonsecaea pedrosoi* are located predominantly in the upper dermis and the sclerotic cells seen in the upper dermis are larger in size than the sclerotic cells found in the deeper portions of the dermis. Those located deeper in the tissues have a tendency to form clusters [57].

In cases of subcutaneous abscesses caused by *Exophiala jeanselmei*, the main fungous elements are hyphae that are faintly brown in color and may be overlooked in hematoxylin and eosin stain sections. A number of fungal elements may be seen in the central portion of the abscess that is surrounded by an epithelioid cell granuloma (Fig. 12).

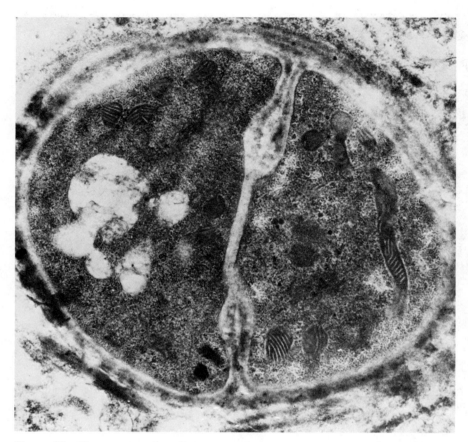

Figure 10 Chromomycosis. Electron microscopical preparation of a dividing sclerotic cell of *Fonsecaea pedrosoi*. 8000X.

A common macroscopical feature of brain lesions caused by dematiaceous fungi are the concentric zones. The central necrotic foci of such lesions are light in color, whereas the peripheral zones are dark black. Histologically, hyphae of the fungi with light brown pigment are sparsely scattered in the central caseous necrotic region. In the peripheral zone, round forms of the fungous cells which are abundantly pigmented are predominant (Fig. 13) in the epithelioid cell granuloma. Most of the fungous cells in this zone are engulfed in multinucleated giants cells.

3. Mycetoma

Mycetoma may be caused by a variety of different species of fungi and actinomycetes. A few of the prominent species of fungal etiologic agents of mycetoma are included in Table 5 [10,20]. The infection is usually confined to the feet and legs [12] and is characterized by localized, indolent, deforming tumefaction with draining sinuses. The lesions involve cutaneous and subcutaneous tissues, fascia, and bone. Histologically, the lesions are composed of numerous abscesses containing grains and surrounded by nonspecific granulomatous changes. The grains are up to 1-5 mm in diameter and are

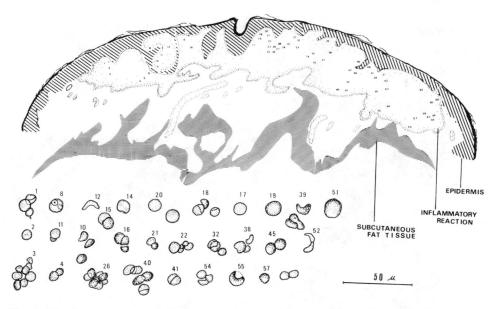

Figure 11 Schematic presentation of cutaneous chromomycosis. Sclerotic cells in a
skin lesion caused by *Fonsecaea pedrosoi* are shown in the lower part. Numbers attached
to the sclerotic cells indicate the location where the sclerotic cells are found.

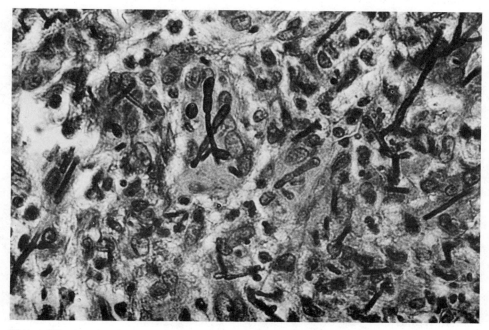

Figure 12 A subcutaneous abscess caused by *Exophiala jeanselmei.* Hyphae are the
main fungal elements; however, single or catenate spores are also recognizable in this
epithelioid cell granuloma. Periodic acid Schiff stain, 574X.

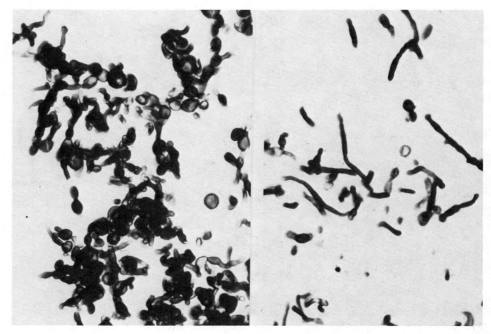

Figure 13 Cerebral phaeohyphomycosis. Left: Round cells of the fungus are the predominant form at the periphery of the lesion. Right: Hyphae of the fungus is the predominant form in the center of the lesion. Grocott's stain, 283X.

Table 5 Some Etiologic Agents of Eumycotic Mycetoma

Black granules
   1. *Madurella grisea*
   2. *Madurella mycetomatis*
   3. *Leptosphaeria senegalensis*
   4. *Leptosphaeria tompkinsii*
   5. *Exophiala jeanselmei*
   6. *Pyrenochaeta romeroi*
   7. *Curvularia geniculata*
   8. *Cochliobolus spicifer*

White to yellow granules.
   1. *Pseudallescheria boydii*
   2. *Acremonium* spp.
   3. *Neotestudina rosatii*
   4. *Fusarum* spp.
   5. *Aspergillus* spp.

Source: Refs. 20,62.

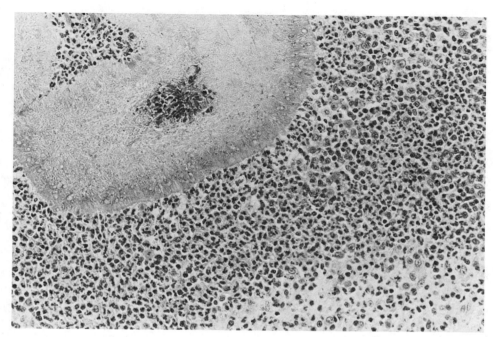

Figure 14 Mycetoma. The grain consists of a conglomerate of fungous filaments and peripheral rounded structures (upper left). The granule is surrounded by numerous polymorphonuclear leukocytes and macrophages. Hematoxylin and eosin stain, 222X.

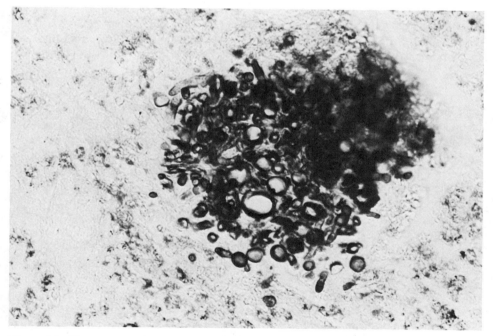

Figure 15 Mycetoma. The grain is composed of a radiating conglomerate of fungous filaments and spore-like structures, some of which are markedly round. Grocott's stain, 566X.

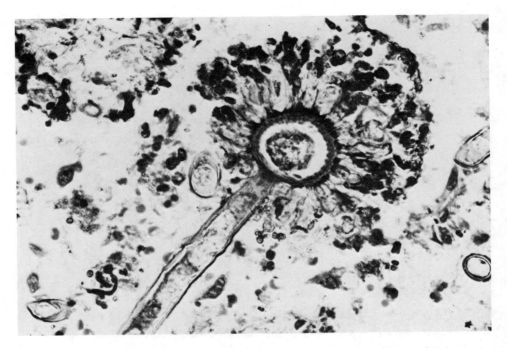

Figure 16 Conidial head of *Aspergillus niger* found in a pulmonary fungus ball. The conidia attached to the phialides are less than 5 μm in diameter and black in color. Hematoxylin and eosin stain, 566×.

surrounded by polymorphonuclear leukocytes and macrophages (Fig. 14). The grains are microcolonies of the etiologic fungus and consist of a conglomerate of radiating filamentous and rounded structures (Fig. 15).

D. Systemic Mycoses

According to Wolstenholme et al. [74], the deep (systemic) fungal infections comprise mycotic disease of the dermis and deeper tissues and include such infections as sporotrichosis, cutaneous chromomycosis, and mycetoma, together with those involving the viscera and producing septicemias, such as histoplasmosis, cryptococcosis, and coccidioidomycosis. For the sake of convenience, the former group of cutaneous and subcutaneous infections was already described in the section on the inoculation mycoses, and therefore only the latter group of visceral mycoses and septicemias will be considered in this section.

1. Aspergillosis

Aspergillosis may be defined as any infection or colonization of the tissues and cavities by fungi in the genus *Aspergillus* [59]. The genus *Aspergillus* is comprised of fungi that are among the most ubiquitous of airborne fungi. The disease may involve the skin, the external ear, the nasal sinuses, the orbit, the eye, the bronchopulmonary systems, or indeed, any organ of the body by hematogenous dissemination. Among the various forms of disease, bronchopulmonary aspergillosis is the most common.

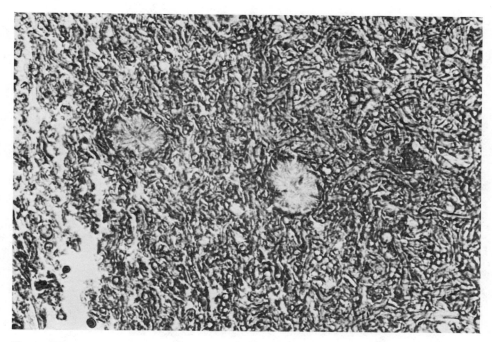

Figure 17 Calcium oxalate crystals in a pulmonary fungus ball caused by *Aspergillus niger*. The colorless crystals are arranged in a radiating pattern. Hematoxylin and eosin stain, 566X.

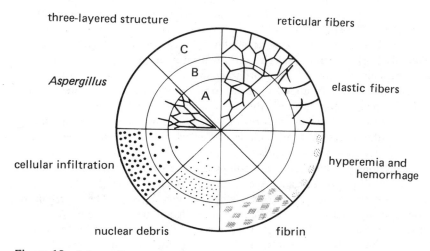

Figure 18 Schematic presentation of the principal histological structures within a focus of acute bronchopulmonary aspergillosis: A. Zone of central coagulative necrosis. B. Zone of peripheral necrosis. C. Zone of perifocal inflammation. (From Ref. 54.)

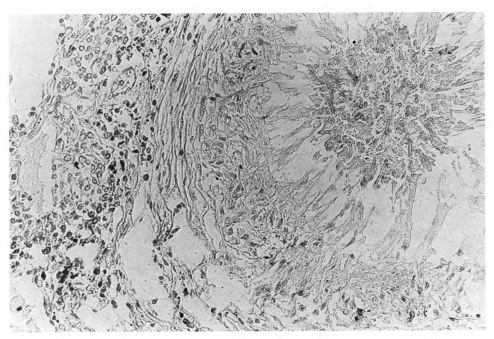

Figure 19 Granulomatous pulmonary aspergillosis. The center of the lesion is necrotic and hyphal elements of *Aspergillus* are recognizable (upper right). The growth of the fungus is surrounded by epithelioid cells and fibrosis. Periodic acid Schiff stain, 223X.

In cases of colonization of cavities by *Aspergillus* hyphae (often called a fungous ball), the tissue reaction is minimal and nonspecific. Calcium oxalate crystals have been found in pulmonary aspergillomas caused by *Aspergillus niger* [24,41]. The same substance is also detectable in colonization of the other body cavities such as paranasal sinuses by *Aspergillus niger* (Figs. 16 and 17).

In cases with acute bronchopulmonary aspergillosis, three zones are recognizable in the lesions (Fig. 18) [54]. Such lesions exhibit a central zone of coagulation necrosis surrounded by a variable number of polymorphonuclear leukocytes that are often necrobiotic. The lesions are surrounded by a perifocal outer zone with hyperemia and hemorrhage. Occasionally, suppuration is the predominant type of tissue change. Lesions of this sort may be found in any organ of the body; however, an inflammatory cellular reaction is rather sparse in septicemic lesions in which vascular involvement by hyphae in the form of a thrombotic angitis is common.

Granulomatous lesions of aspergillosis are composed of a central necrosis surrounded by epithelioid cells, multinucleated giant cells, and an outer fibrosis (Fig. 19). A granulomatous fibrosis simulating sarcoidosis has been reported [68]. The aspergilli in tissue always occur as hyphae which are usually basophilic and well-stained by the hematoxylin and eosin stain. The basophilic appearance of the hyphae is reduced in old foci [47]. Transverse sections of hyphae are seen as empty rings containing central cytoplasmic structures. The hyphae, which vary somewhat in shape (Fig. 20) [53], are septate, have an almost uniform width of about 7-10 μm in diameter, branch dichotomously at an angle of approximately 45°, and show "Y" or antler patterns (Fig. 21).

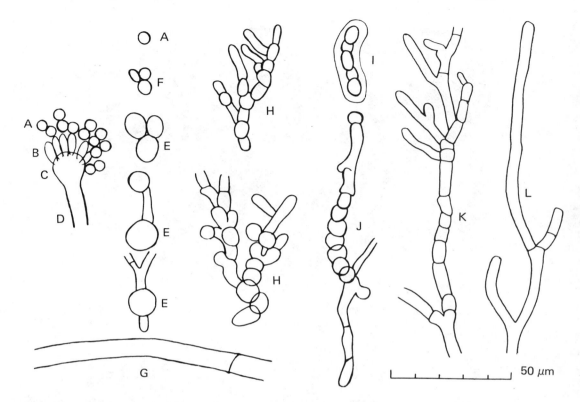

Figure 20   Camera lucida drawings of *Aspergillus* in tissue. A. Conidia. B. Phialides.
C. Vesicle. D. Conidiophore. E. Large spore. F. Intermediate type of spore (between
A and E). G. Foot cell 9?). H. Short, septate, branching hyphae. I. Pseudohyphal
pattern with perihyphal material. J. Arthroconidium-like structure. K. Multiseptate
hyphae. L. Septate hyphae. (From Ref. 53.)

The fruiting heads of the *Aspergillus* are occasionally found in aerated cavities or tracheal
lesions and are, of course, pathognomonic of the disease (Figs. 16, 20, 22).

2. Blastomycosis

Blastomycosis is caused by *Blastomyces dermatitidis* and is characterized by the formation
of suppurative and granulomatous lesions in any part of the body, but with a predilection
for the lungs, skin, and bones [14]. The tissue reaction is predominantly suppurative in
the acute form and granulomatous with epithelioid and giant cells and central necrosis in
chronic disease. Skin lesions are comprised of pseudoepitheliomatous hyperplasia of the
epidermis and chronic inflammation composed of multinucleated giant cells, epithelioid cells,
plasma cells, and lymphocytes with scattered microabscesses (Fig. 23).

The visceral lesions closely resemble tuberculosis, except that perifocal pleural changes
are usually localized and the perifocal tissue reaction is somewhat less intense than it is in
tuberculous foci. Central caseous necrosis or suppurative change are constant features
of the deep-seated lesions.

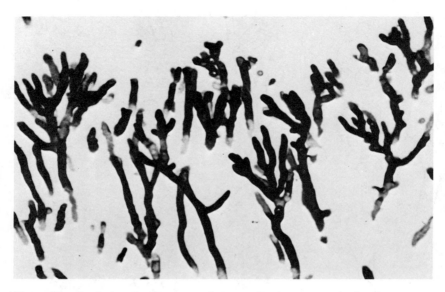

Figure 21 Typical growth pattern of *Aspergillus* in tissue. The hyphae are septate, have an almost uniform size, branch dichotomously, and show an antler-like pattern. Grocott's stain, 377X.

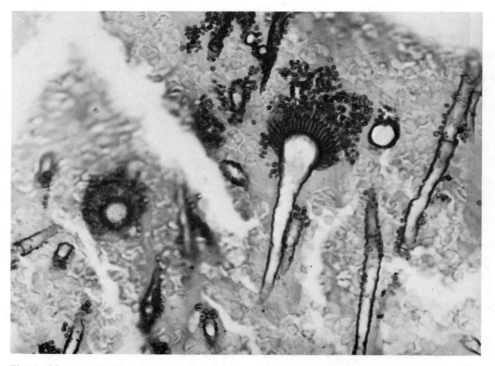

Figure 22 Conidial heads of *Aspergillus fumigatus* found in a necrotizing tracheal lesion. The conidia attached to a single row of phialides are less than 3 μm in diameter. Septa in the conidiospores are seen at the right. Periodic acid Schiff stain, 601X.

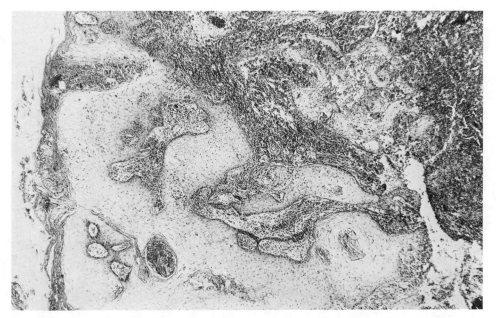

Figure 23 Blastomycosis. Pseudoepitheliomatous hyperplasia and intraepidermal abscess. Heavy inflammatory cell infiltration with microabscess formation is recognizable in the dermis. Hematoxylin and eosin stain, 36X.

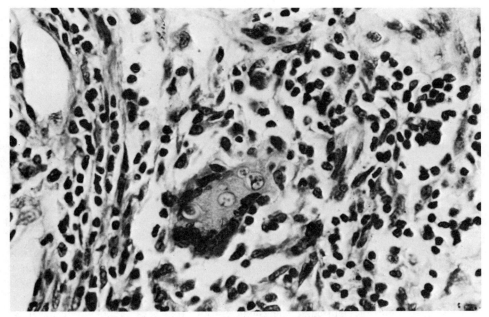

Figure 24 Cutaneous lesions of blastomycosis. Yeast-like cells of *Blastomyces dermatitidis,* some of which are budding, are seen in a multinucleated giant cell. Intracellular granular material in the yeast cells is obvious. The cellular reaction is composed of epithelioid cells, giant cells, small round cells, and polymorphonuclear leukocytes. Hematoxylin and eosin stain, 574X.

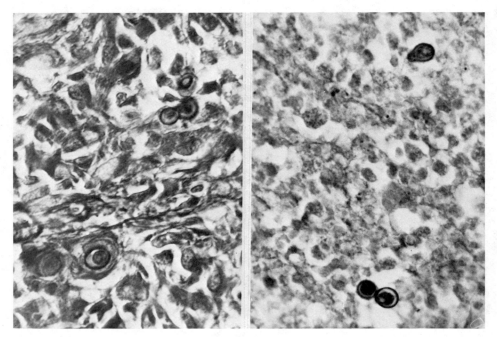

Figure 25 Blastomycosis. Left: A pulmonary lesion with cells of *Blastomyces dermati-tidis*. A broad base separates the bud from the parental budding cell in the upper left portion of the photograph. Right: A cutaneous lesion. An early stage of budding is seen in the upper portion of the photograph. Thick-walled, round, yeast cells, which contain cytoplasmic material, can be seen at the bottom of both the pulmonary and cutaneous lesions. Periodic acid Schiff stain, 329✕.

Blastomyces dermatitidis appears as thick-walled, relatively large yeast cells that occur singly or in clusters with occasional budding. The characteristic appearance of budding cells is that of a bud attached to the parent cell with a broad base (Figs. 24 and 25). Round, relatively distinct, intracytoplasmic structure are found in most of the yeast cells.

3. Candidiasis

Candidiasis (candidosis) is a primary or secondary infection caused by *Candida albicans* or other members of the genus *Candida*. Most cases of candidiasis are diseases of the diseased [73] and *Candida* spp. are among the most common opportunistic fungous infections. Involvement of the skin, vagina, digestive tract, bronchopulmonary system, and occasionally other organ systems may be observed. Chronic mucocutaneous candidiasis has been observed in patients with genetic immune defects.

Thrush is a very common manifestation of candidiasis, and lesions of the digestive tract are usually multiple, lenticular, shallow ulcerations that have a tendency to develop on the top of the mucosal rugae. The saprophytic growth of *Candida* is observed not infrequently on the necrotic surface of gastrointestinal malignancies and ulcers. Acute bronchopulmonary candidiasis cannot be distinguished from the usual bacterial bronchopneumonias. In cases of systemic or septicemic candidiasis, embolic lesions may be found in any organ of the body, and large valvular vegetations are a characteristic finding in fungal endocarditis. In these situations, the presence of *Candida* infection cannot be determined

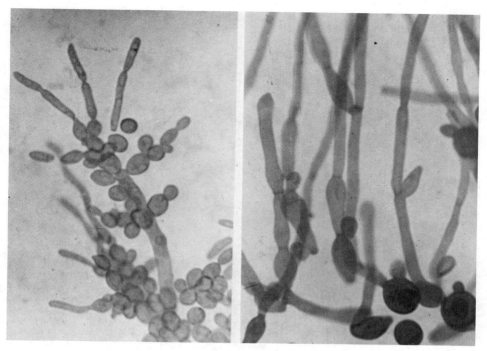

Figure 26 Typical growth of *Candida*. Growth of *Candida albicans* in serum-containing glucose peptone agar. Left: Round to oval spores and pseudohyphal elements. The blastoconidia attach at the point of constriction of the hyphae which look like sausages. Right: The hyphal elements at slightly greater magnification. The growth pattern shown is essentially similar to that seen in lesions. Periodic acid Schiff stain, 859X.

grossly, and histopathological examination with special stain, such as Grocott's or the PAS procedure, are required [55].

Histopathologically, *Candida* lesions of oral and laryngeal mucosa show desquamation of stratified epithelium and scanty inflammatory cell infiltration. In the esophageal lesions, the affected epithelial cells disintegrate into coagulation necrosis with little tendency of desquamation. In the lesions of gastrointestinal mucosa, the mucosal glands necrose and are obviously contracted. The principal tissue reaction in acute bronchopulmonary lesions is purulent, whereas a giant cell reaction is sometimes seen in subacute or chronic infections. In the septicemic foci of any organ, cellular reaction is usually scanty. The most characteristic histopathological findings of candidiasis is the presence of *Candida* spp. in the infected foci.

The typical tissue phase of *Candida* spp. is pseudohyphal growth with associated round-to-oval blastoconidia (Figs. 26 and 27) [55]. In the fresh lesions, yeast-like cells may be faintly stained with hematoxylin, but the fungous cells usually cannot be disclosed with the hematoxylin and eosin stain. *Candida* cells in old lesions are reduced in size and become round, small cells that are phagocytized by histiocytes (Fig. 28) [76]. There is a tendency for the PAS reaction of the fungous cells to become weak in older lesions. This same tendency is observed in gram-stained sections.

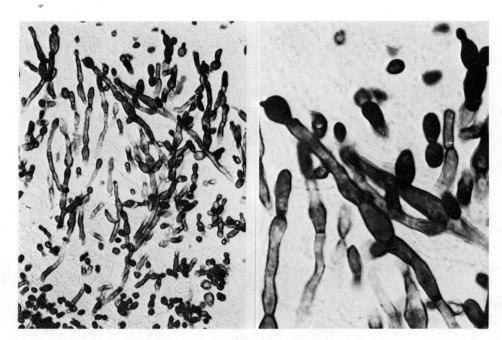

Figure 27 Esophageal candidiasis. Left: Clustered, round-to-oval spores of *Candida* attached to pseudohyphal elements at point of constriction. Grocott's stain, 313X. Right: High-power view of the pseudohyphal elements with budding spores at their tips. Grocott's stain, 783X.

4. Coccidioidomycosis

Coccidioidomycosis is an endemic disease in the southwestern area of North America and in Central and South America [19]. The disease is caused by the fungus *Coccidioides immitis* which produces an infection that remains inapparent in a large percentage of instances. In those who are sick, the illness ranges from benign to severe, and in a few cases, may be fatal. It is respiratory in origin and in the benign forms of the disease, the lesions are limited to the upper respiratory tract and lungs. In disseminated cases, the disease extends to other visceral organs, to the bones and joints, and to the skin and subcutaneous tissues [17].

Skin lesions show pseudoepitheliomatous hyperplasia of the epidermis and cutaneous granulomatous reaction with purulent changes. Usually multinucleated giant cells are a constant component of the lesions. Tissue changes are indistinguishable from those seen in blastomycosis and in paracoccidioidomycosis. In comparison with pulmonary tuberculous foci, pulmonary fungal lesions caused by any of the fungi show scanty perifocal reaction, and the pleural involvement tends to be localized just beneath the pulmonary lesion. These generalizations are also observed in coccidioidomycosis (Fig. 29).

In tissue, the organisms are nonbudding, round cells that have thick, double-contoured cell walls and often contain cytoplasmic material. The pathognomonic form of the fungus in tissue is the spherule, which is a round, double-walled structure containing a number of endospores that are usually 2-5 μm in diameter (Fig. 30).

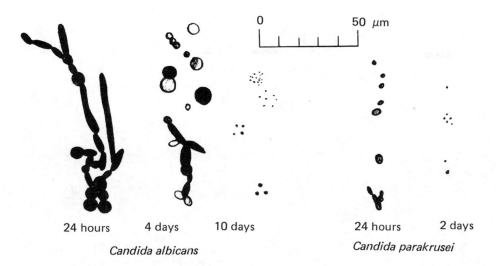

0   50 μm

24 hours   4 days   10 days   24 hours   2 days

Candida albicans   *Candida parakrusei*

Figure 28 Variation of the form and size of *Candida* cells observed in peripancreatic tissue of experimental candidiasis in mice. Experimental *Candida albicans* infections induced by intraperitoneal inoculation. A pseudohyphal growth pattern predominates at 24 hr. After 10 days, the majority of the fungous cells become round and small and are phagocytized by histiocytes. Experimental *Candida parakrusei* infection induced by intraperitoneal inoculation. The majority of the fungous cells are yeast-like by 24 hr, but only coccus-like, small, round elements are recognizable after 2 days. The latter must be confirmed as fungal elements by fluorescent antibody techniques. (From Ref. 76.)

5. Cryptococcosis

Cryptococcosis is caused by *Cryptococcus neoformans*. This fungus has a mucinous capsule that is especially obvious in fresh lesions and is a very characteristic and unique feature among the pathogenic fungi. *Cryptococcus neoformans* is an ubiquitous fungus in nature that is acquired by inhalation. The lungs are primarily involved [37] from whence the fungus may disseminate to other organs. When it does disseminate, the fungus has a marked predilection for the central nervous system.

As with other fungous infections, the tissue reaction to *C. neoformans* varies considerably from case to case and from organ to organ. Early lesions are gelatinous and suppuration is rare [37]. In cases with acute pneumonia, with meningoencephalitis, or in fresh foci in any organ system that arise from hematogenous dissemination, the paucity of cellular reaction is a remarkable and consistent finding (Fig. 31). Alveolar lumen, meningeal spaces, cystic cerebral lesions, and fresh foci in any organs are filled with the fungous cells and their mucinous capsular materials. Histiocytic infiltration and a granulomatous reaction are common in relatively old lesions. Sometimes calcification may occur. The giant cells that appear in granulomatous lesions are very peculiar. Fungous cells, most of which have lost their mucinous capsular material, are located at the periphery of the giant cells, and an eosinophilic, condensed cytoplasmic material collects in the central portion of the giant cells (Fig. 32).

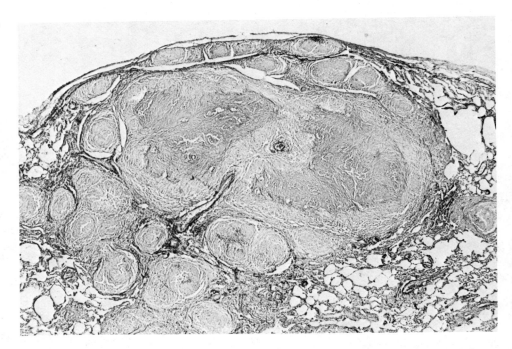

Figure 29 Coccidioidomycosis. Pulmonary lesion consisting of a conglomerate of smaller granulomatous foci with central necrosis. Perifocal reaction and pleural involvement are rather scanty. The fungous cells occur in the center of these granulomas. Gridley's stain, 58X.

The fungous cells in infected tissue are usually round yeast cells, 10-15 μm in diameter, with an abundant mucinous capsule. Budding cells are frequently seen. The yeast cells are pale and faintly basophilic in preparations stained with hematoxylin and eosin and are surrounded by an empty halo, which is the mucinous capsular material that does not stain distinctly in such preparations. In preparation stained by the PAS method, the cell wall stains a deep purple red and the capsular material is weakly stained, often showing a radiating configuration. In sections stained with Mayer's mucicarmin stain, the yeast cells, especially their cell walls, and capsular materials are specifically stained. The mucicarminophilic character of fungous cells also occurs in the causative organism of rhinosporidiosis.

There is a remarkable variation in size of the cells of *C. neoformans* in older lesions. The size of fungous cells in foci of short clinical duration are rather uniform in size, whereas the size of cells in chronic, granulomatous lesions is quite variable (Fig. 33). In the latter instances, atypical, aberrant forms of the fungus are not infrequently seen (Fig. 34) [56]. In rare instances, asteroid bodies are found in multinucleated giant cells (Fig. 35).

Microspectrophotometrical study of the secondary fluorescence of the *C. neoformans* cells stained with fluorochrome indicate that the fungus in fresh lesion emits a strong secondary fluorescence, while in old or granulomatous lesions, the cells emit only weak secondary fluorescence [56]. This finding would suggest that the viability among fungous cells in infected tissues can be evaluated.

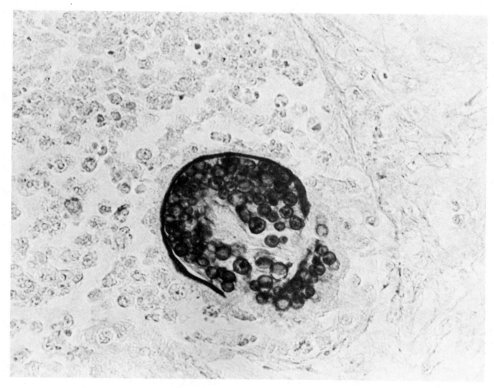

Figure 30 Coccidioidomycosis. Rupturing spherule and extruded endospores of *Coccidioides immitis*. The endosporulating spherule is the diagnostic structure of this fungus in tissue. Gridley's stain, 664X.

6. Geotrichosis

Geotrichosis is an infection caused by *Geotrichum candidum*. Oral, bronchial, and bronchopulmonary forms of geotrichosis are endogenous in origin and have little tendency to hematogenous dissemination. Cutaneous geotrichosis is limited to the skin [46]. *Geotrichum candidum* is an ubiquitous fungus, but confirmed cases of geotrichosis are relatively rare [14,62].

Tissue reactions show suppuration with necrosis. The appearance of the fungus has been described as a mixture of yeast-like cells and septate hyphae with oval and spherical arthroconidia. Histological diagnosis of geotrichosis is very difficult; therefore identification by culture of the fungus is essential for correct diagnosis.

7. Histoplasmosis

Histoplasmosis is a very common granulomatous disease of world-wide distribution caused by *Histoplasma capsulatum*. A clinically distinct form of histoplasmosis, which notably occurs in Africa, is caused by *Histoplasma capsulatum* var. *duboisii*. The former is an endemic disease in the Mississippi and Ohio River valleys in the United States, but cases are observed worldwide. The portal of entry of the organism is the lungs, where a primary focus is formed that is commonly arrested and becomes calcified [65,66,70]. Probably

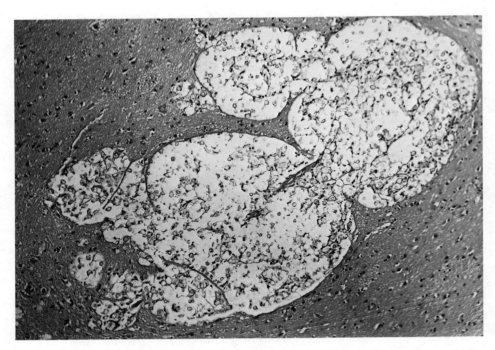

Figure 31 Cryptococcosis of the brain. Abundant growth of *Cryptococcus neoformans* separated by mucinous capsular material in perivascular spaces. Tissue reaction is devoid of cellular infiltration. Hematoxylin and eosin stain, 130X.

more than 95% of all primary infections are benign and self-limited, or completely asymptomatic. The rare disseminated form of the disease that involves the reticuloendothelial system is seen in infants. Cavitary lesions and the solitary tumor-like lesions, i.e., histoplasmomas, are seen in middle-aged individuals [65,70].

The primary lesion of the lungs is usually a calcified focus and is situated just beneath the pleura. The overlying pleura shows fibrous thickening which is always circumscribed. *Histoplasma capsulatum* is invisible in hematoxylin and eosin-stained section, whereas it can be easily detected in the central necrotic foci by Grocott's stain, which is the best method for detection of the fungus. The PAS and Gridley's stains are unsuitable for the detection of the organism in old foci (Fig. 36). Epithelioid cell granuloma are observed in lesions of the gastrointestinal tract.

In the foci of disseminated histoplasmosis and in mucosal lesions, the causative organisms are readily seen in hematoxylin and eosin-stained materials when they come from acute stages of infection. *Histoplasma capsulatum* occurs in histiocytes or phagocytic cells of the reticuloendothelial system as small spherical or oval cells, approximately 3 μm in diameter and surrounded by a clear halo (Fig. 37). Differentiation of *Histoplasma capsulatum* from *Leishmania* and *Toxoplasma* is relatively easy because the latter two protozoans are not stained by any of the fungous stains such as Grocott's or PAS stains.

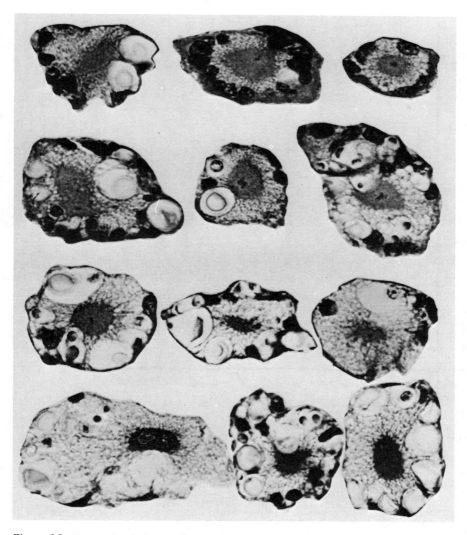

Figure 32 Example of giant cells seen in cryptococcal granulomas. Condensed eosinophilic cytoplasmic materials collect at the center of the cells. Many *Cryptococcus* cells are located in the peripheral portion of the giant cells. Hematoxylin and eosin stain, 400X.

African histoplasmosis, caused by *Histoplasma capsulatum* var. *duboisii,* is a rare disease in which nodular and ulcerative lesions of the skin and bone are seen. The appearance of the fungus and the tissue reaction is similar to that of *H. capsulatum* in both human and experimental infections. The fungous cells vary remarkably in size according to the tissue involved and the duration of the disease (Fig. 38) [59]. The tissue reaction is predominantly histiocytic in nature, and there is a marked tendency to form huge giant cells. Simultaneous occurrence of small, medium-sized, and large forms of yeast cells is usual.

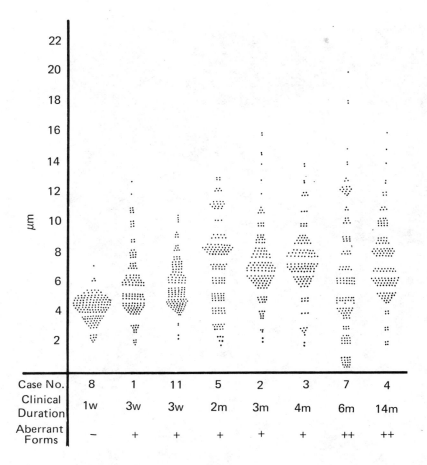

Case No.	8	1	11	5	2	3	7	4
Clinical Duration	1w	3w	3w	2m	3m	4m	6m	14m
Aberrant Forms	−	+	+	+	+	+	++	++

Figure 33 Size and appearance of aberrant forms of cryptococcal cells in a human cerebral lesion. One hundred yeast cells were measured by micrometer in each case, and the individual sizes were plotted as a function of the duration of clinical disease. Size variation among yeast cells is more prominent in older cases. Aberrant forms of the fungus also appear in older cases.

8. Mucormycosis

Mucormycosis is generally an acute, less commonly chronic, and rapid developing infection of a compromised host caused by various species of the order Mucorales [62]. The disease has been divided into deep-seated (cranial, pulmonary, gastrointestinal, disseminated), cutaneous, and focal forms [8].

Massive hemorrhagic infarction of tissue or parts of organs is a common finding of this infection. The tissue reaction is nonspecific, but penetration through tough, arterial walls by the fungus and thrombus formation are characteristic features for this disease (Fig. 39).

The fungus in infected tissue appears as broad, nonseptate (coenocytic) hyphae, which are recognizable in hematoxylin and eosin preparations. The branching pattern

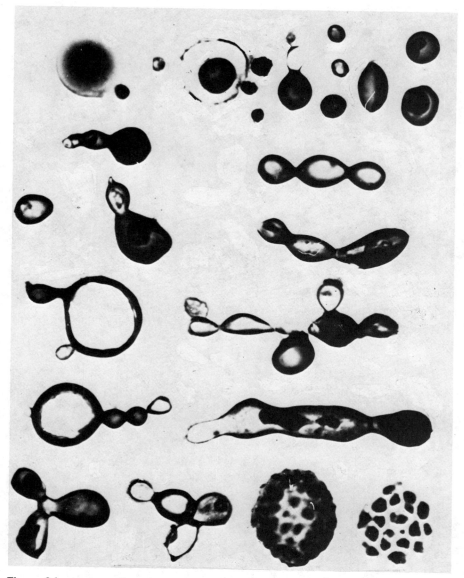

Figure 34 Aberrant forms of *Cryptococcus neoformans* in infected foci. In the top row, the morphologically typical forms of the fungus are shown. Giant, spherical yeast cells, small chains of budding cells, multiple budding cells, and pseudohyphal forms are illustrated in succeeding rows. Periodic acid Schiff stain, 1000×.

is usually at right angles or nearly at right angles, but even a haphazard branching of hyphae can be seen (Fig. 40).

In cases with subcutaneous zygomycosis, the appearance of *Basidiobolus* and *Conidiobolus* in biopsy specimens is simlar to the Mucorales described above.

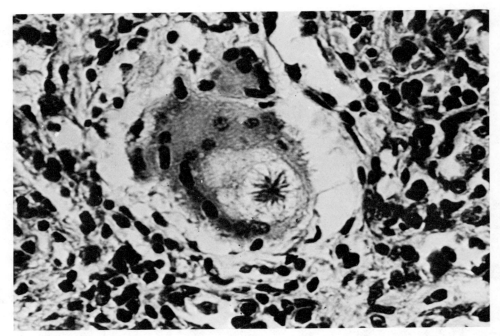

Figure 35 Pulmonary cryptococcosis. An asteroid body in a multinucleated giant cell, which is surrounded by a granulomatous cellular reaction. Hematoxylin and eosin stain, 588X.

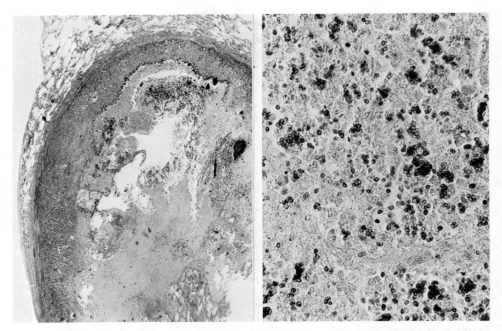

Figure 36 Histoplasmosis. Left: Calcified histoplasmosis of the lung. The subpleural lesion is surrounded by a thin layer of hyalinized, fibrous tissue. The scanty perifocal tissue reaction is characteristic. Dark areas are calcification. Hematoxylin and eosin stain, 52X. Right: High-power view of the center of the lesion showing cells of *Histoplasma capsulatum*. The organisms are oval to spherical in shape and 2-3 μm in diameter. Grocott's stain, 327X.

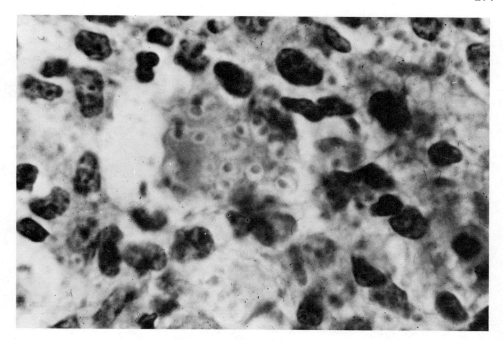

Figure 37 *Histoplasma capsulatum* in tissue. Intracellular, small, yeast-like cells are surrounded by a clear halo. Tissue reaction is predominantly histiocytic. Hematoxylin and eosin stain, 1270X.

9. Paracoccidioidomycosis

Paracoccidioidomycosis is limtied to South and Central America. This disease is a chronic, often fatal mycosis caused by *Paracoccidioides brasiliensis* and is characterized by primary, pulmonary lesions with dissemination to visceral organs and by conspicuous, ulcerative granulomas of the buccal and nasal mucosa with extensions to the skin. The lymphadenopathy is very marked, especially in the region of the neck [17].

The gross and microscopic changes of the infection are granulomatous, with purulent inflammation or central necrosis, and are very similar to those seen in cases of blastomycosis and coccidioidomycosis.

In infected tissues, the fungous cells vary greatly in size. Most of the cells are seen as spherical forms, 5-15 μm in diameter, which appear empty or contain cytoplasmic material (Fig. 41). The characteristic and pathognomonic stage of this organism in tissue is thick-walled, multiple budding yeast-like cell. Multiple budding can be observed as minute dot-like projections from the capsule of parent cell or as large peripheral buds (Fig. 42).

10. Penicillosis

Penicillosis is an infection caused by fungi belonging to the genus *Penicillium* and is relatively rare. Bronchopulmonary lesions are the type of disease that has been most frequently reported [28].

Interspersed basophilic body and vacuoles of hyphae of *Penicillium* have been reported [28]. However, the identical structure can be found in hyphae of *Aspergillus*.

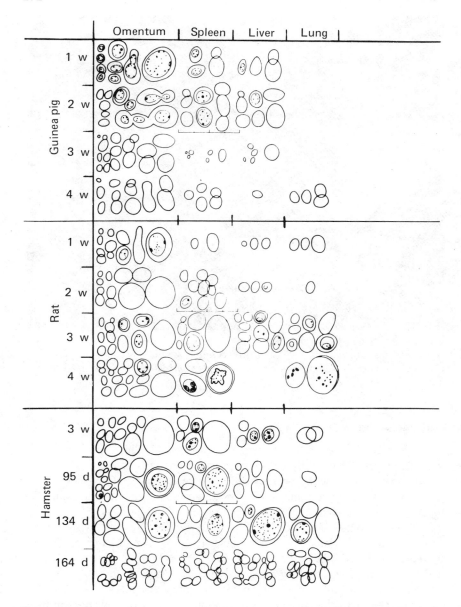

Figure 38 *Histoplasma capsulatum* var. *duboisii* in tissues from experimentally infected guinea pigs, rats, and hamsters. The size and form of the organisms vary considerably not only according to the organ involved, but also with reference to duration of infection, and to animal species. Scales in this figure are 5 μm. (From Ref. 50.)

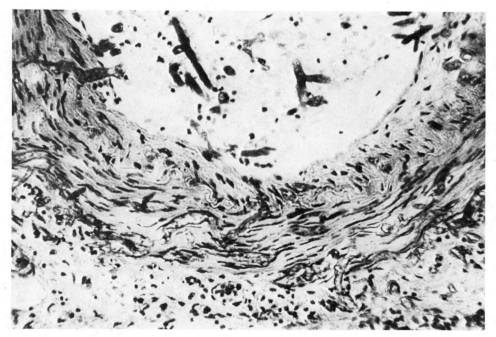

Figure 39 Gastric mucormycosis. Thick wall of an artery penetrated by hyphae of the fungus. In the arterial lumen, basophilic, thick hyphae with right angle branching are seen. Hematoxylin and eosin stain, 231X.

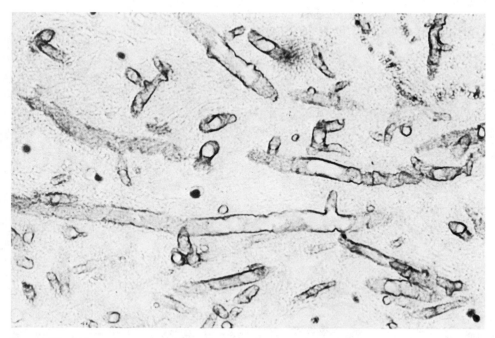

Figure 40 Pulmonary mucormycosis. Hyphae found in a thrombosed pulmonary artery. Thin-walled, broad, nonseptate hyphae with right angle branching are characteristic of members of the Mucorales in tissue. In the center of the right half, a septum-like structure is seen. This is presumed to be a fixation artifact. Grocott's stain, 589X.

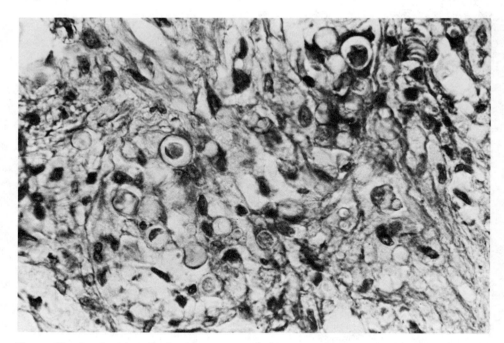

Figure 41 Cerebral lesion of paracoccidioidomycosis. A number of round forms of *Paracoccidioides brasiliensis* is shown. The fungous cells vary greatly in size, and some of them contain round cytoplasmic material. Hematoxylin and eosin stain, 574X.

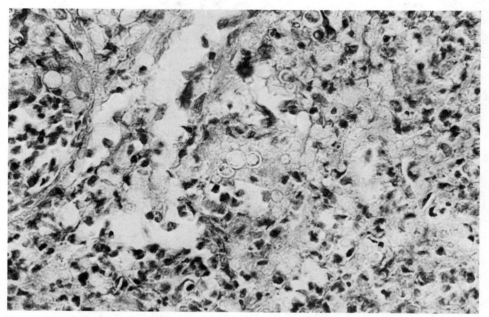

Figure 42 Cerebral lesion of paracoccidioidomycosis. In the center of this figure, a parent cell with large multiple buds is demonstrated. Tissue reaction is rather suppurative. Hematoxylin and eosin stain, 574X.

Appearance of this fungus in tissue seems to be closely similar to that of *Aspergillus*. Differentiation between *Aspergillus* and *Penicillium* should be based on cultural isolation of the etiologic agent.

11. Miscellaneous Mycoses

Rare fungous infections such as adiaspiromycosis, lobomycosis, and rhinosporidiosis are not covered in this chapter. Descriptions of the histopathology of these infections are provided in most textbooks of medical mycology [8,10,14,17,20,62].

IV. SOURCES OF ERROR

A. Artifacts

Artifacts may find their way into tissue preparations to be examined for fungi. These artifacts may be inert substances that take fungous stains or extraneous contamination of sections and fluids. A few examples are given.

Tissues may be contaminated with starch powder from surgical gloves used by the pathologist at the autopsy table. These starch granules are PAS-positive and birefringent [5].

When deparaffinized tissue sections are stored in running water for 4-5 days, bacteria or yeast-like organisms may grow on the tissue sections. Yeast-like organisms will grow

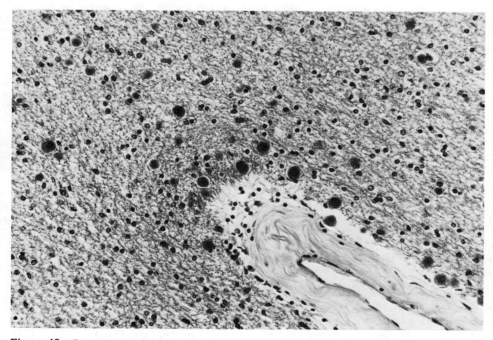

Figure 43 Corpora amylacea in the brain. Round bodies are seen in perivascular tissue. The outline of the corpora amylacea is somewhat indistinct and some of the bodies are laminated. No glial or inflammatory reaction is seen around them. Hematoxylin and eosin stain, 226X.

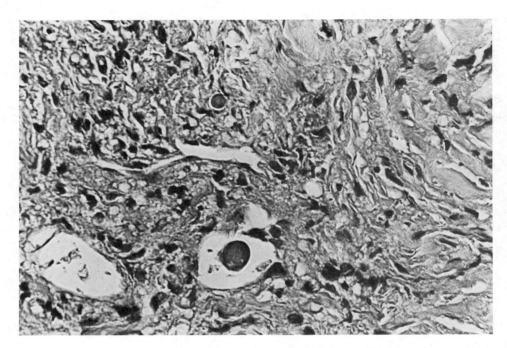

Figure 44 A Russel body and an unidentified round body. A Russel body comprised of homogenous globular material is demonstrated in the center of upper half of the photograph. A round body in a clear space is seen in the center of the lower half of the photograph. The latter is brown in color in a hematoxylin-eosin stain, and the nature of it has not been determined so far. Hematoxylin and eosin stain, 574X.

in Mayer's egg albumin which is used for attachment of paraffin sections to glass slides. Filamentous fungi are occasionally encountered in paraffin sections stored for a long time. The growth pattern of such contaminating, filamentous fungi is identical to that of fungi on a slide culture. In such instances, the microorganisms can be recognized as an extraneous contaminant because there is no tissue reaction and because the surrounding portions of the sections will show fungal growth.

B. Histological Structures Resembling Fungi

Numerous tissue structures, particularly those forms with corpuscular appearance often resemble fungous cells. Salfelder [63] has beautifully demonstrated these structures, which include peripheral nerve cells, Russel bodies, amylaceous bodies, tissue cells with halos, intratubular renal calculi, lentil soup aspiration, cooked cereal particles, aspirated meconium, Michaelis-Guttman bodies, Hamasaki-Wesenberg bodies, anthracotic pigment, cytoplasmic inclusions in tumor cells, lymphoma with dysproteinemia, cytomegalovirus-infected cells, and calcifications in the lung. Anthony [5] has described other structures that may be confused with fungi, e.g., conchoid and asteroid bodies of sarcoid granulomas, vegetable fibers and suture material (particularly when cross-cut), partly laked red cells, nuclear debris, and the like. Some of these structures will be discussed by way of examples.

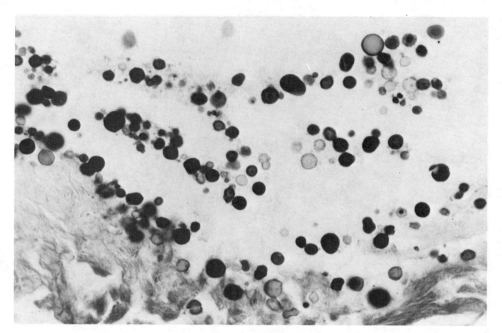

Figure 45 Calculus bodies. The bodies are deeply basophilic, round in shape, variable in size, and in some cases laminated. This material was taken from the wall of an old amoebic liver abscess. Hematoxylin and eosin stain, 581X.

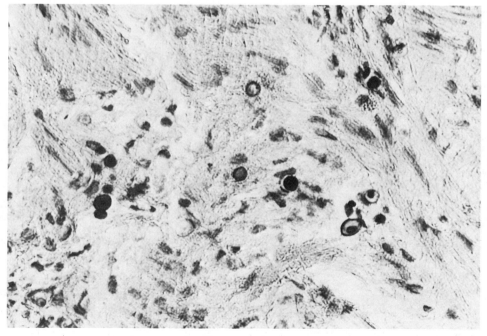

Figure 46 Michaelis-Guttman bodies. Small, round, sometimes laminated, basophilic structures. This photograph was taken from malakoplakia of the urinary bladder. Hematoxylin and eosin stain, 574X.

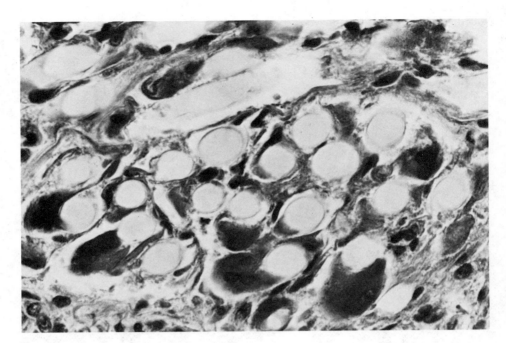

Figure 47 Suture material. Cross-section of suture materials that resemble *Crypto-coccus*. The round sutures are homogenous in structure and almost uniform in size and shape. Most of them are engulfed in foreign-body-type multinucleated giant cells. Hematoxylin and eosin stain, 581X.

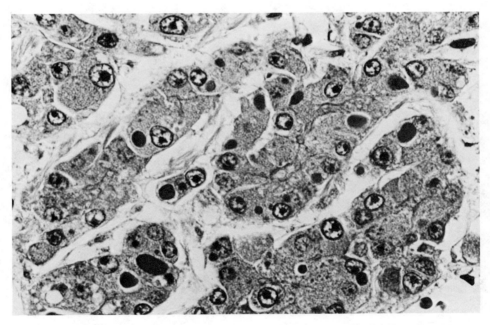

Figure 48 Globular hyalin bodies. Intracellular, globular, hyalin bodies of various sizes. Most of them are surrounded by a clear halo. This photograph was taken from a case of hepatocellular carcinoma. Hematoxylin and eosin stain, 574X.

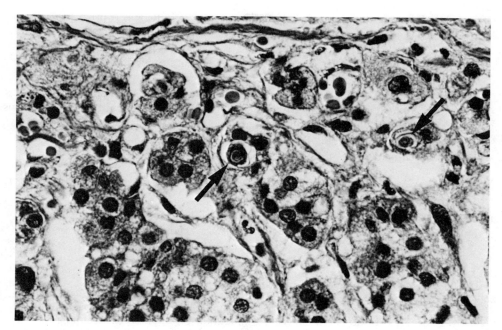

Figure 49 Aldacton bodies. Concentric lamellar bodies (indicated by arrows). This photograph was taken from the adrenals of a patient with cirrhosis of the liver and ascites. Hematoxylin and eosin stain. 581X.

Corpora amylacea are rounded bodies, about 10-15 μm or more in diameter, which are sometimes laminated (Fig. 43). They are often found in elderly people in the white matter adjacent to the ventricles and perivascular tissue, and pial surface of the central nervous tissue. They stain grayish blue in hematoxylin and eosin stain and are PAS positive. No glial cells or inflammatory reaction are found around them.

Russel bodies are eosinophilic, homogenous, globular inclusions of plasma cells (Fig. 44) that are mucoprotein in nature, PAS positive, contain surface gamma globulin, and probably result from condensation of internal cellular secretions.

Calculus bodies are deeply basophilic, rounded bodies (Fig. 45), sometimes laminated, which have indistinct outlines and stain with the von Kossa procedure.

Schaumann bodies are onion-like, layered, basophilic bodies, partially or completely calcified, that are found in sarcoidosis and various other conditions [51].

Michaelis-Guttman bodies, which have been described in malakoplakia, are small, rounded, sometimes apparently laminated basophilic bodies (Fig. 46), that stain for iron and with the von Kossa and PAS procedures, and are believed to be altered bacteria or breakdown products of bacteria that have become mineralized [4].

Suture material, especially when cross-cut, resembles *Cryptococcus* (Fig. 47). Round suture materials are homogenous in structure and almost uniform in size and shape and are birefringent. They are often engulfed in multinucleated giant cells.

Globular hyalin bodies, which vary in size and may be either intracellular or extracellular, are found in hepatocellular carcinoma [22]. Intracellular, globular hyaline is commonly surrounded by a clear halo, is intensely eosinophilic, and is often paranuclear in location (Fig. 48). Such bodies are homogenous in structure and weakly PAS positive.

Aldacton bodies are eosinophilic, concentric, lammelar bodies (Fig. 49) found in cells of the zona glomerulosa of the adrenal in patients with ascites who have been treated with Aldacton A for a long time.

Paneth cells, which are located in the depth of the crypts of Lieberkühn's gland of the intestine, contain a large number of secretory granules. The granules are homogenous in structure and strongly acidophilic in hematoxylin and eosin preparations.

As Salfelder [64] has stated: Particles situated in epithelial and parenchymal cells are hardly ever infective organisms.

ACKNOWLEDGMENT

I am grateful to Dr. Dexter H. Howard, the editor of this monograph, for his kind and complete English revisions of this chapter and for his encouragement.

REFERENCES

1. Ajello, L., L. K. Georg, W. Kaplan, and L. Kaufman. 1966. *Laboratory Manual for Medical Mycology,* 2nd ed., U.S. Government Printing Office, Washington, D.C.
2. Al-Doory, Y. 1972. *Chromomycosis,* Mountain Press, Missoula, Montana.
3. Allen, J. C. (Ed.). 1976. *Infection and the Compromised Host,* Williams & Wilkins, Baltimore.
4. Anderson, W. A. D., and J. M. Kissane (Eds.). 1977. *Pathology,* 7th ed., Mosby, St. Louis.
5. Anthony, P. P. 1973. A guide to the histological identification of fungi in tissues. J. Clin. Pathol. *26*:828-831.
6. Baker, R. D. 1945. *Histopathology of the Mycoses,* American Registry of Pathology, Washington, D.C.
7. Baker, R. D. 1962. Foreword to the International Symposium on Opportunistic Fungus Infections. Lab. Invest. *11*:1017-1018.
8. Baker, R. D. 1971. Mucormycosis (opportunistic phycomycosis). In R. D. Baker (Ed.), *Human Infection with Fungi, Actinomycetes and Algae,* Springer-Verlag, Berlin, pp. 832-918.
9. Cespedes, F. R. 1971. Chromoblastomycosis (chromomycosis). In R. D. Baker (Ed.), *Human Infection with Fungi, Actinomycetes and Algae,* Springer-Verlag, Berlin, pp. 691-700.
10. Chandler, F. W., W. Kaplan, and L. Ajello. 1980. *A Colour Atlas and Textbook of the Histopathology of Mycotic Diseases,* Wolfe Medical Publications, London.
11. Cherry, W. B., M. Goldman, and T. R. Carski. 1960. *Fluorescent Antibody Techniques in the Diagnosis of Communicable Diseases.* Communicable Disease Center, Atlanta, Ga.
12. Chick, E. W. 1961. Acridine orange fluorescent stain for fungi. Arch. Dermatol. *83*:305-309.
13. Chick, E. W., A. Balows, and M. L. Furcolow (Eds.). 1975. *Opportunistic Fungal Infections,* Proceedings of the Second International Conference, Thomas, Springfield, Ill.
14. Conant, N. F., D. T. Smith, R. D. Baker, and J. L. Callaway. 1971. *Manual of Clinical Mycology,* 3rd ed., Saunders, Philadelphia.
15. Coons, A. H., H. J. Creech, R. N. Jones, and E. Berliner. 1942. The demonstration of pneumococcal antigen in tissue by the use of fluorescent antibody. J. Immunol. *45*:157-170.

16. Coons, A. H., and M. H. Kaplan. 1950. Localization of antigen in tissue cells. II. Improvements in a method for the detection of antigen by means of fluorescent antibody. J. Exp. Med. *91*:1-13.

17. Emmons, C. W., C. H. Binford, J. P. Utz, and K. J. Kwon-Chung. 1977. *Medical Mycology*, 3rd ed., Lea & Febiger, Philadelphia.

18. Eveland, W. C., J. D. Marschall, A. M. Silverstein, F. B. Johnson, L. Iverson, and D. J. Winslow. 1957. Specific immunochemical staining of *Cryptococcus neoformans* and its polysaccharide in tissue. Am. J. Pathol. *33*:616-617.

19. Fiese, M. J. 1958. *Coccidioidomycosis*, Thomas, Springfield, Ill.

20. Fukushiro, R. 1979. *Illustrated Atlas of Deep Mycoses* (in Japanese), Tanabe Pharm. Co. Ltd., Osaka.

21. Funder, S. 1961. *Practical Mycology: Manual for Identification of Fungi*, 2nd ed., A. W. Brøggers Boktrykkeri, Oslo.

22. Gibson, J. B., and L. H. Sobin. 1978. Histological typing of tumours of the liver, biliary tract and pancreas. No. 20, p. 22. WHO, Geneva.

23. Grocott, R. G. 1955. A stain for tissue sections and smears using Gomori's methenamine-silver nitrate technic. Am. J. Clin. Pathol. *25*:975-979.

24. Hara, M., D. Ikeda, S. Isahaya, and S. Naoe. 1977. Aspergilloma by *Aspergillus niger* with calcium oxalate deposition. Report of an autopsy case (in Japanese). Jpn. J. Med. Mycol. *18*:102-107.

25. Hicks, J. D., and E. Matthaei. 1958. A selective fluorescence stain for mucin. J. Pathol. *75*:473-476.

26. Hotchi, M. 1967. The application of fluorescent antibody techniques to the identification of pathogenic fungi in tissue specimens. Med. J. Shinshu Univ. *12*:123-139.

27. Hotchi, M., M. Okada, and T. Nasu. 1980. A statistical survey of mycoses in the total autopsy cases in Japan during the period from 1966 to 1975. In E. S. Kuttin, and G. L. Baum (Eds.), *Human and Animal Mycology*, Excerpta Medica, Amsterdam, pp. 26-29.

28. Huang, S., and L. S. Harris. 1963. Acute disseminated penicillosis. Am. J. Clin. Pathol. *39*:167-174.

29. Kanda, M., M. Moriyama, M. Ikeda, S. Kojima, M. Tokunaga, and G. Watanabe. 1974. A statistical survey of deep mycoses in Japan, with particular reference to autopsy cases of cryptococcosis. Acta Pathol. Jpn. *24*:595-609.

30. Kaplan, W., and L. Kaufman. 1961. The application of fluorescent antibody techniques to medical mycology: a review. Sabouraudia *1*:137-144.

31. Kaplan, W., and F. W. Chandler. 1980. Histopathologic diagnosis of fungus infections. In E. S. Kuttin and G. L. Baum (Eds.), *Human and Animal Mycology*, Excerpta Medica, Amsterdam, pp. 149-154.

32. Klainer, A. S., and W. R. Beisel. 1969. Opportunistic infection: a review. Am. J. Med. Sci. *258*:431-456.

33. Klatzo, I., and P. H. Geisler. 1958. Demonstration of *Cryptococcus neoformans* in polarized light. Stain Technol. *33*:55-56.

34. Kuttin, E. S., and G. L. Baum. (Eds.). 1980. *Human and Animal Mycology*, Excerpta Medica, Amsterdam.

35. LeFrock, J. L., and A. S. Klainer. 1976. *Nosocomial infections*, Upjohn, Kalamazoo.

36. Lillie, R. D. 1948. *Histopathologic Technic*, Blakiston Co., Philadelphia.

37. Littman, M. L., and L. E. Zimmerman. 1956. *Cryptococcosis*, Grune & Stratton, New York.

38. Luna, L. G. (Ed.). 1968. *Manual of Histologic Staining Methods of the Armed Forces Institute of Pathology*, 3rd ed., McGraw-Hill Book Co., New York.

39. Lurie, H. I. 1971. Sporotrichosis. In R. D. Baker (Ed.), *Human Infection with Fungi, Actinomycetes and Algae,* Springer-Verlag, Berlin, pp. 614-675.

40. Naoe, S., and Y. Kuroiwa. 1977. Tissue phase of dematiaceous fungi (in Japanese). Jpn. J. Med. Mycol. *17*:241.

41. Nime, F. A., and G. M. Hutchins. 1973. Oxalosis caused by *Aspergillus* infection. Johns Hopkins Med. J. *133*:183-194.

42. Mallory, F. B. 1961. *Pathological Technique,* Hafner Publ., New York.

43. McManus, J. F. A. 1948. Histological and histochemical use of periodic acid. Stain Technol. *23*:99-108.

44. Miyake, M., and M. Okudaira. 1967. A statistical survey of deep fungus infections in Japan. Acta Pathol. Jpn. *17*:401-415.

45. Miyake, M., M. Okudaira, T. Nasu, M. Hotchi, A. Uetsuka, Y. Mine, and K. Hamashima. 1968. Identification of pathogenic fungi in paraffin embedded tissue sections by means of fluorescent antibody technic. Jpn. J. Exp. Med. *38*:95-104.

46. Morenz, J. 1971. Geotrichosis. In R. D. Baker (Ed.), *Human Infection with Fungi, Actinomycetes and Algae,* Springer-Verlag, Berlin, pp. 919-952.

47. Okudaira, M. 1955. Histoplathological differentiation between *Candida albicans* and *Aspergillus fumigatus* in tissue sections. Acta Pathol. Jpn. *5*:117-124.

48. Okudaira, M. 1956. A statistical and histopathological study of mycotic infections. Acta Pathol. Jpn. *6*:207-243.

49. Okudaira, M., T. Ono, T. Araki, and R. Fukushiro. 1959. Sporotrichosis with hyphal element in tissue. Report of a biopsy case (in Japanese with English summary). Trans. Soc. Pathol. Jpn. *48*:254-260.

50. Okudaira, M., and J. Schwarz. 1961. Infection with *Histoplasma duboisii* in different experimental animals. Mycologia *53*:53-63.

51. Okudaira, M., J. Schwarz, and S. M. Adriano. 1961. Experimental production of Schaumann bodies by heterogenous microbial agents in the golden hamster. Lab. Invest. *10*:968-982.

52. Okudaira, M., E. Tsubura, and J. Schwarz. 1961. A histopathological study of experimental murine sporotrichosis. Mycopathologia *54*:284-296.

53. Okudaira, M., and J. Schwarz. 1962. Tracheobronchopulmonary mycoses caused by opportunistic fungi, with particular reference to aspergillosis. Lab. Invest. *11*: 1053-1064.

54. Okudaira, M. 1964. Pathology of pulmonary aspergillosis, a statistical and pathological study (in Japanese). Jpn. J. Med. Mycol. *5*:18-34.

55. Okudaira, M. 1969. Pathology of candidiasis (in Japanese). Jpn. J. Med. Mycol. *10*:108-113.

56. Okudaira, M., and H. Kume. 1975. Pathological studies on cryptococcosis, especially on the morphological change and the estimation of the viability of cryptococcal cells in infected foci. Abstracts of the VIth Congress of the International Society for Humans and Animals, Tokyo, pp. 122-123.

57. Okudaira, M., and H. Kume. 1982. Pathological studies on chromomycosis. In M. Baxter (Ed.), *Proceedings of the VIIIth Congress of the International Society for Human and Animal Mycology,* Massey Univ., New Zealand, pp. 109-112.

58. Okun, M. R., and L. M. Edelstein. 1976. *Gross and Microscopic Pathology of the Skin,* Vol. 1. Dermatopathology Foundation Press, Boston, pp. 258-263.

59. Pena, C. E. 1971. Aspergillosis. In R. D. Baker (Ed.), *Human Infection with Fungi, Actinomycetes and Algae,* Springer Verlag, Berlin, pp. 762-831.

60. Pickett, J. P., C. M. Bishop, E. W. Chick, and R. D. Baker. 1960. A simple fluorescent stain for fungi. Selective staining of fungi by means of a fluorescent method for mucin. Am. J. Clin. Pathol. *34*:197-202.

61. Prier, J. E., and H. Friedman (Eds.), 1974. *Opportunistic Pathogens,* University Park Press, Baltimore.

62. Rippon, J. W. 1982. *Medical Mycology. The Pathogenic Fungi and the Patho-genic Actinomycetes,* Saunders, Philadelphia.

63. Salfelder, K. 1979. *Color Atlas of Deep Mycoses in Man,* F. K. Schattauer Verlag, Stuttgart, pp. 123-131.

64. Salfelder, K., and E. Sauerteig. 1981. *Small Infective Organisms,* Bayer, Germany.

65. Schwarz, J. 1971. Histoplasmosis. In R. D. Baker (Ed.), *Human Infection with Fungi, Actinomycetes and Algae,* Springer-Verlag, Berlin, pp. 67-130.

66. Schwarz, J. 1981. Histoplasmosis, Praeger Publ., New York.

67. Shimamine, T., M. Okudaira, and W. Mori. 1954. Ein Sektionsfall von general-isierter Dermatomykosis, hervorgerufen von Trichophyton purpureum Bang (in Japanese). Trans. Soc. Pathol. Jpn. *43*:501-504.

68. Sugawara, I., T. Shimamine, and M. Okudaira. 1979. Generalized aspergillosis show-ing a granulomatous pattern. Acta Pathol. Jpn. *29*:811-818.

69. Swartz, J. H. 1949. *Elements of Medical Mycology,* 2nd ed., Grune & Stratton, New York.

70. Sweany, H. C. (Ed.). 1960. *Histoplasmosis,* Thomas, Springfield, Ill.

71. The Transvaal Chamber of Mines Co-Ordinating Committee for the Investigation of Sporotrichosis. 1947. Sporotrichosis infection on mines of the Witwatersrand —A symposium. The Transvaal Chamber of Mines, Johannesburg.

72. Toriumi, J., T. Inoue, and M. Ishida. 1959. Histochemical studies on acid muco-polysaccharides. New fluorochromic method. Acta Pathol. Jpn. *9*:343-350.

73. Winner, H. I. 1966. General features of *Candida* infections. In H. I. Winner and R. Hurley (Eds.), *Symposium on Candida Infections,* E. & S. Livingstone Ltd., Edinburgh, pp. 6-11.

74. Wolstenholme, G. E. W., and R. Porter (Eds.). 1968. *Systemic Mycoses,* J. & A. Churchill Ltd., London.

75. Yasaki, Y., M. Miyake, M. Okudaira, J. Toriumi, T. Inoue, and S. Nakajima. 1959. A new histological method for the detection of *Cryptococcus neoformans* and its histopathologic study. Acta Pathol. Jpn. *9*:351-360.

76. Yasaki, Y., M. Miyake, M. Okudaira, J. Toriumi, T. Inoue, and M. Kodama. 1960. A study on the *Candida* group in tissue with the appliance of fluorescence micro-scopy. Acta Pathol. Jpn. *10*:65-73.

8
Routine Culture Techniques
for the Detection of Medically Important Fungi

Glenn D. Roberts / Mayo Medical School, Rochester, Minnesota

I. INTRODUCTION

The fungi are now definitely regarded as significant etiologic agents of serious and often life-threatening infections. The "saprobic fungi" in particular have been consistently associated with an increasing number of deaths among compromised patients. This makes it obligatory for clinicians and microbiologists to consider all fungi as potential pathogens.

Moreover, the clinical microbiology laboratory is obligated to use procedures that have been shown to be optimal for the detection and recovery of fungi from clinical specimens and to correctly identify and promptly report each organism to the clinician. It is only by complete reporting that the significance of fungi recovered from clinical specimens can be determined.

All laboratories are encouraged to use those procedures that will allow them to perform mycologic examinations with accuracy, speed, and ease. The procedures presented in this chapter have been carefully selected or developed for the active clinical mycology laboratory, whether large or small. Obviously every procedure reported in the literature cannot be included; however, appropriate references will guide the reader to alternate procedures when suitable.

II. SPECIMEN REQUIREMENTS

The selection of an appropriate specimen for culture is of utmost importance if the etiologic agent is to be recovered. In many instances, the clinician suspects a specific mycotic infection and Table 1 is designed to serve as a guide for the selection of optimal culture sites. In other instances where a specific infection is not suspected, specimens for culture should be collected from sites that show evidence of infection.

Table 1 Recommended Sites for the Recovery of Fungi from Specific Infections[a]

Infection	Sites to culture
Cutaneous	
Dermatomycosis	Hair
	Skin
	Nails
Subcutaneous	
Chromoblastomycosis	Skin
Mycetoma	Draining sinus tracts
	Bone
	Skin
Sporotrichosis	Aspirate from nodular skin lesions
	Cutaneous ulcers
	Joints
	Maxillary sinuses
	Respiratory secretions
	Bone
Systemic	
Blastomycosis	Respiratory secretions
	Skin
	Gastric washings
	Bone
	Oral mucosa
	Urine
Coccidioidomycosis	Respiratory secretions
	Skin
	Joints
	Urine
	Cerebrospinal fluid
	Gastric washings
	Oral mucosa
Histoplasmosis	Respiratory secretions
	Blood
	Urine
	Gastric washings
	Bone marrow
	Pleural fluid
	Skin
	Cerebrospinal fluid

Table 1 (continued)

Infection	Sites to culture
Opportunistic	
Aspergillosis	Respiratory secretions
	Cornea (mycotic keratitis)
Candidiasis	Blood
	Catheter tips
	Urine
	Skin
	Nails
	Respiratory secretions
	Vagina
	Cornea (mycotic keratitis)
Cryptococcosis	Respiratory secretions
	Blood
	Cerebrospinal fluid
	Urine
	Bone
	Bone marrow
	Pleural fluid
	Skin
Nocardiosis[b]	Respiratory secretions
	Skin
	Gastric washings
	Blood
	Brain abscess
Zygomycosis	Tissue biopsy:
	Nasal area
	Orbital area
	Brain
	Respiratory secretions

[a]Recommended sites for culture are listed in order of specimens most often yielding cultural proof of etiology, except for candidiasis where specimens are listed in order of those most clinically useful. Biopsy specimens are considered best for culture; however, alternative sites as listed in this table provide cultural proof of etiology in most cases.

[b]Although nocardiosis is a bacterial infection, most laboratories recover the etiologic agent on fungal culture media due to the slow growth of the organisms involved.

III. DIRECT MICROSCOPIC EXAMINATION OF CLINICAL SPECIMENS

One of the most important and useful procedures in the clinical microbiology laboratory is the direct examination of specimens for the detection of fungi. In many instances, a tentative diagnosis and frequently a definitive diagnosis can be made shortly after a specimen is submitted to the laboratory. Laboratories are encouraged to observe all specimens microscopically for the presence of fungi.

A. India Ink Preparation

The India ink preparation may be used for the microscopic detection of *Cryptococcus neoformans* in cerebrospinal fluid. The India ink is used as a negative stain and the encapsulated cells of *C. neoformans* are easily visualized against a dark background,

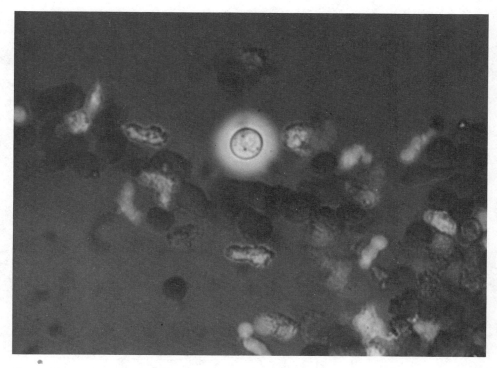

Figure 1 India ink preparation showing *Cryptococcus neoformans* in cerebrospinal fluid. Note large capsule surrounding the spherical yeast cell. 2000X. (From Ref. 8a.)

as shown in Fig. 1. The spherical shape, distinct variation in size of the cells, narrow attachment of the bud to the parent cell, and a capsule, when present, are characteristic of *C. neoformans.*

The India ink preparation is made as follows:

1. Centrifuge specimen for 10 min.
2. Place a drop of sediment on a slide to which a *small* drop of India ink or nigrosin has been added. Mix with an applicator stick and position a coverslip into place.
3. If the cerebrospinal fluid contains erythrocytes, add a drop of 10% potassium hydroxide to the specimen and then add the India ink or nigrosin.
4. Observe using bright-field microscopy for the presence of encapsulated yeast cells.

B. Potassium Hydroxide Preparation

The potassium hydroxide (KOH) preparation has traditionally been used for the microscopic detection of hyphae of dermatophytes in skin, hair, or nails. Since the KOH hastens clearing of tissue and cellular debris, this technique has application for the microscopic detection of other fungi in all types of clinical specimens. Figs. 2-8 are examples of organisms that may be detected in clinical specimens. Accompanying legend descriptions provide the diagnostic characteristics for each organism illustrated.

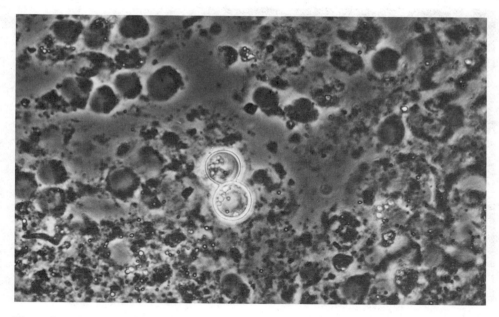

Figure 2 *Blastomyces dermatitidis* in sputum. Characteristic yeast form has budding cell attached by broad base. Also note "double contoured" appearance of cell wall. 2000X. (From Ref. 8a.)

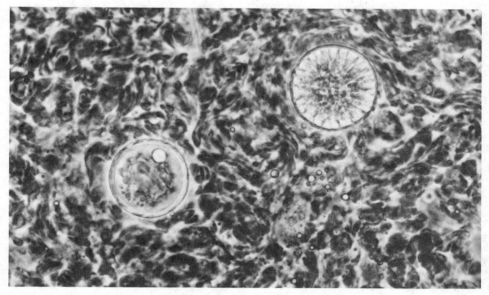

Figure 3 *Coccidioides immitis* in sputum. Large thick-walled spherules with few endospores scattered within interior of spherule or cleavage furrows developing along periphery to form endospores. 2000X. (From Ref. 8a.)

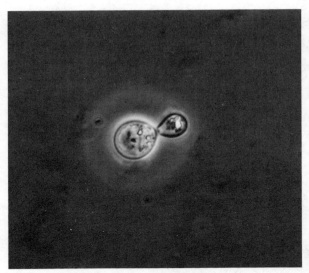

Figure 4 *Cryptococcus neoformans* in sputum. Spherical yeast cell is surrounded by large capsule with small bud arising from parent cell. 2000X.

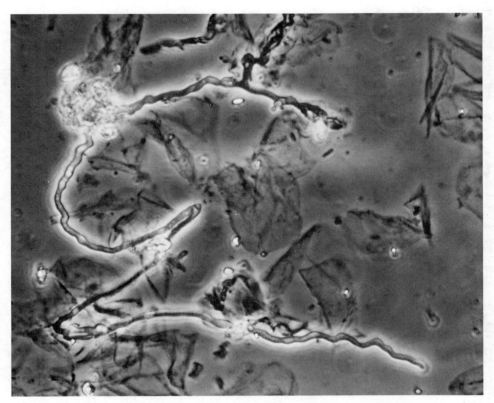

Figure 5 Dermatophyte in skin scraping. Septate hyphae intertwine among squamous cells. 2000X. (From Ref. 8a.)

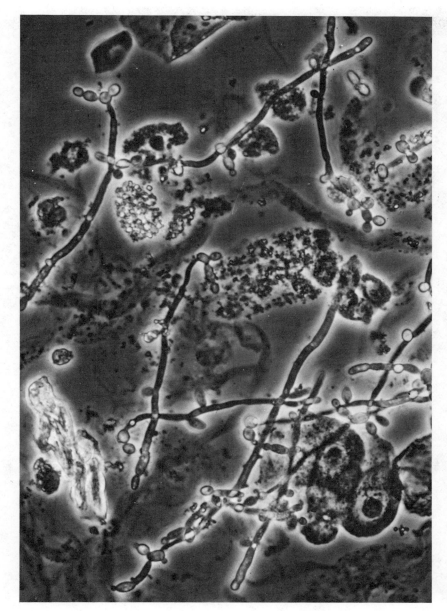

Figure 6 *Candida albicans* in urine. Hyphae, pseudohyphae, and budding yeasts appear among epithelial cells. 2000X. (From Ref. 8a.)

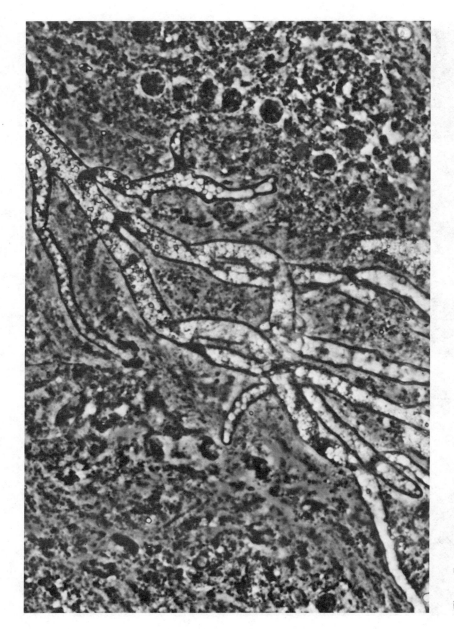

Figure 7 *Mucor* species in pus from skin lesion. The large, branching, ribbon-like aseptate hyphae are indicative of a zygomycete. 2400X. (From Ref. 8a)

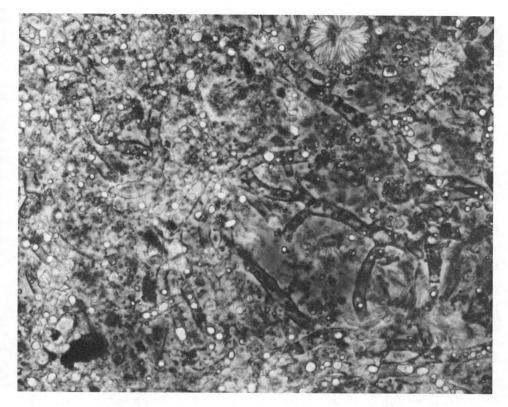

Figure 8 *Aspergillus fumigatus* in sputum. The septate hyphae show dichotomous branching. 2000X. (From Ref. 8a.)

The KOH preparation is made as follows:

1. Place a drop of 10% KOH-glycerin in the center of a microscope slide (see Koneman et al. in general reference section for recipe of this reagent).
2. Place the material to be examined in the KOH.
3. Place a coverslip on the slide and gently heat by passing through a flame. Do not allow to boil.
4. Spread material out by applying gentle pressure to the coverslip with a pencil eraser. Let sit for 5 min and repeat if the material does not spread.
5. Examine under a phase-contrast or bright-field microscope using low and high power. Observe for the presence of fungal elements (hyphae, yeasts, pseudohyphae, or spherules).

C. Interpretation of Results

1. India Ink Preparation

The presence of *C. neoformans* in cerebrospinal fluid is an abnormal and significant finding. When present, it almost certainly represents cryptococcal meningitis. Since other species of cryptococci are found in clinical specimens (rarely cerebrospinal fluid), a definitive identification of *C. neoformans* cannot be made on the basis of the morphologic features observed. However, a statement should be made establishing that the organism observed resembles *C. neoformans*.

The absence of *C. neoformans* in an India ink preparation cannot be used to rule out cryptococcal meningitis since less than 50% of culture proven cases have positive smears.

2. Potassium Hydroxide Preparation

A definitive diagnosis of blastomycosis, paracoccidioidomycosis, coccidioidomycosis, and cryptococcosis may be made when the specific etiologic agent is observed microscopically in a KOH preparation. Tentative diagnoses of aspergillosis, candidiasis, zygomycosis, nocardiosis, and dermatomycosis may also be made if fungal elements resembling the etiologic agents are observed. Cultural proof of etiology is necessary for the confirmation of the tentative diagnoses and is recommended in all instances regardless of the organisms seen in the direct examination.

IV. CULTURING OF CLINICAL SPECIMENS AND EXAMINATION OF CULTURES

A. Storage of Specimens Prior to Culturing

Little has been written about the survival of fungi in clinical specimens during extended storage. However, it is reasonable to assume that specimens contaminated with large numbers of bacteria or yeasts will be overgrown with these organisms when stored at room temperature. Kurung [7] showed that *Histoplasma capsulatum* exhibited a loss of viability in sputum kept at room temperature for greater than 24 h and postulated three causes for this adverse effect: enzymes, bacteria, and variation in pH. He concluded that the rapid death of the organism could not be attributed to any of these factors and recommended that freshly expectorated sputum be used for the recovery of *H. capsulatum*.

Recently, Hariri et al. [2] reported on the effects of time lapsed between sputum collection and culturing on the recovery of clinically significant fungi. The most frequently encountered pathogenic organism, *H. capsulatum*, was recovered most often from fresh clinical specimens but was recovered on some occasions even after 16 days of storage.

Thompson [16] used sputa inoculated with *H. capsulatum, Blastomyces dermatitidis, C. neoformans, Coccidioides immitis,* and *Aspergillus fumigatus* and determined the viability of the organisms after being frozen and stored for 24, 48, and 72 h on dry ice. *A. fumigatus* and *C. immitis* survived with no loss in viability whereas *B. dermatitidis* and *C. neoformans* showed decreased viability after 24 h and *H. capsulatum* was killed after 24 h.

Storage of clinical specimens before culturing is not recommended; however, if necessary, specimens may be kept at 4°C for no longer than 24 h, even though some loss in viability of the fungi present can be expected. Some species of dermatophytes, e.g., *Epidermophyton floccosum* will not survive refrigeration, and specimens of hair, skin, and nails should, if necessary, be stored in a dry container at room temperature to assure adequate recovery of the etiologic agent. The storage of clinical specimens prior to culturing is strongly discouraged and should be resorted to only if unavoidable.

B. Processing of Specimens Prior to Culturing

All specimens received for fungal culture should be considered as potentially contaminated with fungi or mycobacteria since the infections produced by these two groups of etiologic agents are clinically similar. To ensure laboratory safety, all clinical specimens must be handled within a biological safety cabinet.

Techniques useful for the processing of specimens suspected of containing fungi need not be elaborate. The digestion of respiratory specimens with *n*-acetyl-L-cysteine or similar compounds [8] is optional and of questionable value. The addition of 2-4% sodium hydroxide to these compounds is not recommended since it is detrimental to the recovery of fungi [9]. In addition, it is not advisable to add antibiotics to specimens since they may inhibit the growth of nocardiae that are often recovered on fungal culture media. Specific processing information may be found in the section describing the culturing of specimens.

The decision of whether to use culture dishes or tubes must be made by each individual laboratory. Culture dishes are optimal for the recovery of fungi since much more surface area is available for the isolation of discrete colonies. Many investigators, however, recommend that dishes not be used in the clinical laboratory since the open nature of the system provides for an increased chance of laboratory contamination. This concern can now be negated since culture dishes may be taped closed with an oxygen permeable Scotch tape (number 483, Minnesota Mining and Manufacturing Company, Minneapolis, Minnesota). If culture dishes are opened and handled within a biological safety cabinet, then little chance of laboratory contamination exists. Problems with dehydration of media may be overcome by filling dishes so that each contains at least 40 ml of medium.

Culture tubes are less than satisfactory for the recovery of fungi. The total surface area available for the isolation of colonies is small and provides for overgrowth by rapidly growing organisms including bacteria. This is detrimental since some of the pathogenic fungi require an extended incubation period. Oftentimes, lids on the tubes are tightened and inadequate oxygen supply prevents the growth of some organisms. If culture tubes are to be used, they should be as large as possible in size to provide a large surface area and the screw caps should be left slightly loosened during incubation for oxygen exchange to occur.

A reasonable compromise between culture dishes and tubes is the use of a sterile 250-ml tissue culture flask available from several commercial sources. This provides a large surface area optimal for the isolation of colonies and the system is closed. If this method is used, the cap on the flask should be left slightly loosened during incubation.

C. Selection of Media

Media used for the recovery and identification of fungi are numerous and their selection requires careful scrutiny by each laboratory director. The mycological literature lacks well-documented reports of comparative media evaluations. Consequently, most available information is verbal in origin and is based on experience and personal preference of individuals.

1. Primary Recovery Media

a. Routine Cultures: Media commonly used for the primary recovery of fungi from clinical specimens include brain heart infusion agar, brain heart infusion agar containing 5-10% sheep blood, blood agar base containing 5-10% sheep blood, inhibitory mold agar, Mycosel agar (BBL Laboratories, Cockeysville, Maryland) or Mycobiotic agar

(Difco Laboratories, Detroit, Michigan), Sabouraud's dextrose agar, Sabouraud's dextrose agar (Emmons' modification with 2% dextrose), Sabhi agar, yeast extract agar, and Lowenstein-Jensen medium (useful for the recovery of *Nocardia*). Niger seed agar has been shown to be useful for the primary recovery of *C. neoformans*.

Since most clinical specimens submitted for culture contain bacteria and fungi, it is necessary to supplement some of the culture media with antibiotics. Antibacterial antibiotics which have been used with success include the combinations of chloramphenicol (16 μg/ml) and gentamicin (5 μg/ml) or penicillin (20 units/ml) and streptomycin (40 units/ml). The combination of chloramphenicol and gentamicin is preferred because both antibiotics are heat-stable and can withstand autoclaving and in combination have a broad spectrum of activity against gram-negative organisms commonly found in clinical specimens. The combination of penicillin and streptomycin must be added to cooled media and it has a lesser degree of antibacterial activity against bacteria commonly found in specimens. Cycloheximide (Actidione, Upjohn Company, Kalamazoo, Michigan), an antifungal compound, should be added to at least one of the culture media used since it will prevent the overgrowth of slower growing pathogenic fungi (e.g., *H. capsulatum*) by common rapidly growing molds. However, cycloheximide should not be added to all culture media because it causes complete or partial inhibition of the following fungi: *C. neoformans, Pseudallescheria boydii,* most species of *Aspergillus,* and several species of *Candida.* The enrichment of media, e.g., brain heart infusion agar with 5-10% blood, is thought to enhance the recovery of the more fastidious pathogens [2a]. Human blood is not satisfactory since it may contain certain inhibitory substances that may prevent the growth of these pathogens and enrichment with sheep blood is preferred. Generally, media enriched with blood, i.e., brain heart infusion or Sabhi agars, are optimal for the recovery of fungi; however, the sporulation is usually suppressed and it is often necessary to subculture the organism to another medium to induce sporulation.

It is recommended that a battery of at least three culture media be used routinely for the recovery of the etiologic agents of the systemic mycoses. Sabouraud's dextrose agar and Mycosel or Mycobiotic agars are generally regarded as inadequate for this purpose and are not recommended. Any of the other media of preference may be used; however, the following criteria must be met:

1. Media with and without blood enrichment should be used.
2. Media with and without cycloheximide should be used.
3. Media containing antibacterial antibiotics should be used.
4. An antibiotic-free medium should be used if *Nocardia* is suspected.

Any combination of ingredients is satisfactory; a typical battery of media might include:

1. Brain heart infusion agar containing 5-10% sheep blood, 16 μg/ml of chloramphenicol, 5 μg/ml of gentamicin, and 500 μg/ml of cylcoheximide.
2. Brain heart infusion agar containing 5-10% sheep blood, 16 μg/ml of chloramphenicol, and 5 μg/ml of gentamicin.
3. Inhibitory mold agar or a similar medium containing 16 μg/ml of chloramphenicol and 5 μg/ml of gentamicin.

A yeast extract-phosphate agar used with NH_4OH [12] has been shown to be useful for the recovery of *H. capsulatum* and *B. dermatitidis* and may be used to replace the medium that does not contain the blood enrichment. Recommendations of media useful for the culture of specific specimen types are presented in Table 2.

Media useful for the recovery of mycobacteria are not generally recommended for the recovery of fungi. However, *Nocardia asteroides*, which is often identified by the mycology laboratory, grows well on Lowenstein-Jensen medium. It will not grow on most media containing antibiotics, and it is necessary that one medium that contains no antibiotics be used.

Mycosel or Mycobiotic agars both contain Sabouraud's dextrose agar with chloramphenicol and cycloheximide and are useful for the primary recovery of dermatophytic fungi. Dermatophyte test medium and Littman's oxgall agar are satisfactory but are seldom used by most laboratories.

Most commonly used bacteriologic blood culture media are satisfactory for the recovery of fungi from blood if the containers are vented [11]; however, the time for recovery is often delayed enough to make the culture information clinically irrelevant [10]. A lysis-centrifugation method is highly recommended because a higher percentage of recoveries and a decreased recovery time has been recorded with its use [1]. Alternative procedures include the use of a biphasic brain heart infusion bottle [11], the radiometric method [2b], membrane filter method [6], and the direct inoculation of blood onto the surface of a medium that has not been enriched with sheep blood.

In many instances, cultures fail to sporulate or produce characteristic spore arrangements on a primary recovery medium. This commonly occurs with a blood-containing medium, and it is necessary to subculture the recovered organism to another medium to induce sporulation. Commonly used subculture media useful for specific groups of fungi are shown in Table 3.

The definitive identification of *B. dermatitidis*, *H. capsulatum*, *Paracoccidioides brasiliensis*, and *Sporothrix schenckii* is presented elsewhere within this chapter. The exoantigen technique for identifying isolates is described in Sec. IV.G.5.

D. Culturing of Specimens

Procedures for the culturing of clinical specimens vary greatly from one laboratory to another. The procedures presented in this section are those that have proven useful in the Clinical Mycology Laboratory of the Mayo Clinic. The methods are practical and can be easily adapted by most laboratories.

1. Sputum, Induced Sputum, and Delayed Induced Sputum

Specimens are cultured on media shown in Table 2 as follows:

1. Vortex specimen for 20 s; add a small amount of nutrient broth if viscous.
2. Use a wide-bore pipette (sputum pipette) and withdraw 2.0 ml of specimen.
3. Place a 0.5-ml initial streak down the center of each plate.
4. Make several streaks perpendicular to and throughout the length of the initial streak using the pipette tip. When culturing sputum, the most viscous areas or those parts of the specimen that are blood tinged are the most desirable. If not accompanied with other requests, the remaining specimen may be discarded after 14 days.

Table 2 Recommended Media for Culturing of Specimens for Fungi

Specimen		Inhibitory mold agar	Sabouraud's dextrose agar (2%)	Brain heart infusion agar[b]	Brain heart infusion agar[c]	Mycosel or mycobiotic agars	Biphasic BHI medium
Group	Synonyms		Media for recovery of fungi and nocardiae				
Catheter							
Venous		X	X	X	X		
Central venous	cvp	X	X	X	X		
Arterial		X	X	X	X		
Cutaneous[a]							
Skin						X	
Hair						X	
Nails						X	
Eye							
Corneal		X	X				
Feces		X	X	X	X		
Fluids							
Cerebrospinal	Spinal	X	X	X			
	Ventricular	X	X	X			
	Cisternal	X	X	X			
Abdominal	Peritoneal	X	X	X	X		
	Paracentesis	X	X	X	X		
	Dialysis	X	X	X	X		
	Bile	X	X	X	X		
Chest	Pleural	X	X	X	X		
	Thoracentesis	X	X	X	X		
	Empyema	X	X	X	X		
Synovial	Joint	X	X	X	X		
Bone marrow		X	X	X	X		
Blood							X

Specimen					
Gastric washings		X	X	X	X
Genitourinary					
Cervix		X			
Vagina		X			
Urethra		X			
Urine					
Midstream	Clean catch	X	X	X	X
Catheterized		X	X	X	X
Cystoscopic		X	X	X	X
Suprapubic aspirate		X	X	X	X
Respiratory secretions					
Sputum		X	X	X	X
Induced sputum		X	X	X	X
Delayed induced sputum		X	X	X	X
Bronchial washings		X	X	X	X
Transtracheal aspirate		X	X	X	X
Mucous plugs		X	X	X	X
Lung aspirate		X	X	X	X
Tracheal	Endotracheal	X	X	X	X
Ear		X	X	X	X
Nose		X	X	X	X
Nasopharynx		X	X	X	X
Mouth	Oral cavity	X	X	X	X
Tissue		X	X	X	X
Wound	Exudate	X	X	X	X
	Transudate	X	X	X	X
	Drainage	X	X	X	X
	Ulcer	X	X	X	X
	Pus	X	X	X	X
(Swabs)		X	X	X	X

[a]When ordered for dermatophyte culture.

[b]Contains 5% sheep blood, 5 μg/ml gentamicin, and 16 μg/ml of chloramphenicol.

[c]Contains 5% sheep blood, 5 μg/ml gentamicin, 16 μg/ml of chloramphenicol, and 500 = μg/ml of cycloheximide.

Table 3 Subculture Media Useful for Inducing Sporulation of Fungi

Group of organisms	Recommended subculture medium
Dermatophytes	Cornmeal agar
Dimorphic pathogens, e.g., (*Histoplasma capsulatum* and *Blastomyces dermatitidis*)	Yeast extract agar, inhibitory mold agar, Sabouraud's dextrose (2%) agar, Sabhi agar
Dematiaceous rapidly growing molds	Cornmeal agar
Hyaline rapidly growing molds	Inhibitory mold agar, Sabouraud's dextrose (2%) agar, Sabhi agar
Yeasts	Inhibitory mold agar, Sabouraud's dextrose agar, Sabhi agar

2. Bronchial Washings

Specimens are cultured on the media shown in Table 2 and according to the instructions described under sputum specimens above, the specimen may be discarded 14 days after culturing is completed.

3. Transtracheal Aspirations

Specimens are cultured on the media shown in Table 2 and according to the instructions described under sputum specimens above. The specimen may be discarded 14 days after culturing is completed.

4. Mucous Plugs

Sputa, induced and delayed-induced sputa, or bronchial washings submitted to the mycology laboratory with a mucous plug present are treated as follows:

1. Pour the specimen into a sterile petri dish.
2. Examine for viscous, tenacious, and rope-like strands in the specimen.
3. If strands are found, remove one or two from the specimen using a wire hook.
4. Inoculate a portion of each strand onto media according to Table 2.

5. Lung Aspirates and Tracheal Specimens

These specimens are inoculated on the media shown in Table 2 according to the instructions described under sputum specimens. The specimen may be discarded after 14 days.

6. Ear, Nose, Nasopharynx, and Oral Specimens

These types of specimens are often collected on a swab. For culturing purposes, the swab is rolled across the surface of the media shown in Table 2. The specimen may be discarded after 7 days.

7. Cerebrospinal Fluid

If there is less than 2 ml of specimen, proceed as follows:

1. Centrifuge specimen for 10 min.
2. Using only a small amount of sediment, make an India ink or nigrosin preparation as follows:

a. Place a drop of sediment on a slide to which a small drop of India ink or nigrosin has been added. Mix with an applicator stick and position a coverslip.

b. If the CSF contains blood, add a drop of KOH to the specimen and then add the India ink or nigrosin.

c. Observe using bright field microscopy for the presence of encapsulated yeast cells.

3. Resuspend specimen and inoculate a plate of inhibitory mold agar by dropping the fluid in three spots on the surface. *DO NOT STREAK.*

If there is 2-3 ml of specimen, proceed as follows:

1. Centrifuge specimen for 10 min.
2. Make India ink or nigrosin preparation.
3. Resuspend the sediment and filter specimen through a Swinnex filter.
4. Place filter (organism side) down on a medium without cycloheximide or blood. The filter should be moved every other day for the first week, so that colonies underneath the filter may be detected.

If there is more than 3 ml of specimen, proceed as follows:

1. Centrifuge specimen for 10 min.
2. Make India ink or nigrosin preparation.
3. Resuspend sediment.
4. Filter equal amounts of 2 ml or more each through a separate Swinnex filter (Millipore Corp., Bedford, Massachusetts) and place each filter on media shown in Table 2.
5. Move filter every other day for the first week.

8. Body Fluids

All fluids except cerebrospinal fluid are inoculated onto the media shown in Table 2 and according to the instructions described under sputum specimens. Large volumes of fluid should be centrifuged prior to culturing.

Chest, abdominal, and synovial fluids are those most commonly encountered. All body fluids should be kept in the refrigerator until culturing is completed. A direct examination should be made on the sediment of all body fluids. Add a small amount of KOH to hasten clearing of specimen containing blood. The specimen may be discarded after 30 days.

9. Bone Marrow

Equal amounts of specimen should be inoculated onto the media shown in Table 2. Residual amounts of specimens should be kept for 30 days.

10. Blood

The lysis-centrifugation method [1] is currently recommended for fungal blood cultures. If biphasic brain heart infusion bottles are used, the bottles should be vented with a sterile cotton-plugged needle immediately after they are returned to the laboratory.

Be certain that the blood-broth mixture is gently flooded over the agar surface to allow any organisms present to implant on the agar surface. Cultures are incubated at 30°C in an upright position for 30 days.

11. Wounds

Swabs are most commonly submitted for wound culture specimens. The swab is rolled across the surface of the media shown in Table 2. The specimen may be discarded after 7 days.

12. Tissue

1. Specimens are inoculated onto the media shown in Table 2 and according to the description given under sputum specimens.
2. If there is 4 ml or more of material, inoculate 1 ml on each of the media shown in Table 2. Less than 4 ml should be evenly inoculated onto the same media.
3. If a zygomycete infection is suspected, inoculate media with minced tissue. Examples are nasal and eye tissue specimens.

13. Catheters

Catheters are rinsed in nutrient broth, and 0.5 ml of the broth is inoculated onto each of the media shown in Table 2. The specimen may be discarded after 7 days.

14. Eye

Equal portions of the specimen are inoculated onto the media shown in Table 2. If sufficient material is present, inoculate all four media.

15. Vaginal

Specimens are inoculated onto the media shown in Table 2. The specimen may be discarded after 7 days.

16. Cervical and Urethral

Specimens are cultured on the media shown in Table 2 and are discarded after 7 days.

17. Urine

The sediment from centrifuged specimens is inoculated onto the media shown in Table 2.

18. Fecal Material

Specimens are cultured on the media shown in Table 2. Those that are loose and watery may be treated as any other liquid specimen and are streaked directly on the media, using 0.5 ml per medium. Hard specimens should be emulsified with an applicator stick to ensure better distribution for culturing. The specimen may be discarded upon completion of culturing.

19. Gastric Washings

Specimens are cultured on the media shown in Table 2 and according to the description given under sputum specimens.

20. Skin, Hair, and Nails

1. Grind all large pieces of nails or skin in a mortar and pestle.
2. Inoculate all skin, hair, and nails on Mycosel or Mycobiotic agar as shown on Table 2.
3. Specimens are *NOT* to be refrigerated but should be kept in a sterile petri dish at room temperature if culturing is delayed.

E. Incubation Conditions

1. Temperature

The temperature of incubation for fungal cultures is a controversial issue among many laboratory investigators. The range of temperatures used by laboratories is from 25°C to 37°C with 30°C as the most common.

Some laboratories use both 25°C and 37°C as incubation temperatures for all specimens to recover the mold and yeast forms of the dimorphic pathogens independently. Most clinical specimens are heavily contaminated by bacteria that rapidly overgrow the yeast form of the dimorphic pathogens that might be recovered at 37°C. In addition, since the yeast forms of the dimorphic fungi morphologically resemble those of certain monomorphic yeasts, it is necessary to distinguish among them. *B. dermatitidis* is the only dimorphic pathogen that has a characteristic yeast form that may be recovered at 37°C. Reliable criteria are not available for the identification of the yeast forms of the other dimorphic pathogens, and therefore their recovery at an elevated temperature is not helpful.

Many laboratories incubate cultures at 25°C and consider this temperature sufficient. In reality, the temperature may drop to as low as 20°C to 22°C at night within the laboratory and rise up to 24°C to 25°C during the day when normal work activities are resumed. The net overall effect is that growth is slower due to the variation in temperature.

The optimal growth temperature for most pathogenic fungi is 30°C because the growth rate is faster and organisms more readily produce characteristic arrangements of spores needed for a definitive identification.

Most fungi grow best in an environment containing a relative humidity of 40-50%. This may easily be accomplished by placing a pan of water in the bottom of a closed incubator. Other alternative methods include the installation of a power humidifier or the placing of culture dishes within sealed oxygen-permeable plastic bags. If the relative humidity is too low, problems with desiccation of media occur. However, this can be prevented if culture dishes containing additional amounts of media (40 ml/plate) are used in conjunction with humidification.

All clinical specimens should be incubated for a minimum of 4 weeks; however, 6 weeks of incubation is optimal since some isolates of the dimorphic pathogens require this extended incubation period for their recovery.

F. Examination of Cultures

All cultures should be examined daily or at least three times weekly throughout the duration of incubation for the presence of yeasts or filamentous fungi. All organisms should be identified and reported so that their clinical significance may be determined. Specific information is given below.

1. Blood Cultures

Blood cultures should be observed twice daily for the first week and daily thereafter.

2. Cerebrospinal Fluid Cultures

Cerebrospinal fluid cultures should be examined daily for the presence of fungal growth on the agar surface. If a Swinnex filter is used for concentration, it should be gently removed from the agar surface and moved to a new location every other day during the first week of incubation. Thereafter, the filter should be left stationary and cultures examined for the presence of growth.

3. Skin, Hair, and Nail Cultures

All specimens submitted for dermatophyte culture should be examined at least twice weekly for visible evidence of growth.

4. Vaginal Cultures

Vaginal cultures should be examined daily for the presence of fungal growth. Many specimens will exhibit the growth of yeasts within 3-4 days; however, cultures should be examined throughout the duration of incubation.

5. General Cultures

Cultures other than those previously mentioned are regarded as general cultures. It is recommended that these be examined at least three times weekly; however, it is preferable to examine them daily.

G. Identification of Cultures

After a specimen has been cultured and incubated, the identification of organisms present is necessary. The identification process utilizes a number of criteria including the growth rate of the organism, gross colonial morphology, microscopic morphology, and selected biochemical features. It is not within the scope of this chapter to discuss all methods useful for the identification of fungi; however, the following discussion will present, in brief, some descriptive information not commonly found in textbooks. In addition, a list of general references is provided that should direct the laboratorian to specific sources helpful for the laboratory identification of fungi.

1. Growth Rate

The slow growth rate (7-21 days) of the strict pathogenic fungi has long been regarded as a useful criterion for their detection; however, exceptions to this rule have occurred with some frequency. Cultures of *B. dermatitidis* and *H. capsulatum* have been recovered in as short a time as 4-5 days, when a large number of colonies are present. In contrast, single colonies of *B. dermatitidis* and *H. capsulatum* sometimes may be detected only after 21 and 45 days, respectively. Cultures of *C. immitis* usually require an incubation time of 4-5 days before detection, but when large numbers of colonies are present, colonies may be seen within 48 h. Single colonies may require 21 days before visible growth can be detected.

Cultures of *P. brasiliensis* may be recovered within 5-25 days with the usual incubation period of 10-15 days. *C. neoformans* has a usual incubation period of 4-6 days but may be seen as early as 48 h and as late as 45 days of incubation.

The growth rate is often a helpful criterion, but it must be emphasized that it is variable for each isolate and type of medium and incubation conditions used.

2. Gross Colonial Morphology

Common textbooks present descriptions for the fungi that the reader assumes are typical for particular organisms. As is true in other areas of microbiology, tremendous variation in the colonial morphology occurs, commonly due to the type of medium used. One must be aware of this and not rely heavily on colonial morphology for the identification of fungi.

The color of the colony is sometimes helpful but varies widely for many organisms. Colonies of *B. dermatitidis* and *H. capsulatum* are described typically as being fluffy and white with a change in color to tan or buff with age. Some isolates initially appear darkly pigmented with colors ranging from gray to dark brown. A type of colonial variation not often mentioned occurs frequently on blood-containing media. Colonies of these two zoopathogens appear heaped, wrinkled, glabrous, neutral in color, and yeast-like and often exhibit tufts of adherent hyphae that project from the top of the colony. Some colonies may appear pink to red due to the absorbence of hemoglobin from the blood-containing medium.

The typical colonial morphology of *C. immitis* is described as fluffy white with scattered areas of hyphae that are adherent to the agar surface to give an overall "cobweb" appearance to the colony. Huppert et al. [3] reported 70 of 301 isolates as being atypical, with textures ranging from woolly to powdery and pigmentation ranging from pink, lavender, yellow, to brown or buff.

Other variations occur with a number of other fungi that cause infection in man but will not be discussed here. It is important to remember that natural variation occurs and that textbook descriptions are often inadequate.

3. Microscopic Morphology

In general, the microscopic morphological features of fungi are stable and exhibit little variation. More often the problem of identifying one of the pathogenic fungi is a lack of sporulation. Table 3 lists subculture media that are useful for inducing sporulation of the various groups of fungi. It should be reemphasized that a subculture medium is always necessary when a culture is recovered on a blood-containing medium.

The microscopic identification of fungi is based on the characteristic shape and arrangement of spores; however, the size of the hyphae present is often of help in detecting the systemic pathogens. These organisms have septate hyphae 1-2 μm in diameter, and often those of *B. dermatitidis* and *H. capsulatum* are tightly compacted together and resemble synnemata without conidia. The hyphae of *C. immitis* may enlarge to 3-4 μm shortly before arthroconidia are formed.

Typically the conidiospores of *B. dermatitidis* are pyriform and are borne on either short or long conidiophores. Occasionally, an isolate may produce large macroconidia which are 10 μm in diameter and may resemble a smooth macroconidium of *H. capsulatum*. It is not uncommon for an isolate of *B. dermatitidis* to fail to sporulate on most common media, and this prevents a tentative identification from being made.

Most isolates of *H. capsulatum* exhibit large tuberculate macroconidia that are characteristic. Some isolates may exhibit only small microconidia or they may be found in combination with macroconidia. Many isolates produce round, smooth-walled macroconidia that fail to become tuberculate, despite numerous subcultures. Others may produce very echinulate conidia intermediate in size between the microconidia and macroconidia. It is not uncommon for an isolate to produce racquet-shaped tuberculate macroconidia or even two or three macroconidia that remain attached in a chain-like fashion. *H. capsulatum* is known to exhibit a wide variation in sizes and shapes of conidia produced, and the identification of this organism is somewhat simplified if this is considered.

C. immitis typically produces barrel-shaped arthroconidia that have an alternate arrangement along the enlarged spore containing hyphae. Some isolates fail to produce arthroconidia despite numerous subcultures, and this prevents a tentative identification from being made. Huppert et al. [3] reported a variation in the size of arthroconidia produced that ranged from 1.5-7.5 μm and in width and 1.5-30 μm in length while most arthroconidia were 3-4.5 μm in width and 3.12 μm in length. The most common spore shape was rectangular; however, other were rounded, square, curved, or flexuous.

Microbiologists should be aware that variation in the microscopic morphologic features of the fungi does occur and that, again, textbook descriptions may be inadequate. Variation exists to some degree with most fungi and this must be considered as the identification of organisms is being made.

4. Biochemical Features

Biochemical features play little role in the identification of filamentous fungi; however, such attributes are crucial in the identification of yeasts and yeast-like organisms. Useful biochemical features include urease production, carbohydrate utilization, carbohydrate fermentation, nitrate reduction, and phenoloxidase production. Many different methods of performing these tests are available and will not be discussed within this section. The list of general references provides adequate coverage of biochemical methods.

5. Tests for Exoantigens

As emphasized in preceding sections of this chapter, it is not uncommon to encounter isolates of *B. dermatitidis, C. immitis, H. capsulatum,* and *P. brasiliensis* whose gross and microscopic features are not typical. In the past, the definitive identification of the dimorphic pathogens (except for *C. immitis*) has been dependent on the conversion of the mold form of each to the corresponding yeast form. Brain heart infusion agar enriched with 10% sheep blood and cystine heart agar enriched with hemoglobin are suitable for the conversion of dimorphic fungi. However, *B. dermatitidis* is more easily and rapidly converted on a cotton seed agar medium [17]. *Coccidioides immitis* may be converted in vitro to the spherule form using a chemically defined medium [15]; however, this method is of little use to clinical laboratories.

Currently, the effort to convert the dimorphic fungi is not recommended and is replaced by exoantigen testing [4,5,5a,13,14] except for *S. schenckii. B. dermatitidis* is easily converted in vitro and the exoantigen test is optional.

Exoantigen testing is accomplished as follows:

1. A mature fungal culture on Sabouraud's dextrose agar is covered with an aqueous merthiolate solution (1:5000 final concentration) and is allowed to remain in contact with the culture for 24 h at 25°C. The aqueous solution containing the exoantigenic (if present) is filtered through a 0.45 μm filter.
2. Five milliliters of the solution is concentrated to 50X for *H. capsulatum* and *B. dermatitidis* and 5X and 25X for *C. immitis* using an Amicon Minicon Macrosolute B-15 Concentrator (Amicon Corporation, Danvers, Massachusetts).
3. The concentrated solution is used in the immunodiffusion test in wells adjacent to control antigen and is reacted with control antiserum known to have specific antibodies. Tests are read after 24 h at 25°C and are examined for bands of identity [4,5,5a,13,14].

REFERENCES

1. Bille, J., L. Stockman, G. D. Roberts, C. D. Horstmeier, and D. M. Ilstrup. 1983. Evaluation of a lysis-centrifugation system for recovery of yeasts and filamentous fungi from blood. *J. Clin. Microbiol. 18*:469-471.

2. Hariri, A. R., H. O. Hempel, C. L. Kimberlin, and N. L. Goodman. 1982. Effects of time lapse between sputum collection and culturing an isolation of clinically significant fungi. *J. Clin. Microbiol. 15*:425-428.

2a. Howell, A. 1948. The efficiency of methods for the isolation of *Histoplasma capsulatum*. Public Health Rep. *63*:173-178.

2b. Hopfer, R. L., K. Mills, and D. Gröschel. 1979. Improved blood culture medium for radiometric detection of yeasts. J. Clin. Microbiol. *9*:448-449.

3. Huppert, M, S. H. Sun, and J. N. Bailey. 1967. Natural variability of *Coccidioides immitis*. In L. Ajello (Ed.), *Coccidioidomycosis*, Papers from the Second Symposium on Coccidioidomycosis, University of Arizona Press, Tucson, pp. 323-328.

4. Huppert, M., S. H. Sun, and E. H. Rice. 1978. Specificity of exoantigens for identifying cultures of *Coccidioides immitis*. J. Clin. Microbiol. *8*:346-348.

5. Kaufman, L., and P. Standard. 1978. Immuno-identification of cultures of fungi pathogenic to man. Curr. Microbiol. *1*:135-140.

5a. Kaufman, L., and P. G. Standard. 1978. Improved version of the exoantigen test for identification of *Coccidioides immitis* and *Histoplasma capsulatum* cultures. *J. Clin. Microbiol. 8*:42-45.

6. Komorowski, R. A., and S. G. Farmer. 1973. Rapid identification of candidemia. Am. J. Clin. Pathol. *59*:56-61.

7. Kurung, J. M. 1952. The isolation of *Histoplasma capsulatum* from sputum. Am. Rev. Tuberc. *66*:578-587.

8. Reep, B. R., and W. Kaplan. 1972. The use of *N*-acetyl-L-cysteine and dithiothreitol to process sputa for mycological and fluorescent antibody examinations. Health Lab. Sci. *9*:118-124.

8a. Roberts, G. D. 1975. Detection of fungi in clinical specimens by phase contrast microscopy. J. Clin. Microbiol. *2*:261-265.

9. Roberts. G. D., A. G. Karlson, and D. R. DeYoung. 1976. Recovery of pathogenic fungi from clinical specimens submitted for mycobacteriological cultures. J. Clin. Microbiol. *3*:47-48.

10. Roberts, G. D., and J. A. Washington, II. 1975. Detection of fungi in blood cultures. J. Clin. Microbiol. *1*:309-310.

11. Roberts, G. D., C. Horstmeier, M. Hall, and J. A. Washington, II. 1975. Recovery of yeast from vented blood culture bottles. J. Clin. Microbiol. *2*:18-20.

12. Smith, C. D., and N. L. Goodman. 1975. Improved culture method for the isolation of *Histoplasma capsulatum* and *Blastomyces dermatitidis* from contaminated specimens. Am. J. Clin. Pathol. *63*:276-280.

13. Standard, P. G., and L. Kaufman. 1976. Specific immunological test for the rapid identification of members of the genus *Histoplasma*. J. Clin. Microbiol. *3*:191-199.

14. Standard, P. G., and L. Kaufman. 1980. *Manual for the Immunological Identification of Pathogenic Fungus Cultures*, U.S. Dept. Health and Human Services, Public Health Service, Center for Disease Control, Bureau of Laboratories, Mycology Division, Atlanta, Ga., 30333.

15. Sun, S. H., M. Huppert, and K. R. Vukovich. 1976. Rapid in vitro conversion and identification of *Coccidioides immitis*. J. Clin. Microbiol. *3*:186-190.

16. Thompson, L. 1945. Note on a selective medium for fungi. Proc. Staff Meet., Mayo Clin. *20*:248-249.

17. Weeks, R. J. 1964. A rapid, simplified medium for converting the mycelial phase of *Blastomyces dermatitidis* to the yeast phase. Mycopathologia *22*:153-156.

BIBLIOGRAPHY

Balows, A., W. J. Hausler, Jr., and J. P. Truant (Eds.). 1980. *Manual of Clinical Microbiology*, 3rd ed., American Society for Microbiology, Washington, D.C.

Barnett, H. L., and B. B. Hunger. 1972. *Illustrated Genera of the Imperfect Fungi*, 3rd ed., Burgess Publishing Co., Minneapolis.

Beneke, E. S., and A. L. Rogers. 1980. *Medical Mycology Manual*, 4th ed., Burgess Publishing Co., Minneapolis.

Campbell, M. C., and J. L. Stewart. 1980. *The Medical Mycology Handbook*, John Wiley, New York.

Chick, E. W., A. Balows, and M. L. Furcolow. 1975. *Opportunistic Fungal Infections. Proceedings of the Second International Conference*, Thomas, Springfield, Ill.

Conant, N. F., D. T. Smith, R. D. Baker, J. L. Callaway, and D. S. Martin. 1971. *Manual of Clinical Mycology*, 3rd ed., Saunders, Philadelphia.

Emmons, C. W., C. H. Binford, J. P. Utz, and K. J. Kwon-Chung. 1977. *Medical Mycology*, 3rd ed. Lea & Febiger, Philadelphia.

Gilman, C. 1957. *A Manual of Soil Fungi*, 2nd ed., Iowa State University Press, Ames.

Haley, L. D. 1978. *Laboratory Methods in Medical Mycology*. Health, Education and Welfare Publ. No. (CDC) 78-8361.

Hazen, E. L., M. A. Gordon, and F. C. Reed. 1970. *Laboratory Identification of Pathogenic Fungi Simplified*, 3rd ed., Thomas, Springfield, Ill.

Koneman, E. W., G. D. Roberts, and S. F. Wright. 1978. *Practical Laboratory Mycology*, 2nd ed., Williams & Wilkins, Baltimore.

McGinnis, M. R. 1980. *Laboratory Handbook of Medical Mycology*, Academic Press, New York.

Moss, E. S., and A. L. McQuown. 1969. *Atlas of Medical Mycology*, 3rd ed., Williams & Wilkins Co., Baltimore.

Raper, K. B., and D. I. Fennell. 1965. *The Genus Aspergillus*. Williams & Wilkins, Baltimore.

Rippon, J. W. 1982. *Medical Mycology: The Pathogenic Fungi and the Pathogenic Actinomycetes*, 2nd ed., Saunders, Philadelphia.

Wilson, J. W., and O. A. Plunkett. 1965. *The Fungous Diseases of Man*, University of California Press, Berkeley.

9
Fungal Vaccines

John N. Galgiani / Veterans Administration Medical Center and University of Arizona, College of Medicine, Tucson, Arizona

I. INTRODUCTION

Cellular and immunological defenses have long been recognized as critical in the satisfactory resolution of fungal infections. Immunosuppressive diseases and therapies permit overwhelming infection by such fungi as *Candida albicans* and *Aspergillus fumigatus* that are rarely encountered as systemic pathogens in immunocompetent hosts. Other fungi such as *Coccidioides immitis, Blastomyces dermatitidis, Histoplasma capsulatum*, and *Cryptococcus neoformans* cause a broad range of illnesses in humans and other mammals that have no general immunological abnormalities, but even these organisms when infecting immunocompromised hosts characteristically produce more-severe disease [12,17,36,44,76,88]. Our understanding of the determinants of disease caused by fungi is not yet complete. However, the study of fungal vaccines might help to elucidate some of the mechanisms involved. Furthermore, as with many other types of infections, vaccination offers the hope of preventing disease. These two areas will be the principal subjects of this chapter.

In defining the scope of this review, discussion will be limited to vaccines that (1) are derived from the specific fungal species being studied, and (2) are employed as a relatively safe immunization. Thus, the area of immunopotentiating substances or the production of nonspecific resistance, except if the latter bears on the specificity of a particular vaccine, will not be addressed. Furthermore, immunological responses produced by sublethal inoculation of an otherwise virulent agent will generally be beyond the scope of this chapter (see Part B:I of this series).

With these restrictions, vaccines from *Coccidioides immitis* have been studied most extensively. Other mycoses of medical interest that have been studied include *H. capsulatum, Cryptococcus neoformans*, and *B. dermatitidis*. These fungi will be the subject of this review, which will emphasize work of the past two decades. A more extensive discussion of earlier work has been published previously [46]. Several other reviews of the immunology of these fungi also provide additional resources [19, 24,71,80a,94].

II. FUNGAL VACCINES IN EXPERIMENTAL INFECTIONS

A. Coccidioidomycosis

1. Murine

Mice are susceptible to both natural and experimental infection with *Coccidioides immitis*. Originally, mice were challenged intraperitoneally or intracerebrally [23,43], but intranasal injection [92] furnishes a route that more closely mimics that of natural infection. Unless otherwise specified, the subsequent discussion of coccidioidal vaccines will envolve studies in which the intranasal route of challenge was used.

A wide range of disease can be produced by using different-sized inocula. Infection occurs in most animals with as few as a half-dozen viable units, a fact which suggests that perhaps a single viable fungal unit may be sufficient for infection. This is in keeping with the presumed level of exposure in naturally acquired infections. Furthermore, animals usually survive such small inocula. However, mortality increases with larger inocula. The degree of lethality depends significantly on the specific strain of mouse studied. For example, 50% of a commercial strain of white mouse survived for 40 days after 100 arthroconidia were given intraperitoneally, whereas 95% of the NAMRU-strain mice were dead by day 20 [23]. The latter strain has frequently been used in coccidioidal vaccine studies. Furthermore, male mice are approximately two-fold more susceptible than females [56]. Finally, strains of *C. immitis* vary markedly in their virulence [23,57,73].

Smith and co-workers [22] first reported marked protection to a lethal peritoneal challenge by a killed mycelial vaccine administered subcutaneously. This encouraging finding was overshadowed by the greatly diminished protection to an intranasal challenge [75]. Live, attenuated mycelial vaccines were found to prevent death in a large proportion of intranasally challenged animals. However, reversion of the attenuated strain to more virulence appeared to have occurred in certain studies [47,75]. Furthermore, any attenuated strain, even one found to be stable, might be sufficiently virulent to cause progressive disease in particularly susceptible recipients. Because of these concerns, live coccidioidal vaccines have received little further attention.

With the advent of methods that allowed the spherule cycle of *C. immitis* to be grown in synthetic medium [13], killed spherules began to be studied as a protective vaccine. From the earliest studies [55], it was apparent that Formalin-killed spherules as an intramuscular vaccination were more protective than either weight-equivalent killed arthroconidia or mycelial preparations. Only 1 of 29 mice died after spherule vaccination as compared with 11 of 30 deaths in each of the other two vaccine-treated groups when challenged with doses ranging from LD_{80} to LD_{100}. It was also noted that *C. immitis* could be recovered from most of the surviving animals. This finding was examined in greater detail and will be discussed in Sec. IV.B.

The efficacy of spherule vaccines was highest when they were prepared from mature spherules [57]. Spherules and endospores derived from either continuous in vitro cultures or lungs of infected mice produced comparable levels of protection [56], indicating that cultured and in vivo-derived spherules were immunogenically similar.

Although a variety of immunization schedules have been employed, multiple immunization appear to improve protection. After two doses of spherule vaccine, a challenge of 1 log above an LD_{80} reduced mortality to below 20% whereas a single dose of twice as much vaccine showed slightly less protection [57]. Dividing the total dose into thirds (given on days 0, 10, and 20) was equivalent to half doses on days 0 and 10. However, a booster dose given at 10-20 weeks showed further enhancement [51]. The onset of immunity was found to be between 1 and 3 weeks, depending on the size of inocula [57]. One study suggested that a low inocula infection given in the second week after immunization enhanced mortality [56]. However, once established, protection was sustained for many months [49,51].

2. Other Animal Models

A number of mammalian species other than mice are susceptible to *C. immitis*, but relatively few of them have been used in vaccine trials. In studies that antedated the work of Smith and co-workers, Vogel demonstrated that spherules grown on embryonated eggs reduced lesions in guinea pigs after a respiratory challenge [102]. More recently, Cox and co-workers demonstrated protection using fractions of mycelia with adjuvants as a vaccine in guinea pigs [53]. Cynomolgous monkeys have been used with the killed-spherule vaccine in one study that suggested that primates could also be protected by vaccination [58]. No protection by respiratory vaccination with a mycelial preparation was found in dogs [11].

B. Histoplasmosis

There has been some difficulty in identifying a suitable animal model of progressive histoplasmosis [19]. Small laboratory animals are relatively resistant to serious infection, and intracerebral injections were used in many early studies to overcome this problem [81,86]. A lethal infection was produced by intraperitoneal challenge in mice if 10^6-10^8 yeast phase organisms were used [86]. In those studies, 8-week-old mice were approximately twice as susceptible as 14-week-old animals. Intravenous challenge required 1.4×10^7 viable cells of *H. capsulatum* to obtain an LD_{50} in mice. In another series of studies, inocula over 10^6 cells of various strains of *H. capsulatum* were required to produce mortality [97]. Hamsters and guinea pigs are more sensitive to dissemination than mice [80] albeit they also are more expensive for animal studies. Experimental infections have been induced in hamsters, but these animals have not been used in vaccine studies [3]. Also, aerosol-induced pneumonias have been produced in guinea pigs [87]. Such animal models might be useful in future vaccine studies.

Protection against both intraperitoneal and intravenous challenge has been demonstrated with killed preparations of whole yeast cells. Heat-killed cells reduced mouse mortality from an intraperitoneal challenge by more than half [86]. Garcia and Howard [32] found similar protection to an intravenous challenge in mice vaccinated intraperitoneally with merthiolate-killed cells. Recent studies by Tewari and co-workers have indicated protection of mice by vaccination with ribosomal preparations from the yeast phase [21].

C. Cryptococcosis

Although the rabbit has been examined as a model for cryptococcal vaccines [45], this animal appears resistant to intraperitoneal infection and most work has employed mice. Difficulty in demonstrating protection by killed yeast vaccines was encountered in early studies [20,28,41,45,63]. However, Abrahams and Gilleran [2], in systematically examining several variables in the murine model, were able to show significant protection with Formalin-killed *Cryptococcus neoformans*. These authors employed Swiss-Webster albino mice, 2-week immunization schedules, and an intravenous route of challenge with inocula exceeding an LD_{100} that resulted in median survival of 11-14 days in nonvaccinated controls. With these standard conditions, other experimental variables had significant effects on observed protection. Optimal protection was noted with approximately 10^7 Formalin-killed cells/vaccine dose, whereas protection was not evident using a dose of 10^8 cells. Although subcutaneous immunization was significantly protective, intraperitoneal immunization was more so. Immunity was demonstrable within 1 week and persisted for at least 3 weeks, although apparently waning. Pertussis given concurrently with the vaccine potentiated the protective effect [1]. Vaccines prepared from strains with small capsules resulted in greater protection than those from large-capsule strains. This point has been corroborated by the studies of Gadebusch [30,31], which indicated that removal of the polysaccharide capsule results in a more protective vaccine.

Vaccines prepared from attenuated strains have been studied. Louria reported that a strain known to be of low virulence for mice when used as a live vaccine increased the survival after a virulent challenge [61,62]. Similar results have been reported more recently with vaccines prepared from other mutants [26,77]. It should be noted, however, that virulence may be species specific. For example, one of Louria's isolates, which was of low virulence for mice, was also temperature sensitive but nonetheless had been isolated from a human with cryptococcal meningitis. Moreover, a virulent strain may not be lethal when administered by a different route. Moser et al. [68] reported that a virulent strain administered intracutaneously resulted in a localized infection and, in fact, produced protection to a subsequent intravenous challenge.

As with other mycoses that are naturally acquired by the respiratory route, it should be of interest to study the efficacy of cryptococcal vaccines in protecting against a pulmonary challenge. Although infection with *C. neoformans* from both intranasal and aerosol inoculation has been reported [78,90], these methods have not yet been used in vaccine studies.

D. Blastomycosis

Guinea pigs, rabbits, and some strains of mice have been known for some time to be susceptible to *B. dermatitidis* [16,39]. Of these, the murine infection has been used most commonly to study the consequences of vaccination. Intravenous, intraperitoneal, and intranasal challenges can produce progressive forms of disease [9,15,38,52].

Recently, Stevens and co-workers compared the susceptibility of two strains of mice when challenged by intraperitoneal or intranasal routes [65]. Whereas the DBA/1J strain was very sensitive to intraperitoneal challenge, this strain had previously been found to be very resistant to intranasal infection [67]. In contrast, the C34/HeJ strain, which was very susceptible to the intranasal challenge, was resistant to the intraperitoneal infection. Thus, the route of challenge can have a profound effect on outcome, which varies for different strains of mice. These investigators also noted that subcutaneous challenge of either strain did not lead to progressive disease [65].

Although sublethal infection with *B. dermatitidis* has been shown repeatedly to protect from subsequent lethal challenge [40,66,87,91], vaccines made from killed organisms have only recently been reported to afford any degree of protection in mice. Landay et al. reported that a particulate fraction of killed yeast-phase organisms, when given intraperitoneal injection 2 weeks prior to an intravenous challenge of mycelial phase organisms, prolonged survival as compared with saline-injected controls [52]. Although these workers could not demonstrate similar protection to a yeast-phase challenge, Cozad and Chang [15] showed that such protection was achieved by using a subcutaneous immunization given as two doses (separated by 1 week) in Freund's incomplete adjuvant. These investigators also demonstrated equivalent protection to an intraperitoneal challenge. These studies examined the onset and duration of protection after immunization. Protection was not demonstrable before 9 days and appeared to wane by 1 month following the first immunizing injection.

III. IMMUNOGENS IN FUNGAL STRUCTURES

A. Location

As indicated earlier, not all morphological forms of fungi confer resistance to disease. With *Coccidioides immitis*, mature spherule preparations are more protective than immature spherules or mycelia [57]. This could be due to the acquisition of the protective immunogen with spherule maturation or to a difference in antigen presentation related to phase of growth. The latter possibility is discussed in Sec. V.A.

Protection can be localized to the cell wall for *C. immitis*. The spherule wall conferred protection equivalent to whole spherules, whereas the cytosol of disrupted spherules did not [49].

The cell wall of *H. capsulatum* was found to be nearly as protective as whole cells in protecting against an intraperitoneal challenge [32]. Similarly, Salvin and Ribi [81] observed that the cell wall fraction was protective. Other work suggests that a ribosome-rich fraction derived by sodium dodecylsulfate extraction of the yeast phase of *H. capsulatum* also affords protection [86]. It is not clear whether the protection provided by the ribosomal vaccine is produced by the same or a different mechanism than that of cell wall preparations.

The capsular polysaccharide of *Cryptococcus neoformans* appears not to confer protection and, in fact, appears to be associated with lack of protection. However, a protective cell wall component has been observed. Neill et al. [70] found that vaccines made from weakly encapsulated strains were more protective than those made from strains with large capsules. Gadebusch [30] reported that progressive degradation of the cell wall yielded yeast cells that conferred increased protection. Complete removal of the wall led to loss of protection. Subsequently, a similar result was obtained by mechanical methods of wall removal [31]. Graybill et al. [33,35] have recently reported protection by several chromatographic fractions from supernatants of cryptococcal growth, only one of which had detectable capsular polysaccharide.

The particulate fraction of *B. dermatitidis* disrupted by mechanical means was found to be protective [52]. However, this observation was not characterized further, and results with other fractions were not reported.

B. Chemistry

The chemical nature of the spherule-derived immunogen(s) has been difficult to characterize due in part to the resistance of the cell wall to extraction [56]. A chloroform-water extract of spherule walls administered with adjuvants has been found to confer protection against an intranasal challenge of *Coccidioides immitis*. Whether this fraction was a true solution or a colloidal suspension of cell wall fragments was not determined. Treatment with a commercial chitinase diminished protection of the vaccine, but other evidence indicated that the enzyme preparation may not have had precise specificity. Recently, an alkali extract of mycelia administered with Freund's adjuvant has shown protection against intraperitoneal or intranasal challenge [53]. The results of immunization without adjuvant were not reported. The composition of this fraction was suggested to be a large molecular weight polysaccharide-protein complex, of which the protein comprises approximately 20% of dry weight [14] but as yet has not been characterized further.

Dissociation of immunogens from the yeast phase cell wall of *H. capsulatum* has also been difficult. Garcia and Howard [32] reported that of various extraction procedures, only that employing ethylenediamine resulted in a protective vaccine. Other investigators have indicated that a polysaccharide fraction was able to limit spread from the lungs in intratracheally challenged hamsters [4]. The ribosomal vaccine prepared by Tewari and co-workers sedimented as a single peak with a sedimentation coefficient of 77S on a sucrose density gradient [21]. The product contained 55% protein and 45% ribonucleic acid. Treatment of the vaccine with ribonuclease, trypsin, or pronase significantly reduced protection. However, 2-chloroethanol-extracted ribosomal protein, free from ribonucleic acid was highly immunogenic.

Graybill et al. [35] fractionated *Cryptococcus neoformans* and its culture supernatant by ion-exchange and gel-filtration column chromatography. Those fractions that protected mice contained high molecular weight substances, predominantly carbohydrate and distinguishable from the capsular polysaccharide.

C. Specificity

Most of the investigators studying killed spherule vaccines employed a vaccine and challenge with the same strain of *Coccidioides immitis* (Silveira). In one study, a comparable vaccine was made from a second strain (Woodville A-6) and was found equally effective against a Silveira challenge [57]. A subsequent report demonstrated that the Silveira vaccine protected equally against two strains with typical and five strains with atypical colonial morphology [42]. This relatively small sample of cross-strain protection is consistent with the presumed general protection after naturally acquired infection, since second primary infections are recognized only rarely in humans [79]. Nonspecific resistance was not demonstrated to *Cryptococcus neoformans* or *Pseudomonas pseudomallei* [42].

Bauman and Chick [4] examined intraspecies protection to dissemination with cell wall vaccines of *H. capsulatum*. In general, protection to heterologous-strain challenge was obtained; 52 of 60 vaccinated hamsters had sterile spleens as compared with 3 of 20 control animals. Tewari studied intra- and interspecies specificity of his ribosomal vaccine [96]. A vaccine prepared from one strain of *H. capsulatum* protected 90-100% of mice from lethal challenges of three other strains, but no protection was found to lethal challenges of *B. dermatitidis, Candida albicans, Cryptococcus neoformans,* or *Salmonella enteritidis*. However, sublethal infection with *H. capsulatum* has been reported to protect against lethal challenge with *B. dermatitidis* [78a].

The cryptococcal vaccines studies by Louria [61] protected mice from a lethal challenge with *C. neoformans* but did not protect animals from lethal challenges with *Klebsiella pneumoniae, Staphylococcus aureus,* or *Mycobacterium tuberculosis*. However, administration of an endotoxin instead of a vaccine produced similar protection against *C. neoformans* challenge. Also, bacille Calmette-Guérin (BCG) given repeatedly has been found to afford apparently nonspecific protection [64]. More recent work by Graybill and Taylor [37] also demonstrated cross-protection by extracts of *Candida albicans* and *C. (Torulopsis) glabrata* whereas coccidioidin or histoplasmin did not. Although these workers suggested that the protection afforded by the *Candida* preparations was related to antigenic similarities, it may be that their protection was of a less specific nature. *Candida* extracts can have pyrogenic effects, whereas, histoplasmin and coccidioidin which are used as skin-testing reagents usually do not.

The studies of Sethi et al. [89] suggest that sublethal *B. dermatitidis* infection protects mice from subsequent lethal challenge with *H. capsulatum*.

IV. EVENTS THAT ACCOMPANY VACCINATION

A. Histology after Challenge

Fungal vaccines have uniformly failed to prevent infection after challenge and consequent development of infectious lesions. Savage [82] quantitated the histologic changes that occurred in mouse lungs after intranasal challenge of *Coccidioides immitis*. Those vaccinated intramuscularly with the killed spherule vaccine generally showed more rapid but less intense inflammatory changes than did nonvaccinated controls, as evidenced by increased lung weight and leukocytic infiltrates on stained sections of lung. Counts of leukocytes in tracheobronchial washings showed other differences. In vaccinated animals, neutrophils, eosinophils, and lymphocytes were found earlier, whereas macrophages were slower to become evident. The percentage of macrophages from vaccine recipients containing fungi was always lower than it was in those from controls. These findings suggest that vaccination resulted in a more brisk leukocyte response and a more rapid reduction in organisms.

B. Fungal Multiplication

Quantitative differences in cultures of various organs of vaccinated animals as compared with controls have been reported for various vaccines. The spherule vaccine given intra-dermally [48] reduced pulmonary multiplication of *C. immitis* 50- to 500-fold. At low levels of intranasal challenge (7-15 arthroconidia), dissemination to the liver or spleen occurred in 36-40% of control mice but in none of the immunized mice. The yeast wall polysaccharide vaccine of *H. capsulatum* [22] reduced extrapulmonary spread from 85% in controls to 10% in vaccinated hamsters. Similar findings have been obtained with the ribosomal vaccine of *H. capsulatum* [21].

In contrast to the findings after intradermal vaccination, intravenously administered vaccine was much less effective in reducing fungal multiplication or dissemination. The spherule vaccine retarded fungal growth only slightly, a fact that correlates with its lack of protectivity by this route [59,83-85]. With *H. capsulatum*, pulmonary infections were increased in primates after intravenous vaccination [4a].

C. Delayed Hypersensitivity

Delayed hypersensitivity often accompanies acquisition of protective immunity, but whether these developments are different expressions of a common immunological event is a disputed and currently unresolved issue [54,103]. Although delayed hyper-sensitivity is sometimes demonstrable after effective fungal vaccination, generally the correlation is more consistent after natural immunity has been acquired. Intramuscular injection of killed spherules of *C. immitis* resulted in delayed hypersensitivity to coccidioidal antigens in some, but not all, mice [50]. However, this response was transient and almost undetectable after 5 months. Furthermore, reconstitution of ir-radiated mice with lymphocytes from vaccinated animals generally did not confer hyper-sensitivity, although protection to a lethal challenge could be demonstrated [7]. Spherule vaccine if given intravenously evoked little or no dermal hypersensitivity to antigens of *C. immitis* [59]. An alkali-soluble, water-soluble extract of mycelial walls was found to detect delayed hypersensitivity from a prior coccidioidal sensitization in humans and guinea pigs [14,100]. However, it was not reported whether this extract itself induces delayed hypersensitivity.

Graybill and Taylor [37] have demonstrated hypersensitivity associated with pro-longed survival after vaccination against cryptococcosis. Subsequently, this group also demonstrated that fractions of cryptococcal filtrate, that were each protective, elicited a hypersensitivity response. However, capsular polysaccharide also elicted an equivalent dermal response but was not protective [35]. Others have reported suppression of delayed hypersensitivity by capsular polysaccharide [10,69]. Vaccination with an avirulent strain of *Cryptococcus neoformans* has also been noted to produce lympho-cyte stimulation [25,27]. The transient protection of killed yeast cells of *B. dermatitidis* is associated with development and subsequent waning of delayed hyper-sensitivity to related fungal antigens [15]. Cell wall antigens of *H. capsulatum* have also been shown to elicit delayed hypersensitivity [18,93], but the correlation of such hypersensitivity with protection has not been established.

D. Antibody Response

The coccidioidal spherule vaccines administered in a fashion that affords protection
(i.e., by intramuscular injection) have been found to engender detectable tube-precipitin
antibody. However, this antibody response was less than that produced by the same
vaccine given by a relatively ineffective route (intravenous injection) [59]. Antibody
response to cryptococcal vaccines has been noted by several investigators [29-31,34,70]
and in some instances the magnitude has correlated with protection. Antibody to *B.
dermatitidis* is detectable after a sublethal inoculation that also affords protection
against a subsequent lethal challenge [66], However, a role for antibody in protection has
not been established for either *H. capsulatum* or *B. dermatitidis*.

V. MECHANISMS OF PROTECTION

A. Antigen Presentation

One possible reason that the protective antigen has been difficult to dissociate from the
fungal cell wall may be due to adjuvant properties of the particulate matrix. The
particulate coccidioidal vaccines clearly remain at the injection site for considerably
longer than soluble antigens [57], and antigens mixed in adjuvants also delay antigen
clearance. If the spherule wall is ground very finely, this material loses its protectivity.
However, if mixed with an adjuvant, protection is restored [72]. Recently, Lecara et
al. have found that an alkali-soluble mycelial extract showed significant protection when
vaccination included an adjuvant [53]. Thus, it is possible that the increased protection
of the spherule over saprophytic forms could be due to differences in the carrier rather
than specific protective immunogens.

B. Role of Sensitized Lymphocytes

Although little is known about the handling of fungal antigens that leads to immunity,
it is clear that intact T-lymphocyte function is essential. Spleen cells from mice immunized with the killed spherule vaccine, when transferred to other nonimmune mice,
confer protection to a lethal intranasal challenge [7]. Furthermore, spleen cell-mediated
protection was removed if the leukocyte preparation was treated with anti-T-lymphocyte
antiserum. Of interest, treatment of the splenic cells with anti-B-lymphocyte antiserum
enhanced protection, suggesting a possible humoral suppressor mechanism [8]. In none
of these studies, however, was serum from immune mice capable of conferring protection.
Similar studies have indicated that spleen or peritoneal exudate cells from mice immunized with ribosomal fractions of *H. capsulatum* were capable of protecting nonimmune mice from a challenge with that fungus whereas serum could not [95,98,99].
In those studies, viable T lymphocytes also seemed responsible. Adoptive transfer
studies of mice given cryptococcal vaccines have not been reported, although transfer
of some degree of protection has been noted when a virulent sublethal sensitization of
donor animals was used [60].

C. Role of Activated Macrophages

The means by which sensitized T lymphocytes effect protection is not well understood.
A few recent studies suggest that activated macrophages may play some role in coccidioidal infection. By themselves, alveolar macrophages from nonimmune primates or

peritoneal macrophages from either normal or immune mice fail to kill *Coccidioides immitis* [5,6]. However, if preincubated with lymphocytes from immunized mice, this leukocyte mixture is capable of killing endospores. Furthermore, supernatants from immunized lymphocytes stimulated in vitro with coccidioidal antigens induce murine peritoneal macrophages capable of killing *C. immitis* [5a]. Phagocytosis was equivalent in all situations. However, with the stimulated macrophage, phagolysosomal fusion as judged in acridine orange assays was found to be enhanced in lymphokine-stimulated macrophages as compared with unstimulated macrophages. These studies suggest that lymphokine-mediated activation of macrophages may be involved in preventing progressive infection in immunized mice.

VI. PREVENTION OF NATURALLY ACQUIRED INFECTION

A. Human Coccidioidomycosis

The possibility of preventing coccidioidomycosis by vaccination has been a specific goal for over two decades. If such a vaccine could prevent extrathoracic dissemination, it would be of value to all who might be exposed. Because the mechanisms underlying progressive disease are not understood, it is also possible that immunization would not prevent this sort of progression because in those individuals the vaccine would be no more likely to "take" than would a naturally acquired infection. However, a coccidioidal vaccine effective in preventing morbidity associated with the pulmonary infection would be of significant value, particularly to several special groups such as diabetics, those with severe pulmonary disease, and others in whom a severe pulmonary illness would be a particularly great hazard. Such a vaccine might be of value to groups at risk of high-inocula exposure, such as archeologists, laboratory technicians, and those working in earth-moving occupations in the endemic areas.

Recently, a collaborative effort has begun to determine the efficacy of a coccidioidal vaccine in humans. The vaccine consists of Formalin-killed spherules. Preliminary trials to assess acute toxicity of the vaccine have been conducted [74, 101]. In those studies, multiple intramuscular doses of 1.75 mg were found to give mild to moderate pain at the injection site but with no abnormalities in standard hematologic and chemistry surveillance. With higher doses, reactions at the injection site were found to be unacceptable. Skin-test conversion occurred in 55% after three doses of vaccine and 100% had boosting of their lymphocyte transformation to coccidioidal antigens.

Since the initial safety trials, a study was begun in 1981 to test vaccine efficacy. Participants are being enrolled at study sites in Bakersfield, Lemoore and Visalia, California, and Tucson, Arizona. Volunteers between the ages of 18 and 55 are eligible for randomization if negative results are obtained with all coccidioidal skin tests (coccidioidin and spherulin, each at the usual and high test strengths). Those randomized have a chest roentgenograph and are bled for serologic studies before receiving either vaccine or saline intramuscular injections administered in a blinded fashion on days 0, 7, and 49. Two weeks after the last injection, skin tests and phlebotomy are repeated. Participants are then surveyed for the duration of the study for episodes of illness compatible with acute coccidioidomycosis, at which time evaluations are performed to establish a diagnosis. For the purposes of this trial, a case is defined by recovery of *C. immitis* and/or a conversion of coccidioidal serologic tests. The data collected at all study sites is being collated for sequential analysis by a review team at Stanford University. Based on the assumption of a 1% per year detectable case rate, it is expected that 9000 participant-years will need to be accrued in order to test the primary hypothesis satisfactorily.

After 2 years of work, over 4000 volunteers have contributed to nearly 2000 randomized participants (the remainder were found to have at least one positive coccidioidal skin test) and approximately 3000 participant-years of surveillance. The trial is expected to finish enrollment (3000 randomized participants) in 1983 and then proceed for an additional 2 or 3 years.

ACKNOWLEDGMENTS

This work was supported in part by the Veterans Administration. The secretarial assistance of Shirley Johnson is most appreciated.

REFERENCES

1. Abrahams, I. 1966. Further studies on acquired resistance to murine cryptococcosis: enhancing effect of *Bordetella pertussis*. J. Immunol. *96*:525-529.
2. Abrahams, I., and T. G. Gilleran. 1960. Studies on actively acquired resistance to experimental cryptococcosis in mice. J. Immunol. *85*:629-635.
3. Bauman, D. S., and E. W. Chick. 1969. An experimental model for studying extrapulmonary dissemination of *Histoplasma capsulatum* in hamsters. Am. Rev. Respir. Dis. *100*:79-81.
4. Bauman, D. S., and E. W. Chick. 1969. Immunoprotection against extrapulmonary histoplasmosis in hamsters. Am. Rev. Respir. Dis. *100*:82-85.
4a. Bauman, D. S., and E. W. Chick. 1973. Acute cavitary histoplasmosis in rhesus monkeys: influence of immunological status. Infect. Immun. *8*:245-248.
5. Beaman, L., E. Benjamini, and D. Pappagianis. 1981. Role of lymphocytes in macrophage induced killing of *Coccidioides immitis* in vitro. Infect. Immun. *34*: 347-353.
5a. Beaman, L., E. Benjamini, and D. Pappagianis. 1983. Activation of macrophages by lymphokines: enhancement of phagosomes fusion and killing of *Coccidioides immitis*. Infect. Immun. (In press).
6. Beaman, L., and C. A. Holmberg. 1980. In vitro response of alveolar macrophages to infection with *Coccidioides immitis*. Infect. Immun. *28*:594-600.
7. Beaman, L., D. Pappagianis, and E. Benjamini. 1977. The significance of T cells in resistance to experimental murine coccidioidomycosis. Infect. Immun. *17*: 580-585.
8. Beaman, L., D. Pappagianis, and E. Benjamini. 1979. Mechanisms of resistance to infection with *Coccidioides immitis* in mice. Infect. Immun. *23*:681-685.
9. Brass, C., and D. A. Stevens. 1982. Maturity as a critical determinant of resistance to fungal infections: studies in murine blastomycosis. Infect. Immun. *36*:387-395.
10. Breen, J. F., I. C. Lee, F. R. Vogel, and H. Friedman. 1982. Cryptococcal capsular polysaccharide-induced modulation of murine immune responses. Infect. Immun. *36*:47-51.
11. Castleberry, M. W., J. L. Converse, J. T. Sinski, E. P. Lowe, S. P. Pakes, and J. E. Del Favero. 1965. Coccidioidomycosis: studies of canine vaccination and therapy. J. Infect. Dis. *115*:41-48.
12. Cohen, I. M., J. N. Galgiani, D. Potter, and D. A. Ogden. 1982. Coccidioidomycosis in renal replacement therapy. Arch. Intern. Med. *142*:489-494.
13. Converse, J. L. 1957. Effect of surface active agents on endosporulation of *Coccidioides immitis* in a chemically defined liquid medium. J. Bacteriol. *74*: 106-107.

14. Cox, R. A., E. Brummer, and G. Lecara. 1977. In vitro lymphocyte responses of coccidioidin skin test-positive and -negative persons to coccidioidin, spherulin, and a *Coccidioides* cell wall antigen. Infect. Immun. *15*:751-755.
15. Cozad, G. C., and C. Chang. 1980. Cell-mediated immunoprotection in blastomycosis. Infect. Immun. *28*:398-403.
16. Davis, B. F. 1911. The immunological reactions of oidiomycosis (blastomycosis) in the guinea-pig. J. Infect. Dis. *8*:190-240.
17. Diamond, R. D., and J. E. Bennett. 1974. Prognostic factors in cryptococcal meningitis. A study in 111 cases. Ann. Intern. Med. *80*:176-181.
18. Domer, J. E., and H. Ichinose. 1977. Cellular immune responses in guinea pigs immunized with cell walls of *Histoplasma capsulatum* prepared by several different procedures. Infect. Immun. *16*:293-301.
19. Domer, J. E., and S. A. Moser. 1980. Histoplasmosis—a review. Rev. Med. Vet. Mycol. *15*:159-182.
20. Dykstra, M. A., and L. Friedman. 1978. Pathogenesis, lethality and immunizing effect of experimental cutaneous cryptococcosis. Infect. Immun. *20*:446-455.
21. Feit, C., and R. P. Tewari. 1974. Immunogenicity of ribosomal preparations from yeast cells of *Histoplasma capsulatum*. Infect. Immun. *10*:1091-1097.
22. Friedman, L., and C. E. Smith. 1956. Vaccination of mice against *Coccidioides immitis*. Am. Rev. Tuberc. Pulm. Dis. *74*:245-248.
23. Friedman, L., C. E. Smith, and L. E. Gordon. 1955. The assay of virulence of *Coccidioides immitis* in white mice. J. Infect. Dis. *97*:311-316.
24. Fromtling, R. A., and H. J. Shadomy. 1982. Immunity in cryptococcosis: an overview. Mycopathologia *77*:183-190.
25. Fromtling, R. A., R. Blackstock, N. K. Hall, and G. S. Bulmer. 1979. Immunization of mice with an avirulent pseudohyphal form of *Cryptococcus neoformans*. Mycopathologia *68*:179-181.
26. Fromtling, R. A., R. Blackstock, N. K. Hall, and G. S. Bulmer. 1979. Kinetics of lymphocyte transformation in mice immunized with viable avirulent forms of *Cryptococcus neoformans*. Infect. Immun. *24*:449-453.
27. Fung, P. Y., and J. W. Murphy. 1982. In vitro interactions of immune lymphocytes and *Cryptococcus neoformans*. Infect. Immun. *36*:1128-1138.
28. Gadebusch, H. H. 1958. Active immunization against *Cryptococcus neoformans*. J. Infect. Dis. *102*:219-226.
29. Gadebusch, H. H. 1958. Passive immunization against *Cryptococcus neoformans*. Proc. Soc. Exp. Biol. Med. *98*:611-614.
30. Gadebusch, H. H. 1960. Specific degradation of *Cryptococcus neoformans* 3723 capsular polysaccharide by a microbial enzyme. J. Infect. Dis. *107*:406-409.
31. Gadebusch, H. H. 1963. Immunization against *Cryptococcus neoformans* by capsular polysaccharide. Nature *199*:710.
32. Garcia, J. P., and D. H. Howard. 1971. Characterization of antigens from the yeast phase of *Histoplasma capsulatum*. Infect. Immun. *4*:116-125.
33. Graybill, J. R. 1981. Immunization and complement interaction in host defense against murine cryptococcosis. J. Reticuloendothel. Soc. *30*:347-357.
34. Graybill, J. R., M. Hague, and D. J. Drutz. 1981. Passive immunization in murine cryptococcosis. Sabouraudia *19*:237-244.
35. Graybill, J. R., D. C. Straus, T. J. Nealon, M. Hague, and R. E. Paque. 1982. Immunogenic fractions of *Cryptococcus neoformans*. Mycopathologia *78*:31-39.
36. Graybill, J. R., and R. H. Alford. 1974. Cell-mediated immunity in cryptococcosis. Cell. Immunol. *14*:12-21.
37. Graybill, J. R., and R. L. Taylor. 1978. Host defense in cryptococcosis. I. An *in vivo* model for evaluating immune response. Int. Arch. Allergy Appl. Immunol. *57*:101-113.

38. Harvey, R. P., E. S. Schmid, C. C. Carrington, and D. A. Stevens. 1978. Mouse model of pulmonary blastomycosis: utility, simplicity, and quantitative parameters. Am. Rev. Respir. Dis. *117*:695-703.

39. Heilman, F. R. 1947. Experimental production of rapidly fatal blastomycosis in mice for testing chemotherapeutic agents. J. Invest. Dermatol. *9*:87-90.

40. Hill, G. A., and S. Marcus. 1959. Immunization against blastomycosis in mice. In *Bacteriological Proceedings of the 59th General Meeting of the Society of American Bacteriologists,* M 96, p. 87.

41. Hoff, C. L. 1942. Immunity studies of *Cryptococcus hominis* (*Torula histolytica*) in mice. J. Lab. Clin. Med. *27*:751-754.

42. Huppert, M., H. B. Levine, S. H. Sun, and E. T. Peterson. 1967. Resistance of vaccinated mice to typical and atypical strains of *Coccidioides immitis.* J. Bacteriol. *94*:924-927.

43. Karrer, H. E. 1953. Virulence of *Coccidioides immitis* determined by intracerebral inoculation in mice. Proc. Soc. Exp. Biol. Med. *82*:766-768.

44. Kauffman, C. A., K. S. Israel, J. W. Smith, A. C. White, J. Schwarz, and G. F. Brooks. 1978. Histoplasmosis in immunosuppressed patients. Am. J. Med. *64*: 923-932.

45. Kligman, A. M. 1947. Studies of the capsular substance of *Torula histolytica* and the immunologic properties of *Torula* cells. J. Immunol. *57*:395-401.

46. Kong, Y. M., and H. B. Levine. 1967. Experimentally induced immunity in the mycoses. Bacteriol. Rev. *31*:35-53.

47. Kong, Y. M., and H. B. Levine. 1967. Loss and recovery of virulence of arthrospores and spherule-endospores of *Coccidioides immitis* live vaccines. In L. Ajello (Ed.), *Coccidioidomycosis,* Papers from the Second Symposium on Coccidioidomycosis, University of Arizona Press, Tucson, pp. 189-195.

48. Kong, Y. M., H. B. Levine, S. H. Madin, and C. E. Smith. 1964. Fungal multiplication and histopathologic changes in vaccinated mice infected with *Coccidioides immitis.* J. Immunol. *92*:779-790.

49. Kong, Y. M., H. B. Levine, and C. E. Smith. 1963. Immunogenic properties of nondisrupted and disrupted spherules of *Coccidioides immitis* in mice. Sabouraudia *2*:131-142.

50. Kong, Y. M., D. C. Savage, and L. N. L. Kong. 1966. Delayed dermal hypersensitivity in mice to spherule and mycelial extracts of *Coccidioides immitis.* J. Bacteriol. *91*:876-883.

51. Kong, Y. M., D. C. Savage, and H. B. Levine. 1965. Enhancement of immune responses in mice by a booster injection of *Coccidioides* spherules. J. Immunol. *95*:1048-1056.

52. Landay, M. E., M. Hotchi, and N. Soares. 1972. Effect of prior vaccination on experimental blastomycosis. Mycopathol. Mycol. Appl. *46*:61-64.

53. Lecara, G., R. A. Cox, and R. B. Simpson. 1983. *Coccidioides immitis* vaccine: potential of an alkali-soluble, water soluble cell wall antigen. Infect. Immun. *39*:473-475.

54. Lefford, M. J. 1975. Delayed hypersensitivity and immunity in tuberculosis. Am. Rev. Respir. Dis. *111*:243-245.

55. Levine, H. B., J. M. Cobb, and C. E. Smith. 1960. Immunity to coccidioidomycosis induced in mice by purified spherule, arthrospore, and mycelial vaccines. Trans. N.Y. Acad. Sci. *22*:436-449.

56. Levine, H. B., J. M. Cobb, and C. E. Smith. 1961. Immunogenicity of spherule-endospore vaccines of *Coccidioides immitis.* J. Immunol. *87*:218-227.

57. Levine, H. B., Y. M. Kong, and C. E. Smith. 1965. Immunization of mice to *Coccidioides immitis*: dose, regimen and spherulation stage of killed spherule vaccines. J. Immunol. *94*:132-142.

58. Levine, H. B., R. L. Miller, and C. E. Smith. 1962. Influence of vaccination on respiratory coccidioidal disease in cynomolgous monkeys. J. Immunol. *89*:242-251.

59. Levine, H. B., and G. M. Scalarone. 1971. Deficient resistance to *Coccidioides immitis* following intravenous vaccination. III. Humoral and cellular responses to intravenous and intramuscular doses. Sabouraudia *9*:97-108.

60. Lim, T. S., and J. W. Murphy. 1980. Transfer of immunity to cryptococcosis by T enriched splenic lymphocytes from *Cryptococcus neoformans*-sensitized mice. Infect. Immun. *30*:5-11.

61. Louria, D. B. 1960. Specific and nonspecific immunity in experimental cryptococcosis in mice. J. Exp. Med. *111*:643-665.

62. Louria, D. B., T. Kaminski, and G. Finkel. 1963. Further studies on immunity in experimental cryptococcosis. J. Exp. Med. *117*:509-520.

63. Marcus, S., and F. R. Rambo. 1955. Comparative aspects of the immunization of mice against systemic mycosis. In *Bacteriological Proceedings of the 55th General Meeting of the Society of American Bacteriologists*, M 100, p. 92.

64. Monga, D. P. 1981. Role of macrophages in resistance of mice to experimental cryptococcosis. Infect. Immun. *32*:975-978.

65. Morazumi, P. A., E. Brummer, and D. A. Stevens. 1981. Strain differences in resistance to infection reversed by route of challenge: studies in blastomycosis. Infect. Immun. *34*:623-625.

66. Morazumi, P. A., E. Brummer, and D. A. Stevens. 1982. Protection against pulmonary blastomycosis: correlation with cellular and humoral immunity in mice after subcutaneous nonlethal infection. Infect. Immun. *37*:670-678.

67. Morazumi, P. A., J. W. Halpern, and D. A. Stevens. 1981. Susceptibility differences of inbred strains of mice to blastomycosis. Infect. Immun. *32*:160-168.

68. Moser, S. A., F. L. Lyon, J. E. Domer, and J. E. Williams. 1982. Immunization of mice by intracutaneous inoculation with viable virulent *Cryptococcus neoformans*: immunological and histopathological parameters. Infect. Immun. *35*:685-696.

69. Murphy, J. W., and J. W. Moorland. 1982. Regulation of cell-mediated immunity in cryptococcosis. I. Induction of specific afferent T suppressor cells by cryptococcal antigen. J. Immunol. *128*:276-283.

70. Neill, J. M., I. Abrahams, and C. E. Kapros. 1950. A comparison of the immunogenicity of weakly encapsulated and of strongly encapsulated strains of *Cryptococcus neoformans* (*Torula histolytica*). J. Bacteriol. *59*:263-275.

71. Nickerson, D. A. 1981. Immunoregulation in disseminated histoplasmosis: characterization of splenic suppressor cell populations. Cell. Immunol. *60*:287-297.

72. Pappagianis, D., R. Hector, H. B. Levine, and M. S. Collins. 1979. Immunization of mice against coccidioidomycosis with a subcellular vaccine. Infect. Immun. *25*:440-445.

73. Pappagianis, D., and G. S. Kobayashi. 1960. Approaches to the physiology of *Coccidioides immitis*. Ann. N.Y. Acad. Sci. *89*:109-121.

74. Pappagianis, D., and H. B. Levine. 1975. The present status of vaccination against coccidioidomycosis in man. Am. J. Epidemiol. *102*:30-41.

75. Pappagianis, D., H. B. Levine, C. E. Smith, R. J. Berman, and G. S. Kobayashi. 1961. Immunization of mice with viable *Coccidioides immitis*. J. Immunol. *86*:28-34.

76. Recht, L. D., S. F. Davies, M. R. Eckman, and G. A. Sarosi. 1982. Blastomycosis in immunosuppressed patients. Am. Rev. Respir. Dis. *125*:359-362.

77. Reiss, F., and E. Alture-Werber. 1976. Immunization of mice with a mutant of *Cryptococcus neoformans*. Dermatologica *152*:16-22.

78. Ritter, R. C., and H. W. Larsh. 1963. The infection of white mice following an intranasal instillation of *Cryptococcus neoformans*. Am. J. Hyg. *78*:241-246.

78a. Salfelder, K., and J. Schwarz. 1964. Cross reactions to *H. capsulatum* in mice. Sabouraudia *3*:164-166.

79. Salkin, D. 1967. Clinical examples of reinfection in coccidioidomycosis. In L. Ajello (Ed.), *Coccidioidomycosis*, Papers from the Second Symposium on Coccidioidomycosis, University of Arizona Press, Tucson, pp. 11-18.

80. Salvin, S. B. 1954. Cultural and serologic studies on nonfatal histoplasmosis in mice, hamsters, and guinea pigs. J. Infect. Dis. *94*:22-29.

80a. Salvin, S. B., and R. Neta. 1982. Immunopathology of mycotic infections. In N. R. Rose and B. V. Siegel (Eds.), *The Reticuloendothelial System*, Vol. 4, Plenum, New York, pp. 145-199.

81. Salvin, S. B., and E. Ribi. 1955. Antigens from the yeast phase of *Histoplasma capsulatum*. II. Immunologic properties of protoplasm vs. cell walls. Proc. Soc. Exp. Biol. Med. *90*:287-294.

82. Savage, D. C., and S. H. Madin. 1968. Cellular responses in lungs of immunized mice to intranasal infection with *Coccidioides immitis*. Sabouraudia *6*:94-102.

83. Scalarone, G. M., and H. B. Levine. 1969. Attributes of deficient immunity in mice receiving *Coccidioides immitis* spherule vaccine by the intravenous route. Sabouraudia *7*:169-177.

84. Scalarone, G. M., and H. B. Levine. 1971. Deficient resistance to *Coccidioides immitis* following intravenous vaccination. I. Distribution of spherules after intravenous and intra-muscular doses. Sabouraudia *9*:81-89.

85. Scalarone, G. M., and H. B. Levine. 1971. Deficient resistance to *Coccidioides immitis* following intravenous vaccination. II. Evidence against an immune tolerance mechanism. Sabouraudia *9*:90-96.

86. Schaefer, J., and S. Saslaw. 1954. Some factors affecting resistance of mice to experimental histoplasmosis. Proc. Soc. Exp. Biol. Med. *85*:223-225.

87. Schlitzer, R. L. 1981. Primary acute histoplasmosis in guinea pigs exposed to aerosolized *Histoplasma capsulatum*. Infect. Immun. *33*:575-582.

88. Schwarz, J., and K. Salfelder. 1977. Blastomycosis, a review of 152 cases. Curr. Top. Pathol. *65*:165-200.

89. Sethi, K., K. Salfelder, and J. Schwarz. 1964. Cross reactions to *Blastomyces dermatitidis* in mice. Mycopathol. Mycol. Appl. *24*:70-72.

90. Smith, C. D., R. Ritter, H. W. Larsh, and M. L. Furcolow. 1964. Infection of white swiss mice with airborne *Cryptococcus neoformans*. J. Bacteriol. *87*:1364-1368.

91. Spencer, H. D., and G. C. Cozad. 1980. Cell-mediated immuno-protection in blastomycosis. Infect. Immun. *28*:398-403.

92. Tager, M., and A. A. Liebow. 1942. Intranasal and intraperitoneal infection of the mouse with *Coccidioides immitis*. Yale J. Biol. Med. *15*:41-59.

93. Taylor, M. L. 1980. Immunology of histoplasmosis: humoral and cellular activity from a polysaccharide-protein complex and its deproteinized fraction in experimentally immunized mice. Mycopathologia *71*:159-166.

94. Tenenbaum, M. J., and T. M. Kerkering. 1982. Blastomycosis. Crit. Rev. Microbiol. *9*:139-163.

95. Tewari, R. P. 1982. Blastogenic responses of lymphocytes from mice immunized by sublethal infection with yeast cells of *Histoplasma capsulatum*. Infect. Immun. *36*:1013-1018.

96. Tewari, R. P. 1975. Immunization against histoplasmosis. In E. Neter and F. Milgrom (Eds.), *The Immune System and Infectious Diseases*, Fourth International Convocation of Immunology, Karger, Basel, pp. 441-452.

 97. Tewari, R. P., and F. J. Berkhout. 1972. Comparative pathogenicity of albino and brown types of *Histoplasma capsulatum* for mice. J. Infect. Dis. *125*:504-508.

 98. Tewari, R. P., D. K. Sharma, and A. Mathur. 1978. Significance of thymus-derived lymphocytes in immunity elicited by immunization with ribosomes or live yeast cells of *Histoplasma capsulatum*. J. Infect. Dis. *138*:605-613.

 99. Tewari, R. P., D. Sharma, M. Solotorovsky, R. Lafemina, and J. Balint. 1977. Adoptive transfer of immunity from mice immunized with ribosomes or live yeast cells of *Histoplasma capsulatum*. Infect. Immun. *15*:789-795.

100. Ward, E. R., R. A. Cox, J. A. Schmitt, Jr., M. Huppert, and S. H. Sun. 1975. Delayed-type hypersensitivity responses to a cell wall fraction of the mycelial phase of *Coccidioides immitis*. Infect. Immun. *12*:1093-1097.

101. Williams, P. L., S. P. Sorgen, D. L. Sable, D. Pappagianis, H. B. Levine, S. K. Brodine, and D. A. Stevens. 1980. Immunologic responsiveness and safety associated with the *C. immitis* spherule vaccine in volunteers of white, black and Filipino ancestry. In *Proceedings of the Twenty-Fifth Annual Coccidioidomycosis Study Group Meeting*, A12.

102. Vogel, R. H., B. F. Fetter, N. F. Conant, and E. P. Lowe. 1954. Preliminary studies on artificial active immunization of guinea pigs against respiratory challenge with *Coccidioides immitis*. Am. Rev. Tuberc. *79*:498-503.

103. Youmans, G. P. 1975. Relation between delayed hypersensitivity and immunity in tuberculosis. Am. Rev. Respir. Dis. *111*:109-118.

ADDENDUM

10

The Taxonomic Structure of *Exophiala*

G. S. de Hoog / Centraalbureau voor Schimmelcultures, Baarn, The Netherlands

I. INTRODUCTION

Despite various taxonomic treatments [3,5,14-19], the species of the black yeast genus *Exophiala* Carmichael are still not clearly delimited, and therefore remain difficult to identify. The authors of the references noted above all held different opinions on the best classification of these fungi, and discussions on isolated taxonomic decisions are still going on.

The main source of dispute is the tremendous phenotypic plasticity of the fungi concerned. The individual strains are highly variable, and each strain shows a pattern of variation slightly different from any other strain. Several more or less stable characters are available, but these are often discordant, so that clear-cut subdivisions can be made only arbitrarily.

Exophiala species show greatly varying degrees of differentiation. The genus is generally accepted as comprising hyphal species producing conidia from annellated zones on either undifferentiated hyphae or differentiated conidiophores. In most strains, the *Exophiala* state is accompanied by budding cells, frequently also by a sympodial state, and sometimes by phialides and sclerotic bodies. Since these states, except for the phialidic anamorph, are capable of propagating independently, they are often classified in separate anamorph genera. It is recommended, however, that such names be used only for monomorphic strains, and in cases of pleomorphism to select the most differentiated anamorph [6]. The pleomorphism, the pigmentation, the slow cultural growth

327

rate, and the ecological similarities suggest that this complex of anamorphs constitutes a biological entity. The delimitation from *Phialophora* Medlar, however, is problematic.

Cultures of black yeasts grow well on most routine media. On oatmeal agar, growth is rather poor but differentiation is optimal. Fresh transfers on media such as 2% malt agar and cherry decoction agar show abundant budding and growth, but the outer parts of the colonies often are composed mainly of sterile hyphae. Budding of poor cultures is sometimes improved if poured onto 2% malt agar after lyophilization. As will be explained below, yeast-like growth is observed in young subcultures, but more or less differentiated conidiophores on hyphae usually develop at a later stage. Preparations should therefore be made at several stages of development.

In the present chapter, I intend to elucidate the interrelationships of the black yeasts, as a supplement to Chap. 7, Part A, of this series [4].

II. THE GENUS *EXOPHIALA*

A. Variability

Variability within the genus is often seemingly random. Various transfers of a single strain under identical conditions can differ morphologically because of the conditions of the inoculum. For comparison, subcultures should therefore be made from young transfers of stock cultures. In addition, freshly isolated strains may differ considerably from those maintained for longer periods on artificial media, even though the sporulation capacity may have remained unaltered. The amount of degeneration or change is strain-dependent, and consequently transfers from stock cultures of different ages may contain artificially induced differences. Rechecking of previously studied strains can give results different from what was seen initially. Even factual remarks on a single strain given by various authors can therefore be different. In general, it is difficult to obtain comparable sets of strains for taxonomic study. It is obvious, therefore, that morphological taxonomy and identification of these organisms is a rather frustrating exercise.

B. Development

Transfers usually show a marked morphological change during maturation. Two main developmental states are customarily distinguished, viz., yeast-like budding with restricted growth, and a subsequent, expanding, hyphal phase with or without differentiated conidiophores. Cells of each of these parts of the colony may go through various developmental stages. Every strain shows only a selection of the entire kaleidoscope of possible development, and this selection may change during maintenance, as explained above. Due to this pattern selection, biologically related cultures may have few common morphological characters. The gamut of possible development is summarized as follows.

Young conidia may inflate, round off, often becoming somewhat thick-walled and olivaceous brown prior to conversion into "germinating cells" [3]. (Since no true germination takes place, the more neutral indication "giant cells" will be used in the present chapter.) Later-formed conidia often inflate similarly, but then the process ceases at an earlier stage; in old cultures, most conidia are therefore roundish. Occasionally some multiplication takes place by multilateral budding. Sometimes giant cells form by detachment of immature conidiogenous cells from monilioid conidiophores.

The giant cells, which can be regarded as a basic structural unit in *Exophiala,* show the following types of development:

1. Conidia

Conidia can be formed from a fixed or slightly progressive locus. Three basic types of conidiogenesis can be distinguished:

a. Sympodial: The first conidial bud is detached as a propagule; each subsequent conidium is produced next to or slightly above the previous one. This type of conidiogenesis is rare on giant cells. The scars are mostly very inconspicuous.

b. Annellidic: The first conidial bud is detached as a propagule; each subsequent conidium is produced through the scar of the previous one. Usually each later abstriction scar is located at a somewhat higher level than the preceding one, thus leading to an annellated zone [11]. Sometimes later scars are formed at the same level. Such "repetitive scars" are recognized with difficulty under the light microscope. Whether or not they have produced several conidia should be confirmed with time-lapse studies; annellations can also be visualized with scanning electron microscopy (SEM) [4,9]. Cells with repetitive scars have been termed "phialides without collarettes" by McGinnis [15], and cells each with several such scars in black yeasts have been referred to as "polyphialides" by Cole and Samson [2]. In *E. mansonii* (Castell.) de Hoog, cells with flat repetitive scars and cells with elongating annellated zones are common in the same strain. As the rate of elongation is extremely variable, the distinction of nonelongating and elongating scars has no taxonomic significance. They are, however, clearly distinct from cells with collarettes which may also be present (see under Sec. II. B.1.c). The use of the term "phialide" for cells that do not form collarettes in any stage of their development is therefore confusing.

c. Phialidic: The first conidial bud deteriorates at the tip and forms an open collarette, thus liberating the first, endogenously formed, conidium. Subsequent conidia are formed in basipetal order. These true phialides occur locally and with irregular frequence in several genera of human-pathogenic dematiaceous fungi (e.g., *Rhinocladiella* Nannf. sensu de Hoog, *Cladophialophora* Borelli), and are rather stable in their morphology. Phialides as well as the above described repetitive scars are quite common in old subcultures of the type strain of *E. dermatitidis,* CBS 207.35 (Fig. 1a-e). Conidia from phialides are small, hyaline, (sub)globose, whereas those from repetitive scars are larger, subhyaline, and often somewhat truncate at the base. The collarettes are extremely fragile, and often visible only for a short period of time after liberation of the first conidium. Older phialides with deteriorated collarettes are often distinguished with difficulty from annellides. The possibility cannot be excluded that phialides develop into repetitive scars with larger conidia in a later stage. In general, the phialides of *E. dermatitidis* are globose and darker than the rest of the conidiophore. Recently an undescribed species was encountered that closely resembled the little-differentiated *Exophiala* species but had phialides only; this species is an intermediate between *Exophiala* and *Phialophora*.

2. Resting Cells

Giant cells may become thick-walled and dark olivaceous brown, thus functioning as resting cells. They may become muriform, leading to small sclerotial bodies. At

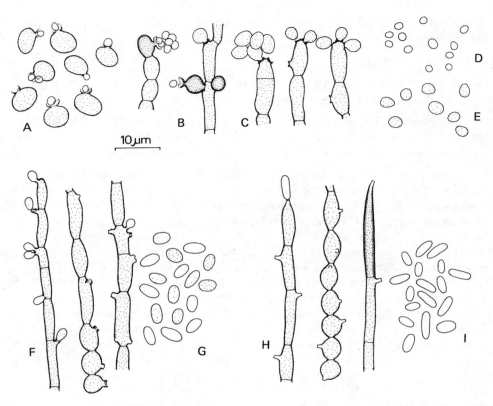

Figure 1   (A-E) *Exophiala dermatitidis*, CBS 207.35. A. Giant cells with collarettes.
B. Hyphal phialides. C. Hyphal annellidic cells. D. Phialoconidia. E. Annelloconidia.
F,G. *Exophiala mansonii*, CBS 158.58. H,I. *Exophiala jeanselmei*, various strians.

transference, the single cells mostly shed their outer walls and liberate the inner cell
which has sometimes duplicated. This endosporulation is similar to that described in
Phaeotheca Sigler et al. [20] .

3. Globose Giant Cells

Globose giant cells can reproduce, leading to coherent chains of inflated cells, usually
referred to as torulose or monilioid hyphae.

4. Hyphae

Hyphae are formed either directly from giant cells, or from torulose hyphae in which
each last-formed cell is narrower than its subtending cell. The hyphae show basically
the same process of conidium production as the giant cells. Annellidic (repetitive)
and sympodial conidiogenesis are prevalent though mostly mutually exclusive. Phialidic
conidiogenesis is only rarely seen. Conidia may be formed from either undifferentiated
hyphal cells or from differentiated, branched or nonbranched conidiophores, largely
depending on the physiological state of the strain. Catenate sympodial conidia are
rarely formed by *Exophiala* strains. This so-called *Cladosporium*-state is somewhat
hygrophobic, in contrast to the hygrophilic yeast-like states at the center of the colony.

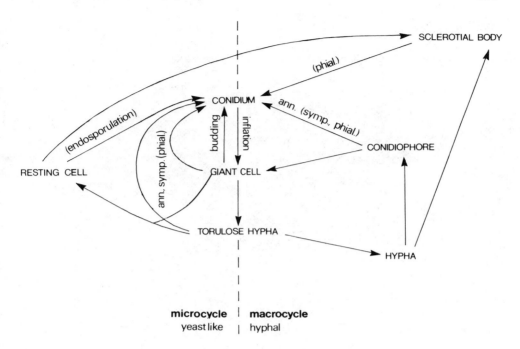

Figure 2 Diagram of possible ways of development of *Exophiala* strains. Abbreviations: ann. = annellidic; symp. = sympodial; phial. = phialidic.

5. Broad Hyphae

In old strains, broader hyphae may be formed that become profusely septate. Occasionally inflation takes place and longitudinal and oblique septa are formed, eventually leading to sclerotial bodies (anamorph genus *Phaeosclera* Sigler et al.). These occasionally sporulate with phialides [21].

The above types of development are summarized in Fig. 2. Two approximate cycles of propagation can be distinguished. Conidia developing into giant cells, which again produce conidia, form a microcycle. Cells in all stages of this cycle, including thick-walled resting cells, are single. This part of the organism shows restricted growth and is yeast-like and hygrophobic. Strains with mere microcycle development fit the anamorph genus *Phaeococcomyces* de Hoog. Conidia producing conidia via giant cells and hyphae with or without differentiated conidiophores, form a macrocycle. With this cycle, the colony is expanding, hyphomycetous, dry, and somewhat hygrophobic, particularly the sympodial-catenulate state. A macrocycle with annellidic conidiogenesis is referred to the anamorph genus *Exophiala,* and with sympodia conidiogenesis to *Rhinocladiella* or rarely *Ramichloridium* Stahel ex de Hoog. The taxonomic structure of *Exophiala* and related genera and the distribution of some forms of propagation is schematically represented in Fig. 3.

Several authors have recently reestablished *Fonsecaea* Negroni for *Rhinocladiella pedrosoi* (Brumpt) Schol-Schwarz and *R. compacta* (Carrión) Schol-Schwarz, both species showing no microcycle development. The phialidic conidiogenous cells in *Fonsecaea* and in both cycles of *Exophiala,* fit the anamorph genus *Phialophora,* but

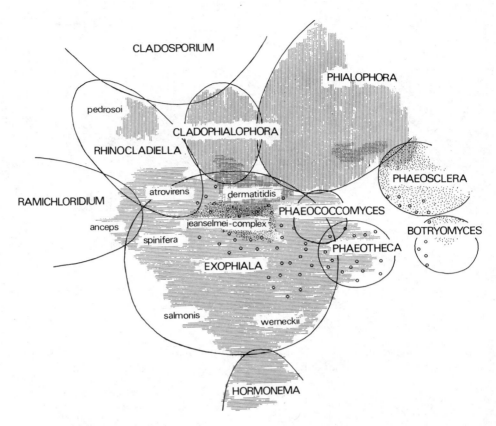

Figure 3 Schematic representation of taxonomic structure of *Exophiala* and related genera, with distribution of some types of conidiogenesis. ≡≡≡ , Budding cells; ||||||| , phialides; ∘∘∘∘ , discrete resting cells; ∴∵∴ , sclerotial bodies.

their occurrence is usually too restricted to be denominated separately. Known pathogenic *Phialophora* species (see Ref. 4) do not have accompanying *Exophiala* states. Borelli [1] accommodated a strain with the rare combination of abundant phialides and acropetal conidial chains in *Cladophialophora*.

C. Key Characters

The following groups of taxonomic parameters are in current use for the distinction of species:

1. Colonies

Some undescribed *Exophiala*-like strains maintained in the CBS culture collection have whitish colonies, but all known species are grayish black or olivaceous black. *Exophiala dermatitidis* sensu stricto is brownish black on standard media and rust-brown on Sabouraud's glucose agar. Several species grow moderately rapidly (up to 22 mm/14 days), particularly *E. salmonis* Carm.; others, e.g., *E. mansonii,* are restricted in growth and often mucous at the center. *Exophiala jeanselmei* mostly takes an intermediate position. When this species forms moderately spreading, lanose, aerial mycelium, a *Rhinocladiella* anamorph is often formed in a later stage. A strain described by Jotisankasa et al. [10] as *Phialophora dermatitidis*, CBS 670.80, now has become very restricted with compact, moriform colonies, characteristic for chlamydosporic genera such as *Botryomyces* de Hoog & Rubio. In the latter, a patchwork of light and dark cell aggregates is often observed. Recently a *Phaeosclera*-like strain, CBS 518.82, with similar colonies was found to produce local phialides. The strain exudes a marked blue pigment into the agar, which is rarely seen in *Exophiala*. Whether or not this pigment has any taxonomic significance is, as yet, unclear.

2. Hyphae

Exophiala werneckii (Horta) von Arx is characterized by broad, profusely septate hyphae and was thus suspected by Hermanides-Nijhof [8] to be related to *Hormonema* Lagerberg & Melin. Relatively broad hyphae are also found in a few *Exophiala* strains, particularly in the anamorph of *Dictyotrichiella mansonii* Schol-Schwarz.

3. Conidiophores

Conidiophores can be suberect and brown with thickened walls. In *E. spinifera*, they arise orthotropically from creeping hyphae; in the *Rhinocladiella* state of *E. jeanselmei*, they are part of an ascending conidial apparatus. In other species (e.g., *E. moniliae* and the *Phialophora* state of *E. dermatitidis*), branched systems composed of short, swollen cells are formed. Differentiated conidiophores can also be absent, the culture remaining hyphal (*E. jeanselmei* var. *lecanii-corni*) or yeast-like (*E. jeanselmei* var. *heteromorpha; Phaeococcomyces*). These taxa have only practical significance for the accommodation of strains that have a possibly divergent relationship, but in which more diagnostic structures could not be induced.

4. Conidiogenesis

Formation of a clearly sympodial *Rhinocladiella* synanamorph in the aerial mycelium is indicative for *E. jeanselmei*. Annellated zones can become sympodial in a later stage in *E. werneckii* and in *E. spinifera*, but without formation of specialized conidiogenous cells. The characters of the annellated zone are important for the distinction of the variable taxa around *E. jeanselmei*. In *E. jeanselmei*, the annellations are invariably inconspicuous on slightly tapering butts (Fig. 1, h and i). In *E. mansonii* and the anamorph of *Dictyotrichiella mansonii*, they are cylindrical and somewhat flaring, sometimes absent (Fig. 1, f and g). In *E. dermatitidis* (Fig. 1, a-e), they are generally nonelongating, broad, and conspicuously flaring. In *E. werneckii*, they are up to 2 μm wide, cylindrical, and flaring.

5. Conidia

The species with septate conidia are easily recognizable; preparations should be made at the center of mature colonies. *Exophiala pisciphila* strains mostly have some one-septate conidia. Shapes and sizes of young conidia of fresh *Exophiala* cultures are also applicable as additional characters for the distinction of taxa within the *E. jeanselmei* complex [5].

Table 1 A Synoptic Key to *Exophiala* and Related Human and Animal Pathogens

Character	Description	Species[a]
Colony appearance	Slimy	1,2,4,5,7,8,11,12,13,19
	Powdery to hairy	3,5,6,8,9,10,11,14,15, 16,17,18
Colony color	Gray to olivaceous black	1,3,4,5,6,7,8,9,10,11,12, 13,15,16,17,18,19
	Brownish black	2,14
Colony diameter	1-6 mm	1,7,8,13,17
(aotmeal 14 days)	6-16 mm	4,5,6,9,10,11,12,13,14, 16,18,19
	Over 16 mm	6,9,15
Brown	Present	1
Undifferentiated hyphae	Over 2.5 μm wide, with cubic cells	12
	Over 2.0 μm wide, with swollen cells	19
Torulose hyphae	Present	1,2,3,4,5,7,8
Differentiated conidiophores	Absent	1,2,3,4,6,7,10,13,19
	Swollen, with loose penicillate branching	8,9,10
	Swollen, with loose torulose branching	8,19
	Acicular, aseptate	5
	Cylindrical acuminate, septate	11
	Cylindrical	14,15,16,18
	Stipe with compact penicillus	17
Annellated zones	Absent	14,15,17,18
	Flat, flaring	2
	Flat or cylindrical, flaring, rel. narrow	1,3,7,8,9,10,13,19
	Cylindrical, flaring, rel. broad	12
	Tapering, mostly smooth	4,5,6,8,11,13,14,16
Collarettes	Deteriorating	2
	Persistent	17,18
Sympodial rachids	Composed of few flat scars	17
	Elongate, denticulate	14,15,16
	Composed of few cylindrical denticles	18
Conidial shape	Globose to guttuliform	8,14
	Ellipsoidal	1,2,4,5,7,9,10,11,12, 13,15
	Cylindrical	3,5,6,16,18,19
	Doliiform	17
Conidial septation	0-1 septate	9,12
	0-3 septate	10

[a]1. *Exophiala alcalophila;* 2. *E. dermatitidis;* 3. *E. dopicola;* 4. *E. jeanselmei* var. *heteromorpha;* 5. *E. jeanselmei* var. *jeanselmei;* 6. *E. jeanselmei* var. *lecanii-corni;* 7. *E. mansonii;* 8. *E. moniliae;* 9. *E. pisciphila;* 10. *E. salmonis;* 11. *E. spinifera;* 12. *E. werneckii;* 13. *Phaeococcomyces exophialae;* 14. *Ramichloridium anceps;* 15. *Ram. cerophilum*: 16. *Rhinocladiella atrovirens*: 17. *R. compacta*: 18. *R. pedrosoi;* 19. *Dictyotrichiella mansonii.*

6. Pathogenicity

A major issue to be investigated is whether the ecology of the organisms correlates with the above distinguished taxa. *Exophiala salmonis* and *E. pisciphila* have been described as pathogens on fish, though strains resembling the latter species are commonly recovered from soil. The human-pathogenic species also occur in soil and on rotten wood. It is striking that the strains assembled as *E. jeanselmei* in the literature have two markedly different ecological backgrounds. In strains from humans, the sympodial state is rare, whereas this state is predominant in strains from rotten wood in the Northern temperate zone. *Exophiala jeanselmei* mostly causes mycetomas, whereas the other species usually are agents of chromomycosis, though they have also been reported from phaeohyphomycosis or keratomycosis, and sometimes show neurotropism. *Exophiala werneckii* is a clear taxonomic entity. It is the causative agent of tinea nigra palmaris and has been recovered from beach sand.

7. Additional Characters

Lach and workers [12,13] described several black yeast taxa as varieties of *Nadsoniella nigra* Issatchenko, an older synonym of *E. jeanselmei* [4]. Both varieties, however, were described invalidly, without Latin diagnoses or indication of type material. The authentic strain of var. *hesuelica*, CBS 519.82, fits the anamorph genus *Phaeococcomyces*. Goto et al. [7] described *Exophiala alcalophila* Goto & Sugiyama (type culture: CBS 520.82) with restricted colonies in which the *Phaeococcomyces alcalophilis* Goto & Sugiyama anamorph easily becomes predominant. The species is further characterized by its capacity to grow on alkaline media and by a rust-brown exudate in the agar.

D. A Synoptic Key

A synoptic key to *Exophiala* and related species is presented in Table 1 (p. 334).

REFERENCES

1. Borelli, D. 1980. Causal agents of chromoblastomycosis (Chromomycetes). In *Proceedings of the Fifth International Conference on the Mycoses,* Pan. Am. Health Organ. Sci. Publ. No. 396, Washington, D.C., pp. 334-335.
2. Cole, G. T., and R. A. Samson. 1979. *Patterns of Development in Conidial Fungi,* Pitman, London.
3. de Hoog, G. S. 1977. *Rhinocladiella* and allied genera. In *Studies in Mycology,* Vol. 15, Centraalbureau voor Schimmelcultures, Baarn, pp. 1-140.
4. de Hoog, G. S. 1982. On the potentially pathogenic dematiaceous hyphomycetes. In D. H. Howard (Ed.), *The Fungi Pathogenic for Humans and Animals,* Part A, Dekker, New York, pp. 149-216.
5. Domsch, K. H., W. Gams, and T.-H. Anderson. 1980. *Compendium of Soil Fungi,* Academic, London.
6. Gams, W. 1982. Generic names for synanamorphs? Mycotaxon *15*:459-464.
7. Goto, S., R. Aono, J. Sugiyama, and K. Horikoshi. 1981. *Exophiala alcalophila,* a new black, yeast-like hyphomycete with an accompanying *Phaeococcomyces alcalophilus* anamorph and its physiological characteristics. Trans. Mycol. Soc. Soc. Jpn. *22*:429-439.
8. Hermanides-Nijhof, E. J. 1977. *Aureobasidium* and allied genera. *Studies in Mycology,* Vol. 15, Centraalbureau voor Schimmelcultures, Baarn, pp. 141-177.

9.   Hironaga, M., S. Watanabe, K. Nishimura, and M. Miyaji. 1981. Annellated co-
     nidiogenous cells in *Exophiala dermatitidis,* agent of phaeohyphomycosis.
     Mycologia *73*:1181-1183.

10. Jotisankasa, V., H. S. Nielsen, and N. F. Conant. 1970. *Phialophora dermatitidis:*
     its morphology and biology. Sabouraudia *8*:98-107.

11. Kendrick, B. (Ed.) 1971. *Taxonomy of Fungi Imperfecti,* University of Toronto
     Press, Toronto.

12. Kozlova, T. M., and S. P. Lach. 1981. The morphology and ultrastructure of
     the black yeast *Nadsoniella nigra* var. *psychrophilica.* Mikrobiologiya (Moscow)
     50:279-284.

13. Lach, S. P., and E. L. Ruban. 1970. Antarctic "black yeasts" *Nadsoniella nigra*
     var. *hesuelica* (Characteristics and identification of strain 365). Izv. Akad Naud.
     SSR, Ser. Biol. *4*:581-592.

14. McGinnis, M. R. 1977. *Exophiala spinifera,* a new combination of *Phialophora*
     spinifera. Mycotaxon *5*:337-340.

15. McGinnis, M. R. 1977. *Wangiella,* a new genus to accommodate *Hormiscium*
     dermatitidis. Mycotaxon *5*:353-363.

16. McGinnis, M. R. 1978. Taxonomy of *Exophiala jeanselmei* (Langeron) McGinnis
     and Padhye. Mycopathologia *65*:79-87.

17. McGinnis, M. R. 1979. Taxonomy of *Exophiala werneckii* and its relationship to
     Microsporum mansonii. Sabouraudia *17*:145-154.

18. McGinnis, M. R., and A. A. Padhye. 1977. *Exophiala jeanselmei,* a new combina-
     tion for *Phialophora jeanselmei.* Mycotaxon *5*:341-352.

19. Schol-Schwarz, M. B. 1968. *Rhinocladiella,* its synonym *Fonsecaea* and its relation
     to *Phialophora.* Antonie Leeuwenhoek J. Microbiol. Serol. *34*:119-152.

20. Sigler, L., A. Tsuneda, and J. W. Carmichael. 1981. *Phaeotheca* and *Phaeosclera,*
     two new genera of dematiaceous hyphomycetes and a redescription of *Sarcinomyces*
     Lindner. Mycotaxon *12*:449-467.

21. Wang, C. J. K. 1964. Studies on *Trichosporium heteromorphum* Nannfeldt. Can.
     J. Bot. *42*:1011-1016.

Author Index

Numbers in brackets are reference numbers and indicate that an author's work is referred to although his name may not be cited in the text. Italicized numbers give the page on which the complete reference is listed.

A

Subject Index

Illustrations are indicated by italicized page numbers.

A

Absidia
    diseases caused by, 138, 214, 215
    peptidofucomannans of, 80
Absidia cylindrospora, peptidofucomannans of, 80
Absidia ramosa, diseases caused by, 138
N-Acetylglucosamine, 59, 64-68, 90
N-Acetylglucosaminidases, 64
O-Acetylserine sulfhydrylase, 27
Achlya, 22
Acid phosphatase, 13, 69, 82, 91, 136
Acidic carboxyl proteinase, 69, 91
Acrasis rosea, conservation of cultures of, 157
Acremonium, diseases caused by, 252
Acremonium falciforme, diseases caused by, 211
Acremonium kiliense, 211
Acremonium recifei, diseases caused by, 211
Actinomadura, 211
Actinomadura madurae, diseases caused by, 211
Actinomadura pelletieri, diseases caused by, 211
Actinomyces israelii, stained by Grocott's method, 233
Actinomycosis, 196
Adiaspiromycosis, 275
Aeration, 20
Aerobes, 20
African histoplasmosis, 266, 267
Agaricus biosporus
    dieback disease of, 104, 109
    virus-like particles of, 104, *105,* 109, *110*
Allomyces, 22
Alternaria, conservation of cultures of, 155
Alternaria kikuchiana, mannans of, 76

Alternaria zinniae, galactomannans of, 76
Amidolyase, 33
p-Aminobenzoic acid, 9
Anaerobes, 20
Antibody-dependent cellular cytotoxicity (ADCC), 134
Antimetabolites, 9
Appearance of fungi in tissue (see also individual fungus or mycosis), 241-280
    aberrant forms (see individual fungus)
    artifacts that resemble fungi, 275, 276
    asteroid bodies, 244, 245, *247*
    India ink preparation, 231, 287, 288, 293, 294, 300, 301
    potassium hydroxide (KOH) preparation, 230, 288-294, 301
    structures resumbling fungi, *275-279,* 280
Armillaria mellea, paramylon from, 62
Arthroderma benhamiae, 22
    respiratory-deficient mutants of, 33
Arthroderma simii, 22
Ascobolus, 22
Ascomycetes, 22
Aspergillosis, 124, 130, 137, 138, 196, 198-200, 211, 254-258, 271, 294, 309
    demography of, 199
    ecology of, 198
    geographic distribution of, 199
    murine, 137
    pathology of, *254-258*
    predisposing factors in, 198-200
Aspergillus, 4, 16
    appearance of in tissue, *254-258*
    cell wall, comparative composition of, 83
    conservation of cultures of, 157, 158